THE AMERICAN PHYSICAL THERAPY ASSOCIATION

Book of
Body Maintenance
and Repair

THE AMERICAN PHYSICAL THERAPY ASSOCIATION

Book of
Body Maintenance
and Repair

by Marilyn Moffat, PT, PhD, FAPTA, and Steve Vickery
Illustrations by Terry Boles

A Round Stone Press Book

An Owl Book
Henry Holt and Company
New York

THIS BOOK is not intended as a substitute for the advice of a
physician or a physical therapist. Readers who suspect they may have
specific medical problems should consult a physician or physical
therapist regarding any of the suggestions made in this book.

Henry Holt and Company, LLC
Publishers since 1866
115 West 18th Street
New York, New York 10011

Henry Holt® is a registered trademark of Henry Holt and Company, LLC.

Library of Congress Cataloging-in-Publication Data
Moffat, Marilyn.
Book of body maintenance and repair/
by Marilyn Moffat and Steve Vickery; illustrations by Terry Boles.
p. cm.
ISBN 0-8050-5571-1 (pbk.)
1. Exercise. 2. Physical fitness. 3. Physical therapy.
I. Vickery, Steve. II. American Physical Therapy Association (1921–).
III. Title. IV. Title: At head of title.
RA781.V53 1999   98-32103
613.7—dc21   CIP

Henry Holt books are available for special promotions and premiums.
For details contact: Director, Special Markets.
First Owl Books Edition 1999

A ROUND STONE PRESS BOOK
Directors: Marsha Melnick, Susan E. Meyer, Paul Fargis
Editorial Director: Nick Viorst
Editor: Judy Pray
Illustrations: Terry Boles
Design Concept: Steve Vickery and Laura Smyth
Production Design: Laura Smyth

Printed in United States of America

10   9   8   7

Contents

A Word from APTA

We would all like to be physically fit, but what does "fitness" really mean? What amount of activity is "enough"? Do we all need to follow the same fitness program? How will exercise affect our back, hips, or knees? People of all ages want to understand more about how to keep this miraculous machine, the human body, in peak condition, how this elixir called exercise affects the body, and how to avoid injury when we put our bodies in motion.

Physical therapists are health care professionals who examine, evaluate, and treat people with health conditions resulting from injury or disease. Most physical therapists hold master's degrees and all have extensive education in anatomy and body mechanics; many also specialize in one or more specific areas, including cardiopulmonary, clinical electrophysiology, geriatrics, neurology, orthopedics, pediatrics, and sports physical therapy.

Physical therapists can help individuals increase and maintain muscle strength and endurance, restore and improve range of motion in joints, increase coordination, increase cardiovascular endurance, and decrease muscle and joint pain. Just as important, physical therapists can help people prevent injury in the first place.

Physical therapists know how the musculoskeletal system works, yet recognize that each individual is unique. They can determine an individual's level of fitness and suggest the types of exercises and activities—including both sports and daily life activities— that are right for him or her.

It is in this spirit that the American Physical Therapy Association (APTA), the national organization that represents physical therapy professionals in the United States, presents *The American Physical Therapy Association Book of Body Maintenance and Repair*. This is the first such volume ever offered by APTA.

We invite you to explore these pages and learn more about how your body works; how exercise affects your body; how to increase your strength, endurance, and flexibility; and how to avoid injury. We hope that the book will help you to maximize your body's ability to work for you and, most important, help you to achieve your "personal best."

Body Maintenance & Repair

If you are one of the thousands of people who have benefited from the expertise of a physical therapist, then you know that "physical therapy" is not a generic term. It refers to a profession that makes use of a wide range of noninvasive interventions to reduce pain and restore function in individuals dealing with injury, disability, or disease. For decades, physical therapists have demonstrated their power both in treating existing conditions and in helping to prevent their recurrence. Physical therapists—and the tools they use—are an integral, and increasingly important, part of modern health care.

The tools of physical therapy take a variety of forms, but certainly the most commonly used are therapeutic exercise; mobilization and manipulation; massage; heat; cold; water; ultrasound; and electrical stimulation. Even more important for treatment than the tools is the unique appreciation that physical therapists have for the workings of the human body. And it is primarily this understanding that *The American Physical Therapy Association Book of*

Body Maintenance and Repair draws on to provide lay readers with a basic, practical education in the essentials of getting and staying as physically fit as possible.

What This Book Offers

Body Maintenance and Repair is a health care manual, a fitness guide, and an exercise book in one—a reflection of physical therapists' own broad expertise.

Physical therapists spend much of their time treating physical ailments of one sort or another. They understand both the physiology of the disorders they treat and the most useful means of treating them. And they know which problems require the attention of a physical therapist and which can simply be addressed at home. Providing a survey of this information is a central part of the mission of *Body Maintenance and Repair.*

With this in mind, the book will help you to identify many common and not-so-common injuries and dysfunctions—from low back strain to tennis elbow, arthritis to bursitis, myofascial pain disorders to iliotibial band

syndrome—with an eye toward helping you determine how to deal with them. While there's no one-size-fits-all prescription for every problem and every patient, in this book you can often find the information necessary to let you make a preliminary evaluation of your symptoms. And when it is clear that home treatment can be helpful, the book takes you step-by-step through just how to help yourself: with exercises, massage, rest, ice, heat, and other simple approaches. For this reason alone, this book can meet many of your important home health care needs.

Physical therapists frequently find that the problems they treat could easily have been prevented had the patient taken some relatively simple precautionary steps. And indeed, taking these preventive steps is an important part of ensuring that the injury or dysfunction does not recur. This is especially true of such common workplace injuries as carpal tunnel syndrome or low back problems. The lesson of this for people who are currently healthy is that they should follow these same preventive steps to avoid trouble.

The vast majority of common ailments occur simply in the course of conducting everyday life: doing the laundry, working at a computer, taking a walk. This is because people often perform these actions in ways that place excessive strain on the body's machinery. And an injury that may seem to come out of nowhere, in the course of doing something you've done countless times before, may be the cumulative result of years of doing that thing improperly.

Preventing injury, then, requires learning how to do things properly. It also requires the presence of adequate strength, endurance, and flexibility in the body's muscles, tendons, and ligaments. Without these qualities, the body is particularly susceptible to problems resulting from such simple actions as lifting a child off the ground, climbing a flight of stairs, or playing a set of tennis.

Body Maintenance and Repair provides the necessary instruction. The book addresses a variety of interrelated subjects, including posture (the way you stand, sit, and lie down), gait (the way you walk and run), and body mechanics (the way you use the body to perform everyday activities), among others. All of these are essential to good body maintenance. *Body Maintenance and Repair* also provides advice to help you develop the strength, endurance, and flexibility your body needs to face the challenges of everyday life, including casual sports and the demands of the workplace. Insofar as fitness can be measured by your ability to face the challenges of everyday life with little fear of injury—rather than the ability to function at the level of a high-powered athlete—this is very much a fitness guide.

Certainly the most widely used tool in the physical therapist's toolbox is a familiar one: exercise. Exercise—which helps bring the strength, endurance, and flexibility of an injured body part up to appropriate levels—is the central component of the rehabilitative program for almost any injury or dysfunction. The exercises developed and used by physical therapists combine physical therapists' unique knowledge of movement science with their knowledge of physiology and anatomy. As it turns out, many of these same exercises may also be used for prevention reasons by people who are currently free from injury, as a way to keep the body in a condition that minimizes the risk of future problems.

Body Maintenance and Repair features dozens of these exercises. For anyone looking for a selection of easy-to-follow exercises from which to put together a regular home conditioning regimen, the offerings in this book are plentiful. (On the other hand, serious bodybuilders will want to look elsewhere, because the exercises in this book are geared to a lesser intensity.) And because these exercises are so commonly used by physical therapists, this book can serve as a useful resource—for both you and your physical therapist—if you ever have occasion to need physical therapy.

Although *Body Maintenance and Repair* can benefit just about anyone, it is perhaps most valuable to individuals over the age of 30. As midlife approaches, the aging process and increasing inactivity can transform many everyday physical activities into minefields of potential aches, pains, and injuries. To counter this altogether natural development, *Body Maintenance and Repair* gives you the information you need to develop an aggressive strategy for taking care of your body.

As valuable a resource on matters of body maintenance as *Body Maintenance and Repair* may be, there are limits to the advice it offers. The book's attention is focused on the musculoskeletal system—the body's core machinery, made up of bones, joints, muscles, tendons, ligaments, and related structures. Remember that complete body maintenance requires that the heart, lungs, and other vital organs be well cared for too. Physical therapists do practice in such areas as cardiopulmonary, neurological, geriatric, pediatric, and women's health care, and topics such as proper diet and cardiovascular conditioning are briefly touched on in *Body Maintenance and Repair*, but they are not addressed in great depth. Nevertheless, you are strongly urged to seek out current information on these issues through your physical therapist or physician or through the many excellent books on these subjects.

Body Maintenance and Repair is also not a substitute for professional health care. As much as you can do for yourself, there are times, as this book often points out, when care provided at the hands of a physical therapist is called

for. Physical therapists have the tools and the specialized knowledge that are essential to proper rehabilitation. And no book, no matter how exhaustive, can replace hands-on attention. With your physical therapist's authorization, however, *Body Maintenance and Repair* may well be used in conjunction with your prescribed rehabilitation program.

How This Book Works

Body Maintenance and Repair is divided into three principal sections (and two brief appendices). Each section has a unique focus, but the three are closely interrelated.

Part I consists of nine chapters, each devoted to a distinct part of the body: the back, neck, jaw, shoulder, elbow, wrist/hand, hip, knee, and ankle/foot. Each of the body parts covered is a relatively common site for injury, ranging from mild soreness and stiffness to strains, sprains, and worse. The individual chapters are designed to provide practical advice on how to deal with such injuries when they do strike—including what you can do for yourself and when you need to consult with a physical therapist or physician.

Equally important, these chapters

also offer advice on how to prevent injuries from occurring in the first place. (This advice draws heavily on Part II, where prevention matters are addressed more thoroughly.) These chapters also feature information on the general functioning of the body part in question and a survey of common problems and their causes. This information is meant both to make the treatment and prevention advice easier to understand and to make you a more informed patient in those instances when seeing a professional is called for.

Part I is designed to serve principally as a reference section. The individual chapters are primarily to be consulted when you experience pain or injury in a specific part of the body. (Readers may also wish to use these chapters more proactively for the information they provide on preventing pain and injury in a specific body part.) The nine chapters can certainly be read straight through; indeed, together they offer a thorough education in body maintenance and repair. But because the individual chapters are essentially self-contained—and because different parts of the body experience many similar problems—there is some overlap from one body part chapter to the next.

Part II functions quite differently. The eight chapters that make up this section are meant to be read in their entirety, regardless of whether you have experienced pain or injury. Together, they deliver a sound basic education in body maintenance, the essential principles of preventing injury. This section contains individual chapters on subjects relating to human physiology and kinesiology that physical therapists have long recognized as key in determining the body's overall well-being: posture, gait, body mechanics, footwear, and body weight.

Even more important, this section features a chapter devoted to building strength and endurance in the body's muscles, and flexibility in the body's muscles, tendons, and ligaments—qualities that, developed through regular exercise, are the very cornerstone of health. Part II also includes a chapter on how to avoid problems when playing sports and another on avoiding problems in the workplace, whether your job is active or sedentary.

Part III is an illustrated compendium

of nearly 200 exercises, broken into two chapters: one contains exercises for building and maintaining strength and endurance in every part of the body, and the other focuses on building and maintaining flexibility. These exercises have been refined through decades of use by physical therapists and have proven consistently safe and sound. Although some of the exercises call for a pair of hand or ankle weights, most require no special equipment.

Together, the exercises constitute a broad spectrum from which anyone can put together the sort of conditioning program that is essential for good body maintenance. The flexibility exercises can also be used to prepare the body for the challenges of sports and work. As vital elements in keeping the body free of injury, these exercises should be used in association with the relevant chapters in Part II.

The exercises can also play a role in body repair, helping restore the body to good working condition in the wake of injuries. Except in the case of simple soreness or stiffness (matters addressed in Part I), however, exercises should be used for this purpose only under the supervision of a physical

therapist or a physician. Otherwise, you put yourself at risk of further injury.

However you decide to use these exercises, be sure to read the introductions to the chapters before attempting any of them. The introductions contain important cautions and other information essential to proper performance of the exercises.

This book also features two appendices. One provides quick-reference first aid information for dealing with injuries. The other offers some useful tips on cardiovascular conditioning, an important part of overall health.

One final point: Physical therapy, like many areas of health care, is an ever-evolving field, with new approaches continually being developed and applied. As a result, there are occasionally differences of opinion among physical therapists about particular diagnoses and treatments. The material in this book is no exception. Nevertheless, *The APTA Book of Body Maintenance and Repair* represents a general consensus among the APTA's Editorial Review Board, staff consultants, and co-author Marilyn Moffat, PT, PhD, FAPTA.

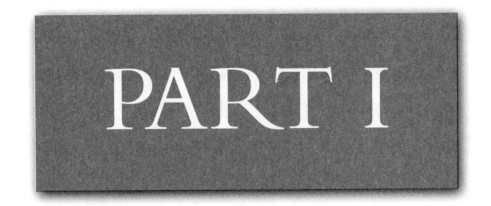

PART I

CHAPTER ONE

The Back

If your back hurts right now, you probably don't care that back pain is the most common cause of "loss of activity" for adults under 45…or that it's estimated that as many as 80 percent of American workers suffer back pain at some time during their careers…or that back pain is the most frequent medical complaint in America next to the common cold…or that back pain costs us $60 billion annually in medical expenses and lost productivity.

What you care about is that your back hurts.

No one can promise miracles. But reading this chapter and following its recommendations—and, if necessary, working with a physical therapist—just might soothe your aching back.

And if you happen to be one of the lucky people who've never "thrown their back out," you have even more reason to read on. Preventing back problems is a lot easier and cheaper than treating them.

How the Back Works

The back functions as the central link of a kinetic chain that includes the head, jaw, neck, upper back, shoulders, and arms at one end and the legs and feet at the other. All of these different areas of the body are interrelated and depend on each other for correct functioning and movement. This is one reason why a healthy back is so important: it affects virtually every other part of the body in one way or another.

The **spinal column,** which runs the length of your back, provides basic structural stability to your body. Both your rib cage and pelvis are anchored to the spine, and you depend on the spine for the ability to perform some of the body's most essential movements: bending forward, backward, and to the side, and twisting or rotating.

The main section of the spine is constructed of 24 cylindrical bones, or **vertebrae,** extending from the back of the head to the pelvis. When looked at from the side, the stacked vertebrae form three natural curves from head to pelvis, with the neck at the top forming a gentle "C" curve, the upper back a gentle backward "C" curve, and the low back another gentle "C" curve. Pairs of bony projections called **facets** connect the rear sections of each vertebra to form a series of interlocking joints. The

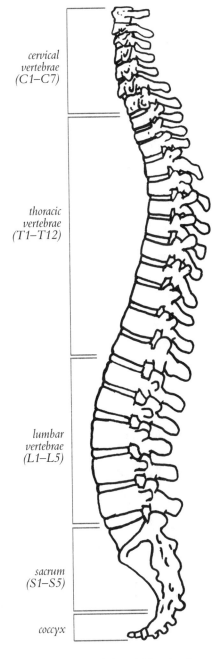

cervical vertebrae (C1–C7)

thoracic vertebrae (T1–T12)

lumbar vertebrae (L1–L5)

sacrum (S1–S5)

coccyx

Spine (side view)

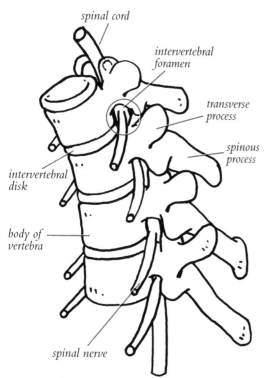

spinal cord

intervertebral foramen

transverse process

spinous process

intervertebral disk

body of vertebra

spinal nerve

Detail of spine

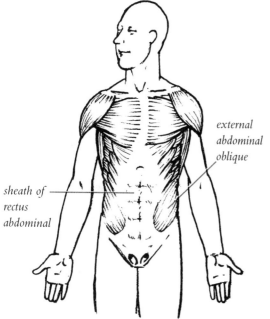

external abdominal oblique

sheath of rectus abdominal

Muscles of abdomen

vertebrae are the building blocks of the spinal column. Each facet joint has its own **synovial membrane** that surrounds the joint and secretes a tiny amount of lubricating **synovial fluid.** And the joint surfaces are covered with a smooth **articular cartilage** that facilitates movement in the region.

The major portion of the spine is divided into three sections of vertebrae: the 7 **cervical vertebrae** in the neck region; the 12 **thoracic vertebrae** of the upper and middle back; and the 5 **lumbar vertebrae** of the low back. The cervical vertebrae, which are the smallest, are discussed in detail in **Chapter 2—The Neck.** The thoracic vertebrae, to which the ribs are attached, are midway in size between the cervical and lumbar vertebrae.

The thick, stronger lumbar vertebrae are the largest vertebrae and are designed to take the great stresses of weight, support, and movement put on the low back. The lumbar region usually takes the most "punishment" (for example, through improper lifting) of any area of the back.

At the very end of the spinal column are the **sacrum** and the **coccyx.** The sacrum is a fusion of five vertebrae that attaches the spine to the pelvis; the point of attachment (to a part of the pelvis known as the **ilium**) is called the **sacroiliac joint.** The coccyx, also known as the "tailbone," is a fusion of three to five very small vertebrae at the very base of the spine.

Between the vertebrae are shock-absorbing **disks.** They vary in thickness and size. Each disk is made up of a jelly-like center and a thick outer sheath of tough fibrocartilage.

Carved out within the bodies of the vertebrae is a sheltering canal (the **spinal canal**) for the **spinal cord**—the nerve impulse transmitter between the brain and the rest of the body. Major nerve roots branch off from the spinal cord and pass through openings in the vertebrae called **foramina.** These nerves allow our muscles to contract and allow us to perceive sensations such as touch, temperature, and pain. One of the most significant of these is the **sciatic nerve**—actually made up of five nerve roots coming from the lumbar spine—which runs all the way down the leg, from the low back and through the buttock to just below the ankle. (Because of this, pain in the hip, buttock, and leg is sometimes the symptom of a problem in the back.)

Muscles in the back, neck, and abdominal region, as well as the shoulder and leg muscles, all work together to keep the spine stabilized and aligned properly while still giving the back mobility. Among the more important of these are the **erector spinae** group, a deep layer of muscles running along each side of the spine. These are aided by other, even deeper muscles in the back. Flexible fibrous cords of tissue called **tendons**—technically, extensions of the muscle—attach the back muscles to the spine and the abdominal muscles to the rib cage and pelvis.

Ligaments, tough bands of fibrous tissue, provide stability and reinforcement by binding each pair of vertebrae together; several long ligaments run the entire length of the spinal column, both in front and back. The spine is further reinforced by **joint capsules,** fibrous and connective tissue material that surrounds the facets.

What Can Go Wrong

When people complain of a "bad back," they're usually talking about problems in the low back (lumbar region). And for good reason: your low back bears the brunt of bending, stooping, sitting, and especially, lifting. In addition, the lumbar area is very flexible. This flexibility, while essential, leaves the low back particularly susceptible to injury. The thoracic spine is not entirely invulnerable; indeed, due to a loss of bone mass, it can become increasingly fragile as we grow older. The sacrum and coccyx do suffer bruises and (occasionally) fractures due to falls, but though painful, they're rarely serious.

While some back problems may arise as the result of a specific traumatic incident—a fall, sports injury, or car accident—others seem to appear out of nowhere. In cases where there's no obvious cause for pain, the culprit is often the cumulative stress, strain, and abuse from years of poor posture and bad body mechanics. The triggering incident may be so trivial as to go unnoticed. This can make diagnosis of a specific back ailment tricky even for health professionals. While many back problems are often associated with aging, younger people also endure their share of back troubles—whether they stem from injuries, poor posture, or poor body mechanics. Disease and infection, too, can sometimes strike young backs just as it does more commonly older ones.

Back pain comes in many varieties. It can be dull, sharp, constant, intermittent, shooting, tingling like "pins and needles"—even a burning sensation. It is also highly variable, ranging from mild discomfort to agonizing pain. And although pain may strike just the back itself, a number of back problems are accompanied by irritation of the sciatic nerve, which sends hot shooting pain into the hip, buttock, or leg. This particular variety of pain, called **sciatica,** may come on quickly and usually affects only one side of the body.

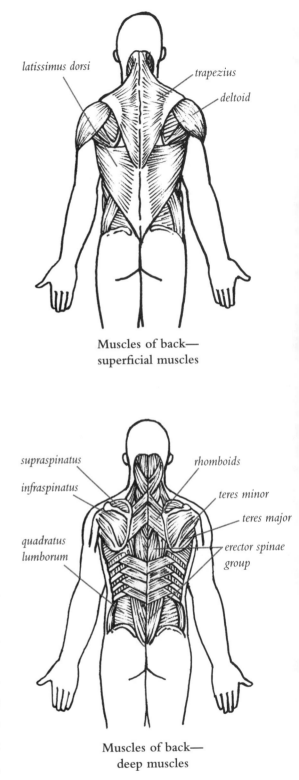

latissimus dorsi
trapezius
deltoid

Muscles of back—
superficial muscles

supraspinatus
infraspinatus
rhomboids
teres minor
teres major
quadratus lumborum
erector spinae group

Muscles of back—
deep muscles

Some back conditions, such as mild strains and sprains (see pages 16–17), call for simple home treatments like rest and ice. Others demand more advanced physical therapy techniques: carefully and scientifically tailored exercises to strengthen the back and improve range of motion; adjustments of the posture; mobilization; and perhaps approaches (modalities) like ultrasound and electrical stimulation as well. Still other problems require surgery or other major interventions, although these, too, are usually complemented with an exercise program designed by a physical therapist as part of the rehabilitation stage. In every instance, however, you should look to your physician or physical therapist to make a diagnosis and determine treatment.

Muscles in the back (especially those in the low back) are frequent sites of back dysfunction. Certainly the mildest such dysfunction, if it can even be called that, is the tendency of these muscles—like muscles throughout the body—to become stiff or tight in response to heavy back activity. Similar **muscle tightness,** especially in the low back, may be produced by simple emotional stress. The result is usually minor, short-term achiness and may be no cause for concern. (On the other hand, muscle tightness does diminish the back's range of motion, which, unless the muscles are warmed up and stretched, puts the back at risk of injury when called upon to push beyond that range.)

More worrisome is the accumulation of excess lactic acid and other chemicals in the back muscles whenever they are subject to excessive stress over prolonged periods of time, whether it be from poor posture, from leaning over a computer, or from holding the back in a fixed position. The cellular and chemical responses to excessive stress almost inevitably lead to **muscle inflammation,** the development of hard knots of muscle called **trigger points,** and pain. Unfortunately, the effects of such irritation are cumulative over time; what starts out as a mild twinge may wind up as a full-blown backache. And this may strike the lumbar or thoracic region or both.

Tearing of the muscles may result from direct trauma or overuse (as from engaging in sports or some other physical activity) and possibly prolonged poor posture or poor body mechanics. A **muscle strain,** sometimes inaccurately called a "pulled muscle," occurs when the muscle has been overstretched or overexerted and may have microscopic tearing as its cause. When the tearing is more severe, it is called, simply, a **muscle tear,** which may be partial or complete. When a muscle is strained or torn, the blood vessels in the muscle are strained or torn as well, causing inflammation in the surrounding tissue. The symptoms of strains and tears vary only in degree and may include pain, inflammation, bleeding into the surrounding tissues, and muscle spasm (see page 17). Strains, however, are often mild and require little more than a few days of rest.

Strains and tears often trigger **muscle spasm**—the sudden, intense, involuntary contraction of muscle tissue. Although very painful, a muscle spasm is the body's natural mechanism for protecting injured tissue by acting as a brace. In cases of major injury, the spasm may be so intense that the back will lean sharply to one side or flatten the normal curve of the lumbar spine. Because it is a protective mechanism, spasm is present in a wide range of back disorders. Spasm may also be caused by damage to nerves that run through the back.

Not unlike the muscles, the ligaments that support the back's joints can be overstretched—that is, pushed beyond their normal limits—or may sustain tears ranging from microscopic to major. This injury, a **sprain,** can afflict any of the back's ligaments and can be produced by trauma (like a fall), overuse (from activities such as gymnastics or ballet), the cumulative impact of poor posture, or poor body mechanics (like lifting heavy objects incorrectly). One common back sprain appears in the ligaments that bind the facet joints together. As usual, the lumbar region is the most vulnerable, especially to injuries caused by overuse. But the sacroiliac joint is also a frequent site of sprain, especially those due to falls or twisting; in women the ligaments of the sacroiliac joint may become lax during pregnancy or during certain phases of the menstrual cycle. With sprains, the pain may be localized or it may radiate down the buttocks and into the leg. If overstretched ligaments are not holding a joint firmly in place, there may also be a feeling of slippage. Over time the joint may become stiff and restricted.

The facet joints are subject to the degenerative changes associated with **arthritis,** which can lead to both pain and stiffness. This condition can be the result of early trauma to the joints, but there is a wide range of possible causes. One form of arthritis is **rheumatoid arthritis,** a disease whose origin is not fully understood (but which may be the result of autoimmune mechanisms or viral infections). Although some cases of rheumatoid arthritis are relatively benign, in extreme cases the joints become so swollen that they essentially fuse together. This is a serious and often debilitating condition. Physical therapy is necessary to help maintain mobility and flexibility in the region.

A far more widespread form of arthritis in the facet joints is **osteoarthritis,** the degeneration of the articular cartilage and a wearing down of the joint surfaces. In some cases osteoarthritis may result in the buildup of spurs (deposits of bony tissue) on the vertebrae. And if these bone spurs develop in the area occupied by the spinal nerves (a condition known as **spinal stenosis**) and encroach on the spinal cord or the nerves branching off it, the result can be severe pain not just in the back but in the legs as well (especially when standing upright). In older people osteoarthritis can also lead to a forward curvature of the thoracic spine.

Osteoarthritis has a number of possible causes, including trauma, overuse, degenerative disk disease (see page 19), and inactivity. But by far the most common is degeneration of the joint due to age, typical (though not inevitable) among middle-aged individuals. Although it sometimes has no symptoms at all, osteoarthritis may well lead to general stiffness and low back pain from mild to severe.

The osteoarthritis-related degenerative changes to the disks, joints, and vertebrae of the spine, common among people over 40, are known generally as **spondylosis.** This condition requires an X-ray to accurately diagnose. Flare-ups are commonly treated with rest and immobilization of the spine, followed by exercises and postural training provided by a physical therapist. Only in extreme cases is surgery necessary.

Disk problems are perhaps the most familiar of all low back ailments. "Slipped disk" is a catch-all term for **herniated, bulging, protruding, extruded,** or **ruptured disks**—terms that have been used to describe various degrees of a similar problem. Generally speaking, a herniated disk is one whose contents have been pushed beyond the normal boundaries. The pressure of the disk center against its outer sheath can sometimes lead to a bulge of this wall. In severe cases the disk wall actually breaks; the gelatinous contents of the disk then spill into the surrounding area and put pressure on the wall, the ligaments, and the nerve root itself. Sometimes this can lead to nerve inflammation.

Herniated disks often display no symptoms and can go unnoticed by those who have them. But in some cases the result of any herniated disk can be numbness or tingling down the legs (if the nerves are irritated) or even sharp pain. Herniated disks are also the most common cause of sciatica (see page 15). Furthermore, depending on the degree of disk bulging or rupture, part of the protective cushion between the vertebrae in question may be gone permanently. The facet joints may then meet with increased wear and become damaged; this is another contributor to osteoarthritis (see page 17).

Herniated disks often result from poor body mechanics during daily activities (such as poor lifting techniques) and bad posture. Sports injuries are another common cause, particularly from sports that require running,

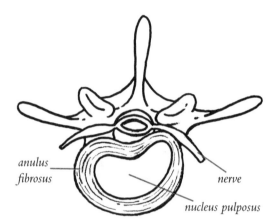

anulus fibrosus

nerve

nucleus pulposus

Bulging disk

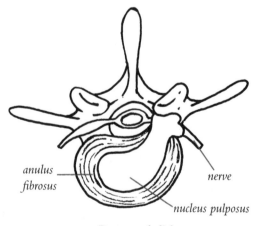

anulus fibrosus

nerve

nucleus pulposus

Ruptured disk

jumping, twisting, or extreme flexibility (such as gymnastics). The loss of disk thickness due to aging or degeneration (see page 17) tends to make the disks more vulnerable.

A herniated disk is usually diagnosed with the help of imaging techniques such as magnetic resonance imaging (MRI). Physicians often recommend rest, medications, and other noninvasive techniques to relieve any pain. Surgery is usually reserved for cases in which all other treatments fail.

The disks are also susceptible to **degenerative disk disease,** which is, like joint degeneration, a typical if not inevitable function of aging. As we reach our late twenties or early thirties, the gelatinous center of the disk begins to dry out and becomes more fibrous. Eventually the disk may dry up completely. Although degenerative disk disease and degenerative joint disease are often a part of the aging process, they don't necessarily produce major symptoms.

The low back may also develop **spondylolisthesis,** in which one vertebra slips forward (subluxates) on top of another. Most often this involves the bottom lumbar vertebra slipping forward over the sacrum, although it can also happen elsewhere in the lumbar region. Spondylolisthesis may be the result of trauma, spinal fracture, or arthritis (see page 17). This malalignment of the spine may produce symptoms ranging from mild low back pain to sciatica (see page 15) to muscle spasm (see page 17)—or it may produce no symptoms at all.

Like all bones, the vertebrae are subject to **fracture** as a result of trauma, like a fall or a collision. Surprisingly, fractured vertebrae may go undetected. Often fractures cause pain (local or radiating) and joint impingement. In some cases fractures can cause damage to the spinal cord, perhaps the most serious injury the back can sustain. For this reason even the suspicion of a spinal fracture should be treated as a major medical emergency demanding immediate professional attention.

Fractures can, of course, happen to anyone, but they are more likely among people who suffer from **osteoporosis.** This disease, most commonly found in older women, causes bones to become weak and brittle. And even those who do not sustain a traumatic back injury sometimes suffer compression fractures, causing a forward curvature of the thoracic spine.

A variety of posture-related back problems—from minor aches and pains to sprains to arthritis—can also be found in people with **scoliosis.** This is a condition in which the spine as a whole, when viewed from behind, is skewed into the shape of a "C" or an "S" instead of displaying a straight vertical line. It first shows up most often in girls and young women aged 9

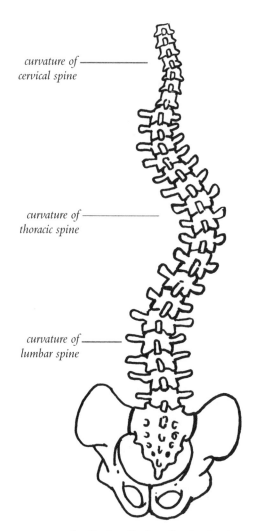

curvature of —————
cervical spine

curvature of —————
thoracic spine

curvature of —————
lumbar spine

Scoliosis of spine (back view)

to 14 who are undergoing growth spurts, though it may occur in boys as well. Its causes are usually not known, although there is more and more evidence of its being an inherited disorder. Early treatment is essential to prevent a mild case of scoliosis from turning into a lifetime of trouble.

Taking Care of Your Back

As with many other parts of the body, **proper posture** is an important factor in maintaining a healthy back. By preserving the straight vertical alignment of the spine, proper posture minimizes stress on the muscles, tendons, ligaments, and disks of the back. Proper posture should be observed as much as possible while standing, sitting, and lying down; those activities that disrupt proper posture for an extended period, or that do so repeatedly, should be avoided. (This admonition should not, however, interfere with normal vigorous activities such as sports, which are in fact much encouraged.)

Although to some people proper posture seems to come almost naturally, for most of us it takes cultivation (and sometimes even professional guidance). For detailed information on recognizing and developing proper posture, see **Chapter 10 — Posture.**

Another important factor in back maintenance is a **proper gait.** The term "gait" refers to your particular manner of walking or running, and a proper gait is a manner of walking or running that displays symmetry, rhythm, and even leg and foot alignment. And while there is no one proper gait, gaits that do not meet these criteria may increase stress on the low back and on other parts of the body (like the hip, knee, ankle, and foot) as well. This is particularly true for serious athletes and anyone else who does a lot of running.

Like proper posture, a proper gait comes naturally to many people, while others may need to cultivate it. In some instances a proper gait is not even attainable without the right tools, like corrective footwear. For more information on identifying and developing a proper gait, see **Chapter 11 — Gait.**

Yet another essential ingredient in maintaining a healthy back is **proper body mechanics** in the various activities of daily life. With regard to the back, proper body mechanics means using the body, and the different parts of the body in ways that are consistent with the smooth functioning of the joints, muscles, ligaments, disks, and other structures of the back. Among other things, this means knowing how to lift and carry heavy objects properly, not holding your back in a fixed position for prolonged periods, and being careful never to twist the trunk when reaching for something.

As with proper posture, proper body mechanics can significantly reduce the risk of many back problems.

Proper body mechanics are by no means always self-evident; occasionally they may even be counterintuitive. For most of us they need to be learned and consciously adopted. For detailed information and instructions on identifying and developing proper body mechanics, see **Chapter 12—Body Mechanics**.

Although they represent slightly different ways of thinking about the body, posture, gait, and body mechanics are closely related phenomena. Indeed, proper posture and a proper gait are practically prerequisites of proper body mechanics, because in their absence you are always undermining the smooth functioning of your joints, muscles, tendons, and ligaments. In fact, some of the poor biomechanical habits most harmful to the back are poor postural and gait habits.

Weight control is a factor that's easily overlooked when it comes to keeping your back healthy. But, in fact, excess weight can significantly magnify the stress on the lumbar spine. That excess weight generally settles around the stomach, and so the muscles that should be working to keep the back in alignment have to support the added pounds as well. To avoid this burden on your back, it's important to remain within your appropriate weight range. (Your weight also has implications for other parts of your body.) For more information, see **Chapter 13—Body Weight**.

Keeping your back healthy also calls for **strength** in the muscles that help to keep the back stable, moving, and well aligned, including not just the back muscles but the leg muscles and especially the abdominals as well. The less developed your muscle strength, the narrower the range of physical activities you are capable of performing—or capable of performing without putting stress on your back. As a result, many common practices of everyday life, from lifting up a child to pushing open a heavy door, become riskier than they should be. Furthermore, a certain amount of strength is necessary simply to hold the back upright, especially with proper posture. A balance of strength in the back, legs, and abdomen is important too so that one area need not compensate for weakness in another.

Endurance in the muscles that support the back is also essential. Endurance is the ability of the muscles to contract (that is, be in use) over time. The less developed a muscle's endurance, the shorter the amount of time it can be called upon to contract before it tires—forcing other, often more vulnerable parts of the body to do its job and putting itself and those other parts at risk of injury. Since a range of common activities, including

Back Inactivity

In one form or another, excessive stress on the back is certainly the most familiar cause of injury to the muscles and joints. Another cause, however, is only slightly less threatening: simple inactivity. Failure regularly to use the muscles of the trunk (back and abdomen) and to bring the spine to the limits of its range of motion through moderately vigorous activity makes the region particularly susceptible to sudden overuse, poor posture, and other kinds of stress. The joints stiffen; ligaments and muscles may contract; good blood flow is inhibited. Even more noteworthy, inactivity may make the back more susceptible to general joint degeneration.

The effects of inactivity tend to be magnified with age. And it is inactivity, more than aging itself, that leads to the conditions generally associated with growing older, like osteoarthritis. Regular exercise—walking, swimming, or golf, for example—may well keep these problems at bay. Indeed, an elderly person who is active may have a "younger" back than an inactive person in his thirties.

many sports and work activities (and even holding the body upright with proper posture), calls upon our muscles to contract over extended periods, a certain level of endurance is absolutely vital.

Flexibility in the muscles, tendons, and ligaments is just as critical as muscle endurance and strength. The less flexible your muscles and ligaments, the more susceptible they are to the natural (and often painful) tightening that comes from everyday activities. And the more susceptible they are to injury when called upon to perform many common practices—from twisting around to look behind you to fielding a ground ball. As with endurance and strength, this flexibility must be distributed among all the muscles that support the back.

Appropriate strength, endurance, and flexibility for your back (and other parts of your body as well) may be achieved through a regular program of exercise. For more information, see **Chapter 15—Strength, Endurance, and Flexibility.**

Although **sports** and other vigorous activities are highly recommended, they do put the back at greater risk of injury, even for those who generally have good endurance, strength, and flexibility in the muscles. The twisting and bending common in many sports and activities, from softball to gardening, make the back vulnerable to a range of minor and major problems. While the risks tend to increase the older you are and the more intense your workout, it is nevertheless a good idea for anyone to fully prepare the back for such a workout: warm up through gentle aerobic activity (such as walking for 5 or 10 minutes, being sure to move the arms) and then stretch the back muscles.

Still, common sense is the best line of defense against injury. If you don't play sports or engage in similar physical activities regularly, it is important not to push yourself too much when you do. And if you do experience any pain in the back, stop what you're doing at once. To try to "play through it" is to risk injury.

For more information on protecting your back and other parts of your body from injury during particular sports, see **Chapter 16—Sports.**

Like sports, many lines of **work** carry considerable risks of back injury due to strain or overuse. Needless to say, just about any sort of heavy labor that involves bending, lifting, and carrying (like construction work or furniture moving) falls into this category. So, too, do jobs that involve standing for long hours or, worse, leaning forward frequently, like drafting, dishwashing, and some assembly-line work. Many back problems are associated with sitting at a desk all day, which places constant stress places on the lumbar spine. If you hold an occupation of this sort—even if your muscle endurance, strength, and flexibility are good—it is a wise precaution to first warm up and then stretch the back muscles before beginning your workday and several times throughout the day.

It's also important as much as possible to configure your physical work environment so that it does not force you to use poor body mechanics. Drafters, for example, might raise their drafting tables; dishwashers or assembly-line workers might put down a low footstool on which to set one foot. If you work at a desk, it is essential that your chair be appropriately supportive and that both chair and desk be at proper heights.

Finally, if your occupation does subject your back to strain and overuse, be sure to take a break of at least several minutes every hour. And if you feel any tightness or stiffness *at all*, stretch the muscles a bit (see below). In fact, to head off problems, you may want to try this routine even if you don't have tightness or stiffness.

For more information on protecting your back and other parts of your body from injury during work activities, see **Chapter 17—Work.**

When Problems Occur

No matter how well you treat your back, **occasional temporary tightness and stiffness** are inevitable, especially as you grow older. After all, everyday life can be grueling on the back; we sit at computer terminals all day, stand for long periods on crowded buses, sleep on too-soft hotel mattresses. One way to ease your discomfort is with a few focused **stretching exercises,** which will bring back some badly needed flexibility and blood flow to your tired or aching muscles. (See the box, **"Quick-Relief Back Stretches,"** at right.)

Massage, which increases blood flow to the region while warming and stretching the back's muscle and soft tissue, may also work nicely. Although electric hand-held massagers and various nonelectric massage rollers are available on the market, you're much more likely to get a sensitive massage from someone just using the hands.

Sometimes a bout of back stiffness or soreness can be traced directly to a particular instance of poor posture or poor body mechanics. This is often the explanation for pain that occurs during a specific activity—brushing your teeth, for example, or stepping into a pair of pants. If this is the case, double-check your posture and body mechanics; you might find that a simple adjustment will quickly eliminate the problem. If discomfort tends to strike just after you've gotten out of bed, it may be an indication

Quick-Relief Back Stretches

The stretches below may ease (and sometimes even head off) common back tightness and stiffness, especially tightness and stiffness caused by repetitive stress or overuse from daily activities. Feel free to do them as often as you wish. Detailed instructions and appropriate illustrations can be found in Chapter 19—Flexibility Exercises. These exercises are especially valuable if you work long hours at a desk. (They may also help with muscle spasm.) If your back tightness and stiffness produce more than minor discomfort, consult your physical therapist before attempting them. Be sure to warm up your muscles prior to doing these exercises by, for instance, getting up and walking around your office.

- Seated Low Back Stretch (p. 228)
- Seated Spinal Twist (p. 231)
- Extended-Arm Side Stretch (p. 233)
- Stretch and Reach (p. 234)

Pain-Relief Devices

The marketplace is loaded with elaborate devices meant to combat back pain—like inversion swings, arc-shaped tables, and oversized rubber balls (for lying down on). While some of these may be effective at times, there is no easy cure for most problems related to the low back. Under no circumstances should you use these products without consulting a health professional.

you need to change bad sleeping habits.

If your back stiffness and soreness persist for more than a week, it's a good idea to have your back checked by a physical therapist or physician.

Beyond temporary soreness and stiffness, it is not unlikely that you will experience **more serious back problems** of one sort or another at some point in your life even if you have a generally healthy back. The normal wear and tear of everyday living has its cumulative effects. Age, too, takes its toll, and with it may come thinning disks (with their associated problems) and possibly osteoporosis and other dysfunctions. Many people will sustain an occasional fall or have an accident that may bring sprains, muscle tears, herniated disks, or even fractures. Anyway, few of us can claim perfect back maintenance, which makes us especially vulnerable to a whole range of back problems.

Because a particular bout of back pain may be a sign of any number of ailments, it is essentially impossible to diagnose a problem yourself—and just as impossible to figure out how to deal with the problem. Instead, it is best to see a physical therapist or physician at the first sign of trouble, no matter how innocent-seeming. This is usually an obvious course of action in the case of a traumatic event, like when your back "goes out" trying to move a piece of furniture or, worse, when you take a bad spill on the ice or down a flight of stairs. In these cases you should seek **immediate professional attention.** In such urgent situations it's also a good idea to know some basics of **first aid.** But because of the possibility of a broken back or spinal cord damage, you should always take a traumatic back injury very seriously. Indeed, one cardinal rule of first aid is, *Never attempt to move a person who has suffered possible spinal trauma.* (See **Appendix A—First Aid Basics**.)

Even if it's not the result of a traumatic event, any case of severe back pain—or of acute pain, numbness, or weakness in the legs, which may indicate a serious back problem—also demands immediate professional attention (and, if appropriate, first aid).

Milder degrees of back pain, if persisting for more than a few days or recurring, should also be evaluated by a physical therapist or physician. This includes the "common cold" of back problems, **minor low back pain,** a dull ache that usually lasts, on and off, for a few days (at least initially). Since minor low back pain is generally the eventual result of back or abdominal muscle weakness and improper body mechanics and poor posture, it can easily develop into a chronic condition if not addressed. Of equal concern is the possibility that minor low back pain is the symptom of a more involved problem. But take heart! Most people recover soon from their episodes of low back pain. In fact, research shows that nine out of ten people recover within one month.

In the meantime, minor back pain may be managed by heeding a few simple tips. **Rest** may provide some relief by allowing strained muscles to heal. Lie down on a firm supporting surface on your back or side, choosing the position most comfortable to you—as long as you maintain the proper alignment of the spine (see **Chapter 10—Posture**). Many people even find it beneficial to lie on the floor with both legs bent and the calves set up on a chair. (Lift your legs gently and one at a time.) This particular position places the least amount of compressive force on your lumbar disks. Sitting certainly is not dangerous, but it generally puts more stress on the back than does standing. So while you're recovering, you may want to spend less time sitting or at least make your sitting more comfortable by supporting the curve of your low back with a pillow or by using a chair that has a slightly reclining back. Prolonged bed rest of more than a couple of days, however, is not recommended; it actually weakens the back and could cause your discomfort to last longer. A gradual return to normal activities is best. Continuing to walk, even in the initial stages, may be helpful.

For the first day or two after the appearance of minor back pain, you may apply **ice** to the affected area. The ice numbs the pain temporarily and may reduce or prevent swelling. One good method for applying ice is to put crushed ice in a sealable plastic bag with a little water, then cover the bag with towels. (A bag of frozen peas or corn works well too; refrigerated towels can be used in a pinch.) To avoid harming the skin or underlying tissues, apply the ice for only 15 to 20 minutes at a time, with 20 to 40 minutes between applications.

After a period of using ice, you may try **moist heat,** applied to the back in a 20-minutes-on/20-minutes-off cycle. Moist heat tends to relax tense muscles, offering some relief from pain and stiffness. Warm showers or warm, moist towels work well for this. Heating pads, although not highly recommended, are also acceptable, but take care that the heat is not too intense for you.

For some people **nonsteroidal anti-inflammatory drugs (NSAIDs)** may be very effective in easing back pain. This class of drugs includes aspirin and ibuprofen, both of which are widely available without prescription. Like all drugs, however, NSAIDs have potentially dangerous side effects. Ask your doctor or pharmacist before taking NSAIDs, and follow the directions on the label.

When you first experience back pain, try to make a mental note of when and where you were and what you were doing when it occurred. This information may be important in helping your physical therapist make a diagnosis. When addressing a particular back problem, your physical therapist has a wide range of techniques to draw upon. But—depending on the physical therapist's examination and evaluation—a back rehabilitation program will almost certainly incorporate strength, endurance, and flexibility exercises; attention to improved postural alignment, gait, and body mechanics; and weight management.

The Neck

Chances are you don't give your neck much thought. It holds your head up. It lets you move your head up and down, left and right…or follow the movements of a fly as it buzzes through a room…or trace the flight of a tennis ball as it arcs over a net.

Then one day something goes wrong: You wake up able to turn your head in only one direction…or you can't concentrate on your work because of a muscle knot…or you have a "minor" car accident that forces you to wear a cervical collar.

In short, you discover the true meaning of the phrase *a pain in the neck.*

This chapter is designed to give you a basic understanding of neck problems and, if possible, how to avoid them. We'll also give you some simple advice on avoiding neck strain in every phase of your daily life: working, playing, and even sleeping.

How the Neck Works

The neck is the uppermost region of the spine, and it's vulnerable to the full complement of back-related ailments (see **Chapter 1—The Back**). And while the lower back (lumbar region) is the most troublesome area of the spine, the neck is a close second due to its wide range of motion, delicate vertebrae, and complex musculature.

As part of the spine, it's not surprising that the neck is composed of the same structural building blocks: vertebrae and disks. The neck, or **cervical spine,** consists of seven cylindrical bones, or **vertebrae,** which run from the base of the head to the large bump at the very top of your back between the shoulders. When looked at from the side, the stacked vertebrae form a gentle, forward-projecting "C" curve.

The bottom five cervical vertebrae are in most respects similar to lumbar vertebrae, although smaller. The topmost cervical vertebra (the **atlas**) conforms to the shape of the **occipital bone**—the bone forming the lower part of the back of head—and allows you to nod your head. The second cervical vertebra (the **axis**) has a large upward projection that creates the pivot about which the head rotates.

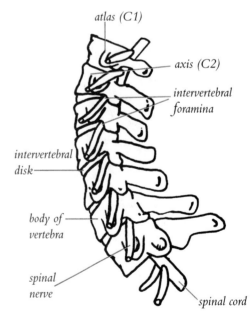

Cervical spine (side view)

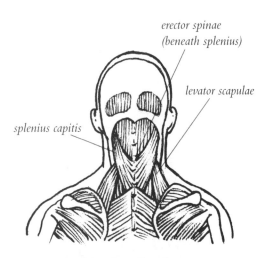

Muscles of neck—
superficial muscles

trapezius

*erector spinae
(beneath splenius)*

levator scapulae

splenius capitis

Muscles of neck—
deep muscles

Pairs of bony projections called **facets** connect the rear portions of the cervical vertebrae to form a series of interlocking **joints.** The facet joints in the neck are surrounded by a **synovial membrane** that secretes tiny amounts of lubricating **synovial fluid.** The joint surfaces also are covered with a smooth **articular cartilage** that facilitates movement in the region.

Between the vertebrae are shock-absorbing cervical **disks.** (There is, however, no disk between the base of the head and the first cervical vertebra or between the first cervical vertebra and the second.) The disks are slightly smaller than the body of the vertebra and, like the disks in the lumbar spine, are slightly thicker toward the front than toward the back. Each disk is made up of a jelly-like center and a thick outer sheath of tough fibrocartilage.

As in the lumbar and thoracic spine, carved out within the bodies of the vertebrae is a sheltering canal (the **spinal canal**) for the **spinal cord**—the nerve impulse transmitter between the brain and the rest of the body. Major **nerve roots** branch off from the spinal cord at all levels of the vertebrae and pass through openings called **foramina.** These nerves allow our muscles to contract and allow us to perceive sensations such as touch, temperature, and pain. One of the most significant of these is the **brachial plexus,** a network of five nerve roots coming from the middle and lower cervical spine. This is very similar to the sciatic nerve in the lumbar spine. The brachial plexus subdivides into three main nerves that run all the way down the arm: the **radial, median,** and **ulnar nerves.** These nerves provide movement and sensation to the arms. (Because of this, shoulder and arm pain is often a symptom of a problem in the neck.)

An elaborate network of **muscles** wraps and supports the spinal column. The muscles in the neck, along with the shoulder and upper back muscles, all work together to keep the cervical spine stabilized and aligned properly. They also allow for fine movement of the head. Among the more important of these is the **erector spinae** group, a deep layer of muscles running along each side of the back of the neck; the **sternocleidomastoid (SCM)** muscles, which run diagonally from just behind the ears to the breastbone; the **scalene** muscles, just below the SCM muscles to the sides of the neck; the **trapezius** muscles, at the back of the neck, on either side of the spine; and the **levator scapulae** muscles, running from the top four vertebrae to the shoulder blade. Strong, flexible, fibrous cords called **tendons**—technically, extensions of the muscles—attach these muscles to the cervical spine and to the nearby shoulder blades, collarbones, upper ribs, lower jaw, and head.

Ligaments, tough bands of fibrous tissue, provide stability and reinforcement by binding each pair of cervical vertebrae together; several long ligaments run the entire length of the spinal column, both in front and back. The cervical spine is further reinforced by **joint capsules,** fibrous and connective tissue material that surrounds the facets.

The neck functions as the part of a kinetic chain that includes the head and jaw at one end and the upper back, shoulders, arms, lower back, and legs and feet at the other. All of these different body areas are interrelated and depend on each other for correct functioning and movement. And as part of the spine, the neck has an effect on many other regions of the body.

What Can Go Wrong

As part of the spine, the neck is subject to many of the same disorders that may afflict the back, from pinched nerves to slipped disks. Adding to the risk of injury is the neck's wide range of motion and flexibility.

While some neck problems may arise as the result of a specific traumatic incident—like a fall or a car accident—they often seem to appear out of nowhere. In cases where there is no obvious cause for pain, the culprit is often the accumulated stress, strain, and abuse from years of poor posture and bad body mechanics. The triggering incident may be so trivial as to go unnoticed. This can make diagnosis of a specific neck ailment tricky even for health professionals. While many neck problems are associated with aging, younger people also endure their share of neck troubles, whether they stem from injuries, poor posture, or poor body mechanics. Disease, too, can sometimes strike young necks just as it does older ones.

Neck pain comes in many varieties. It can be dull, sharp, constant, intermittent, shooting, tingling like "pins and needles"—even a burning sensation. It may be localized in the neck, or radiate down the arm, or both. The degree of pain is also highly variable, from mild discomfort to agonizing pain. And although neck pain may strike just the neck itself, a number of neck problems are accompanied by irritation of the brachial plexus, which sends hot shooting or radiating pain into the shoulder, arm, and hand; this pain comes on quickly and may affect one or both sides of the body. Neck problems may also be associated with headaches.

Some neck conditions, such as mild strains and sprains (see page 30–31), call for simple treatments like rest and ice. Others demand more advanced physical therapy techniques: carefully and scientifically tailored exercises to strengthen the neck and improve range of motion; adjustments of the posture; mobilization; and perhaps approaches (modalities) like ultrasound and electrical stimulation as well. Still other problems require surgery or other major interventions, although these, too, are usually complemented

Headaches and Your Neck

Although headaches have a vast range of possible causes—from eating habits to infections to dehydration—they may also have a cervical origin. Muscle tension in the neck, hyperextension injuries, and cervical disk problems may all refer pain into the head. There is, however, no simple way to determine if and when a particular headache has neck problems as its underlying cause. If your mild headache seems to be associated with tightness in the back of the neck and shoulders, you might try applying a few stretches from the box "Quick-Relief Neck Stretches" on page 37 a couple of times a day. A severe or persistent headache requires the attention of a physician.

with an exercise program designed by a physical therapist as part of the rehabilitation stage. In every instance, however, you should look to your physician or physical therapist to make a diagnosis and determine treatment.

Muscles in the neck are a frequent site of neck dysfunction. Certainly the mildest such dysfunction, if it can even be called that, is the tendency of these muscles—like muscles throughout the body—to become stiff or tight in response to heavy neck activity. A similar **muscle tightness** may be produced by simple emotional stress. The result is usually minor short-term achiness and may be no cause for concern. (On the other hand, muscle tightness does diminish the neck's range of motion, which, unless the muscles are warmed up and stretched, puts the neck at risk of injury when called upon to push beyond that range.)

More worrisome is the accumulation of excess lactic acid and other chemicals in the neck muscles whenever they are subject to excessive stress over prolonged periods of time—whether it be from poor posture, from constantly craning the neck forward, or simply from holding the head in a fixed position. The cellular and chemical responses to excessive stress almost inevitably lead to painful **muscle inflammation** and the development of **trigger points**—sore, hard knots of muscle generally found at the base of the neck, in the upper back, or around the shoulder blades. Sometimes the pain becomes apparent only when you move your head in a particular direction. Sometimes it shows up in the form of headaches. Unfortunately, the effects of such inflammation may accumulate over time; what starts out as a mild twinge may wind up as a full-blown neckache.

The neck's muscles may also suffer from **muscle spasm,** the sudden, intense contraction of muscle tissue. Although very painful, a muscle spasm is the body's natural mechanism for protecting injured tissue by acting as a brace. It often occurs whenever the neck is at serious risk of strain or other injury. Lifting a heavy object or holding the head in an awkward position for too long is sometimes enough to set off a spasm.

Spasm may also be caused by irritation of or damage to nerves in the neck or other traumatic injury. In cases of major injury the spasm may be so intense that the neck will be held rigidly in one place, movable only with difficulty. Muscle spasm may even flatten out the normal curve of the cervical spine, giving a rigid appearance to the neck.

Tearing of the muscles is another cause of muscle spasm and is usually painful in its own right. This tearing may result from direct trauma, overuse (engaging in sports or performing some other physical activity), and possibly prolonged poor posture or poor body mechanics. A **muscle strain,** sometimes inaccurately called a "pulled muscle," occurs when the muscle has been overstretched or overexerted and may have microscopic tearing as its cause. When the tearing is more severe, it is called, simply, a **muscle tear,** which may be partial or complete. When a muscle is strained or torn, the blood vessels in the muscle are strained or torn as well. Besides spasm, the symptoms of strains and tears vary only in degree and may include pain, inflammation, and bleeding into the surrounding tissues. Strains, however, are often mild enough to require little more treatment than rest for a few days.

Muscle strain and tears and the accompanying spasm are common components of the familiar injury known as whiplash (see page 33).

Not unlike the muscles, the ligaments of the neck can be overstretched—that is, pushed beyond their normal limits—or microscopically torn. This injury, a **sprain,** may afflict any of the neck's ligaments and may be produced by trauma (like a fall), overuse (from activities such as gymnastics), the cumulative impact of poor posture, or poor body mechanics (like lifting heavy objects incorrectly). One common neck sprain appears in the ligaments that bind the facet joints together. With a sprain, the pain may be localized or it may radiate down the arm and into the hand. If overstretched ligaments are not holding a joint firmly in place, there may also be a feeling of slippage. Over time the joint may become stiff and restricted. Ligament sprains are also a common component of whiplash (see page 33).

The facet joints are subject to the degenerative changes associated with **arthritis,** which can lead to both pain and stiffness. This condition can be the result of early trauma to the joints, but there is a wide range of possible causes. One form of arthritis is **rheumatoid arthritis,** a disease whose origin is not fully understood (but which may be the result of autoimmune mechanisms or viral infections). Although some cases of rheumatoid arthritis are relatively benign, in extreme cases the joints become so swollen that they essentially fuse together. This is a serious and often debilitating condition. Physical therapy is necessary to help maintain mobility and flexibility in the region.

A far more common form of arthritis in the cervical spine is **osteoarthritis,** the degeneration of the articular cartilage and a wearing down of the joint surfaces. In some cases osteoarthritis may result in the buildup of spurs (deposits of bony tissue) on the vertebrae. And if these bone spurs encroach on the spinal cord or the nerves branching off it, the result may be not just pain and stiffness in the neck but tingling in the arms as well.

Osteoarthritis has a number of possible causes, including trauma, overuse, degenerative disk disease (see page 32), and inactivity. But by far the most common is degeneration of the joint due to age, typical (though not inevitable) among middle-aged individuals. Although it sometimes has no symptoms at all, osteoarthritis may well lead to general stiffness and neck pain from mild to severe.

The osteoarthritis-related degenerative changes to the disks and joints of the cervical spine, common among people over 40, are known generally as **cervical spondylosis.** This condition requires an X-ray to accurately diagnose. Flare-ups are commonly treated initially with rest and immobilization of the cervical spine, followed by exercises and postural training provided by a physical therapist. Only in extreme cases is surgery necessary.

"Slipped disk" is a catch-all term for **herniated, bulging, protruding, extruded,** or **ruptured disks**—terms that have been used to describe various degrees of a similar problem. Generally speaking, a herniated disk is one whose contents have been pushed beyond their normal boundaries. The pressure of the disk center against the outer sheath may sometimes lead to a bulge of the disk wall. In severe cases the wall actually breaks; the gelatinous contents of the disk then spill into the surrounding area and put pressure on the wall, the ligaments, and the nerve root itself. Sometimes this may lead to nerve inflammation.

Herniated disks often display no symptoms and can go unnoticed by those who have them. But the result of any herniated disk can be numbness or tingling (if the nerves are irritated), or even sharp pain. Herniated disks may cause impingement on a nerve root. They may cause headaches as well.

Herniated disks may often result from poor body mechanics during daily activities (such as poor lifting techniques) and poor posture. Sports injuries are another common cause, particularly from sports that require running, jumping, or extreme flexibility (such as gymnastics). The loss of disk thickness due to aging or degeneration (see below) tends to make the disks more vulnerable as we age. Herniated disks may be a common component of whiplash injury (see page 33).

A herniated disk is usually diagnosed with the help of imaging techniques such as magnetic resonance imaging (MRI). Rest, medications, custom-fitted cervical orthoses, postural training, and other noninvasive techniques to relieve any pain are recommended; as pain subsides, a thorough exercise program is essential. Surgery is usually reserved for cases in which all other treatments fail.

Disks are also susceptible to **degenerative disk disease,** which is, like joint degeneration, a typical if not inevitable function of aging. As we reach our late twenties or early thirties, the gelatinous center of the disk begins to

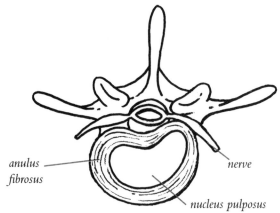

anulus fibrosus

nerve

nucleus pulposus

Bulging disk

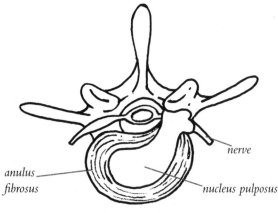

anulus fibrosus

nerve

nucleus pulposus

Ruptured disk

dry out and becomes more fibrous. Eventually the disk may dry up completely. Although degenerative disk disease and degenerative joint disease are often a part of aging, they don't necessarily produce major symptoms.

Like all bones, the neck vertebrae are subject to **fracture** as a result of trauma, like a fall or a collision. Often fractures cause pain (local or radiating) and joint stiffness. In some cases fractures may cause damage to the spinal cord, perhaps the most serious injury the neck may sustain. For this reason even the suspicion of a spinal fracture should be treated as a major medical emergency demanding immediate professional attention.

A variety of posture-related neck problems—from minor aches and pains to joint sprains to arthritis—can also be found in people with **scoliosis.** This is a condition in which the spine as a whole, when viewed from behind, is skewed into the shape of a "C" or an "S" instead of displaying a straight vertical line. It shows up most often in girls aged 9 to 14 who are undergoing growth spurts, though it may occur in boys as well. And while it manifests itself more commonly in the thoracic and lumbar spines, scoliosis may often produce compensatory curves in the cervical spine. Its causes are not known, although there is more and more evidence of its being an inherited disorder. Early treatment is essential to prevent a mild case of scoliosis from turning into a lifetime of trouble.

There is probably no condition more widely associated with the neck than **whiplash.** Whiplash is a diagnostic term that may be applied to a combination of problems resulting from high-speed back-and-forth movement of the neck: severe muscle strain or tears, extreme muscle spasm, severe ligament sprain, and/or herniated disk. (Injuries to the jaw may also be part of this combination.) The typical cause of whiplash—though by no means the only one—is an automobile accident in which an automobile is hit from behind, causing the driver's or passenger's neck to snap too far backward (hyperextension), then too far forward (hyperflexion), then sometimes too far backward again. If a car crashes into an immobile object or has a head-on collision, the sequence is reversed. In most instances of whiplash, pain is felt in both the neck and the arms; even slight movement of the head may be very painful.

Taking Care of Your Neck

As with many other parts of the body, **proper posture** is an important factor in maintaining a healthy neck. By preserving the straight vertical alignment of the spine, proper posture minimizes stress on the muscles, tendons, ligaments, and disks of the neck. Proper posture should be

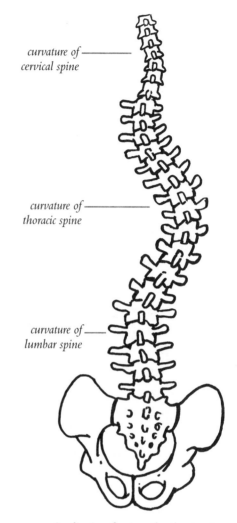

curvature of cervical spine

curvature of thoracic spine

curvature of lumbar spine

Scoliosis of spine (back view)

observed as much as possible while standing, sitting, and lying down; those activities that disrupt proper posture for an extended period, or that do so repeatedly, should be avoided. (This admonition should not, however, interfere with normal vigorous activities such as sports, which are in fact much encouraged.)

Although to some people proper posture seems to come almost naturally, for most of us it takes cultivation (and sometimes even professional guidance). For detailed information on recognizing and developing proper posture, see **Chapter 10—Posture**.

Another important factor in neck maintenance is **proper body mechanics** in the various activities of daily life. With regard to the neck, proper body mechanics means using the body and the different parts of the body in ways that are consistent with the smooth functioning of the joints, muscles, ligaments, and disks of the neck. Among other things, this means knowing how to lift and carry heavy objects properly, not holding the neck in a fixed position for prolonged periods, and being careful never to cradle the telephone between your ear and shoulder. As with proper posture, proper body mechanics can reduce the risk of many neck problems.

Proper body mechanics are by no means always self-evident; occasionally they may even be counterintuitive. For most of us they need to be learned and adopted. For detailed information on identifying and developing proper body mechanics, see **Chapter 12—Body Mechanics**.

Although they represent somewhat different ways of thinking about the body, posture and body mechanics are closely related phenomena. Proper posture is practically a prerequisite of proper body mechanics, because in the absence of proper posture, you are always undermining the smooth functioning of your joints, muscles, tendons, ligaments, and disks. Indeed, quite a few of the poor biomechanical habits harmful to the neck are poor postural habits.

Keeping your neck healthy also calls for **strength** in the muscles that help to keep the neck stable, moving, and well aligned, including not just the neck muscles but the shoulder, upper back, and arm muscles as well. The less developed your muscle strength, the narrower the range of physical activities you are capable of performing—or capable of performing without putting stress on your neck. As a result, many common practices of everyday life, from lifting up a child to pushing open a heavy door, become riskier than they should be. Furthermore, a certain amount of strength is necessary simply to hold the head upright, especially with proper posture. A balance of strength in the neck, shoulder, upper back, and arm muscles is important too so that one area need not compensate for weakness in another.

Endurance in the muscles that support the neck is also essential. Endurance is the ability of the muscles to contract (that is, be in use) over time. The less developed a muscle's endurance, the shorter the amount of time it may be called upon to contract before it tires—forcing other, often more vulnerable parts of the body to do its job and putting itself and those other parts at risk of injury. Since a range of common activities, including many sports and work activities (and even holding the head upright with proper posture for any sustained period of time), calls upon our muscles to contract over long periods, a certain level of endurance is absolutely vital.

Flexibility in the muscles, tendons, and ligaments is just as critical as muscle endurance and strength. The less flexible your muscles and ligaments, the more susceptible they are to the natural (and often painful) tightening that comes from everyday activities. And the more susceptible they are to injury when called upon to perform many common practices—from turning to look over your shoulder to fielding a fly ball. As with endurance and strength, this flexibility must be distributed among all the muscles that support the neck.

Appropriate endurance, strength, and flexibility for your neck (and other body parts) may be achieved through a regular program of exercise. For more information, see **Chapter 15—Strength, Endurance, and Flexibility.**

Like all parts of the body, the neck is generally at greater risk of injury during **sports** or similar physical activities, even for those who generally have good endurance, strength, and flexibility in the muscles. The abrupt and repeated twisting, turning, and bending of the neck common in many sports and activities, from tennis to football, make the neck vulnerable to a range of minor and major problems. While the risks tend to increase the older you are and the more intense your workout is, it is nevertheless a good idea for anyone to fully prepare the neck for such a workout: warm up through gentle aerobic activity (such as walking for 5 or 10 minutes, being sure to move the arms) and then stretch the neck muscles.

Still, common sense is the best line of defense against injury. If you don't play sports or engage in similar physical activities regularly, it is important not to push yourself too much when you do. And if you do experience any pain in the neck, stop what you're doing at once. To try to "play through it" is to risk injury.

For more information on protecting your neck and other parts of your body from injury during particular sports, see **Chapter 16—Sports.**

Like sports, many lines of **work** carry considerable risks of neck injury

Neck Inactivity

In one form or another, excessive stress on the neck is certainly the most familiar cause of injury to the muscles and joints. Another cause, however, is only slightly less threatening: simple inactivity. Failure regularly to use the muscles of the neck and to bring the cervical spine to the limits of its range of motion through moderately vigorous activity makes the region particularly susceptible to sudden overuse, poor posture, and other kinds of stress. The joints stiffen; ligaments and muscles may contract; good blood flow is inhibited. Even more noteworthy, inactivity may make the neck more susceptible to general joint degeneration.

The effects of inactivity tend to be magnified with age. And it is inactivity, more than aging itself, that leads to the conditions generally associated with growing older, like osteoarthritis. Regular exercise—walking, swimming, or golf, for example—may well keep these problems at bay. Indeed, an elderly person who is active may have a "younger" neck than an inactive person in his thirties.

Headrests, Airbags, and Your Neck

One important measure you can take to avoid neck trauma is to use a car outfitted with headrests and airbags. These features offer the best protection against whiplash caused by auto accidents. Your headrest should be raised so that the middle of the back of your head contacts it and, if possible, adjusted so that it corresponds to the curve of your cervical spine.

due to strain or overuse. Needless to say, just about any sort of heavy labor that involves bending, lifting, and carrying (like construction work or furniture moving) falls into this category. So, too, do jobs that involve standing for long hours or, worse, leaning forward frequently, like drafting, dishwashing, and some assembly-line work. Many neck problems are caused by jobs that demand a high degree of concentration, like working at a computer all day, which (among other things) tends to keep the neck in a forward, fixed position for hours on end. If you hold a job of this sort—even if your muscle endurance, strength, and flexibility are good—it may be a wise precaution first to warm up and then to stretch the neck (and related) muscles before beginning your work day and several times throughout the day.

It's also important as much as possible to configure your physical work environment so that it does not force you to use poor body mechanics. Drafters, for example, might raise their drafting tables; dishwashers or assembly-line workers might put down a low footstool on which to set one foot. If you work at a computer, it is essential that your chair be appropriately supportive and that chair, desk, and monitor be at proper heights.

Finally, if your occupation does subject your neck to strain and overuse, be sure to take a break of at least several minutes every hour. And if you feel any tightness or stiffness *at all*, stretch the muscles a bit (see below). In fact, to head off problems, you may want to try this routine even if you don't have tightness or stiffness.

For more information on protecting your neck and other parts of your bod, from injury during work activities, see **Chapter 17—Work**.

When Problems Occur

No matter how well you treat your neck, **occasional temporary tightness and stiffness** are almost inevitable, especially as you grow older. After all, between craning our necks at computer terminals all day and lugging heavy briefcases and purses from place to place, everyday life can be grueling on the neck. One way to ease your discomfort is with a few focused **stretching exercises,** which will bring back some badly needed elasticity and blood flow to your tired or aching muscles. (See the box, "Quick-Relief Neck Stretches," on page 37.)

Massage, which increases blood flow to the region while warming and stretching the neck's muscle and soft tissue, may also work nicely. Because the muscles of the neck and shoulder region are interconnected, you'll get the best results by working both areas. Although electric hand-held massagers and various nonelectric massage rollers are available on the market, you're much more likely to get a sensitive massage from someone just using the hands.

Sometimes a bout of neck stiffness or soreness can be traced directly to a particular instance of poor posture or poor body mechanics. This is often the explanation for pain that occurs during a specific activity—working, reading, or even sleeping. If this is the case, double-check your body mechanics; you may find that a simple adjustment will quickly eliminate the problem. If the discomfort tends to strike just after you've gotten out of bed, it may be an indication that you need to change bad sleeping habits.

If your neck stiffness and soreness persist for more than a week, it's a good idea to have your neck checked by a physical therapist or physician.

Beyond temporary soreness and stiffness, it is possible that you will experience **more serious neck problems** of one sort or another at some point in your life, even if you have a generally healthy neck. The normal wear and tear of everyday living has its cumulative effects. Age, too, takes its toll, and with it may come thinning disks (with their associated problems) and other degenerative conditions. Some people will sustain an occasional fall or have an accident that may bring sprains, muscle tears, herniated disks, or even fractures. Anyway, few of us can claim perfect neck maintenance, which makes us especially vulnerable to a whole range of neck problems.

It is best to see a physical therapist or physician at the first sign of neck trouble, no matter how innocent-seeming. This is usually an obvious course of action in the case of a traumatic event, like when your head has been snapped back and forth in a car accident or when you've suffered a sports-related neck injury. In these cases you should seek **immediate professional attention.** In such urgent situations it's also a good idea to know some basics of **first aid.** But because of the possibility of a broken neck or spinal cord damage, you should always take a traumatic neck injury very seriously. Indeed, one cardinal rule of first aid is, *Never attempt to move a patient who has suffered possible neck trauma.* (See **Appendix A—First Aid Basics.**)

Even if it's not the result of a traumatic event, any case of severe neck pain—or of acute pain, numbness, weakness, or tingling in the arms, which may indicate a serious neck problem—also demands immediate professional attention (and, if appropriate, first aid).

Milder degrees of neck pain, if persisting for more than a few days or recurring, should also be evaluated by a physical therapist or physician. Because minor neck pain is generally the eventual result of weakened muscles and improper posture and body mechanics, it can easily develop into a chronic condition if not addressed. Of equal concern is the possibility that

Quick-Relief Neck Stretches

The stretches below may ease (and sometimes even head off) common neck tightness and stiffness, especially tightness and stiffness caused by repetitive stress or overuse from daily activities. Feel free to do them as often as you wish. Detailed instructions and appropriate illustrations can be found in Chapter 19—Flexibility Exercises. These exercises are especially valuable if you work long hours at a computer terminal. (They may also help with muscle spasm.) If your neck tightness and stiffness produce more than minor discomfort, consult your physical therapist before attempting them. Be sure to warm up your muscles prior to doing these exercises by, for instance, getting up and walking around your office.

- Spine Lengthener (p. 237)
- Seated Neck Nod (p. 237)
- Raised-Arm Neck Flex (p. 238)
- Neck Rotation (p. 239)
- Assisted Lateral Neck Stretch (p. 240)
- Neck Circles (p. 241)

minor neck pain is the symptom of an even more involved problem.

In the meantime, minor neck pain may be managed by heeding a few simple tips. **Rest,** to give the neck muscles a chance to regenerate and heal, is the first item on the agenda. Because all upright activities require constant contraction of the neck muscles, you should lie down on a firm, supporting surface on your back or side, maintaining the proper alignment of the neck (see **Chapter 10—Posture**). Don't stuff too many pillows under your neck—it will only make the problem worse. A contoured cervical pillow is an ideal option. Prolonged bed rest of more than a couple of days is not recommended; a gradual return to normal activities is best.

For the first day or two after the appearance of minor neck pain, you may apply **ice** to the affected area. The ice numbs the pain temporarily and may reduce or prevent swelling. One good method for applying ice is to put crushed ice in a sealable plastic bag with a little water, then cover the bag with towels. (A bag of frozen peas or corn works well too; refrigerated towels can be used in a pinch.) To avoid harming the skin or underlying tissues, apply the ice for only 15 to 20 minutes at a time, with 20 to 40 minutes between applications.

After a period of using ice, you may try **moist heat,** applied to the neck in a 20-minutes-on/20-minutes-off cycle. Moist heat tends to relax tense muscles, offering some relief from pain and stiffness. Warm showers or warm, moist towels work well for this. Heating pads, although not highly recommended, are also acceptable, but take care that the heat is not too intense.

For some people **nonsteroidal anti-inflammatory drugs (NSAIDs)** may be effective in easing neck pain. This class of drugs includes aspirin and ibuprofen, both of which are widely available without prescription. Like all drugs, however, NSAIDs have potentially dangerous side effects. Ask your doctor or pharmacist before taking NSAIDs, and follow the directions on the label.

When addressing a particular neck problem, your physical therapist has a wide range of techniques to draw upon. But—depending on the physcial therapist's examination and evaluation—a neck rehabilitation program will almost certainly incorporate strength, endurance, and flexibility exercises and attention to improved postural alignment and body mechanics.

CHAPTER THREE
The Jaw

For most of us, the jaw is a fairly trouble-free region of the body. But for people who suffer from jaw dysfunction—particularly problems related to the temporomandibular joint, the joint linking the jaw to the skull—the jaw can open a Pandora's box of symptoms. To make matters worse, these symptoms sometimes mimic those associated with a variety of serious ailments.

How the Jaw Works

The **temporomandibular joint (TMJ)** joins the jawbone (mandible) with the lower part of the skull (**temporal bone**). And though it seems to work like a simple hinge, the TMJ is actually a rather complex joint. The end of the mandible features a rounded protrusion called a **condyle,** which glides in and out of a socket called the **fossa** on the underside of the temporal bone. Between the condyle and the fossa lies the **meniscus,** a crescent-shaped disk of shock-absorbing cartilage. The meniscus also serves to separate the joint into two cavities. The joint surfaces are covered with a smooth **articular cartilage** that facilitates movement in the region. This construction allows the jaw a fairly wide range of motion—up and down, side to side, back and forth, even a slight rotation.

Muscles in the head, neck, and jaw all work together to keep the TMJ stable, well aligned, and moving. Among the more important of these are the **masseter,** located directly over the TMJ, and the **temporalis,** located at the temples. **Ligaments,** tough bands of fibrous tissue, provide stability and reinforcement by binding bones together; the most important of these is the **temporomandibular ligament,** which crosses the jaw and binds together the temporal bone and mandible. The joint is further stabilized by a **joint capsule,** fibrous and connective tissue that surrounds it.

Like many other joints, the TMJ has a **synovial membrane** that surrounds the joint and secretes a tiny amount of lubricating **synovial fluid.**

The jaw functions as part of a kinetic chain that includes the head at one end, and the neck, shoulders, back, legs, and feet at the other. The movement and working of all these different body areas are interrelated

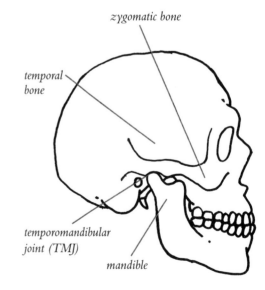

zygomatic bone

temporal bone

temporomandibular joint (TMJ)

mandible

Jaw

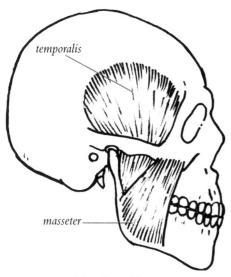

temporalis

masseter

Muscles of jaw

and depend on each other for correct functioning. Other than the teeth, however, no body part has more bearing on the jaw than the neck; see **Chapter 2—The Neck**.

What Can Go Wrong

Jaw problems can be deceptive. We often think of jaw ailments (if we think of them at all) in terms of traumatic injuries—"a sock in the jaw" from a fistfight, for example. But direct trauma represents only a small fraction of jaw problems; most jaw dysfunction is related to the TMJ. In some cases these problems can be acutely painful and debilitating and may cause symptoms that are virtually identical to non-TMJ ailments.

The jaw is vulnerable for a number of reasons: its fairly wide range of motion; its constant use for talking, eating, yawning, swallowing, laughing, and so on; its tendency to become a focal point for emotional stress and muscular tension; and its susceptibility to being influenced by dental problems. In addition, there is always the possibility of trauma, especially from automobile accidents or sports injuries. Many TMJ disorders actually result from multiple, overlapping causes that cannot be easily diagnosed.

Dysfunction in the TMJ can trigger a vast range of symptoms, some of which are quite severe. Common TMJ disorder symptoms include jaw pain, headache, facial pain, stiff neck, ringing in the ears, vertigo, and laryngitis—largely because the jaw is so richly supplied with nerve endings. The relationship between these symptoms and your jaw may seem far-fetched, but the insidious nature of TMJ disorders makes them very real possibilities. Vertigo, for example, may be caused by pain radiating to the inner ear, affecting your balance. And weight loss often occurs simply because it's too painful to chew or because the jaw locks sporadically.

Some jaw conditions call for simple home treatments like rest and ice or heat. Others demand more advanced physical therapy techniques: carefully and scientifically tailored exercises to strengthen the jaw and improve range of motion, adjustments of the posture, mobilization; and perhaps other approaches (modalities) like ultrasound and electrical stimulation as well. Still other problems may require surgery or other dental interventions, although these, too, are usually complemented with an exercise program designed by a physical therapist as part of the rehabilitation stage. In every instance, however, you should look to your dentist or physical therapist to make a diagnosis and determine treatment.

Muscles in the jaw are frequent sites of dysfunction. Certainly the mildest such dysfunction, if it can even be called that, is the tendency of these muscles—like muscles throughout the body—to become stiff or tight in response to heavy jaw activity. Similar **muscle tightness** may be produced by simple emotional stress. The result is usually minor, short-term achiness and may be no cause for concern. (On the other hand, muscle tightnes does diminish the jaw's range of motion, which, unless the muscles are warmed up and stretched, puts the jaw at risk of injury when called upon to push beyond that range.)

More worrisome is the accumulation of excess lactic acid and other chemicals in the jaw muscles whenever they are subject to excessive stress over long periods of time—whether it be from poor posture, from clenching or grinding the teeth (bruxism), from a faulty bite (malocclusion, see page 42), or even from emotional tension. The cellular and chemical response to excessive stress almost inevitably lead to **muscle inflammation,** the development of hard knots of muscle called **trigger points,** and pain. Sometimes the pain shows up in the form of headaches.

The TMJ muscles may also suffer from **muscle spasm,** the sudden, intense contraction of muscle tissue. Although very painful, a muscle spasm is the body's natural mechanism for protecting injured tissue by acting as a brace. It often occurs whenever the jaw is at serious risk of strain or other injury. Resting your jaw in your palm, holding your head in a misaligned position, chewing large bites of food, even yawning, laughing, or otherwise opening the mouth wide are sometimes enough to set off spasm. Spasm may also be triggered by malocclusion (see page 42).

Not unlike the muscles, the ligaments of the jaw can be overstretched— that is, pushed beyond their normal limits—or microscopically torn. This injury, a **sprain,** can afflict any of the jaw's ligaments and can be produced by trauma, overuse, the cumulative impact of poor posture, or poor body mechanics. Pain produced in the TMJ due to a sprain may be localized, or it may radiate into the head or neck. If overstretched ligaments are not holding a joint firmly in place, there may also be a feeling of slippage. On the other hand, the joint may become stiff and restricted. Ligament sprains are also a common component of whiplash (see page 42).

The TMJ is also subject to the degenerative changes associated with **arthritis,** which can lead to both pain and stiffness. This condition can be the result of early trauma to the joints, but there is a wide range of possible causes. One form of arthritis is **rheumatoid arthritis,** a disease whose origin is not fully understood (but which may be the result of autoimmune mechanisms or viral infections). Although some cases of rheumatoid arthritis are relatively benign, in extreme cases the joints become so swollen that they essentially fuse together. This is a serious and often debilitating condition. Physical therapy is necessary to help maintain mobility and flexibility in the region.

A far more widespread form of arthritis in the TMJ is **osteoarthritis,** the degeneration of the articular cartilage and a wearing down of the joint surfaces. In some cases osteoarthritis may result in the buildup of roughened cartilage or spurs (deposits of bony tissue) on the joint surfaces. Osteoarthritis in the TMJ has a number of possible causes, including bruxism, malocclusion (see below), and displaced menisci (see below), but by far the most common is the natural (though not inevitable) degeneration of the meniscus due to aging.

A meniscus may also become **displaced,** slipping out of its position in the fossa. The most obvious symptom is a clicking sound when the jaw opens and closes. Often this is just a temporary condition, but occasionally the condition will worsen: the disk may become displaced and cause the jaw to lock—sometimes intermittently, sometimes for extended periods. The most common cause of meniscus displacement is malocclusion (see below).

Because it is a somewhat unstable joint, the jaw can become **dislocated.** This dislocation can be the result of a blow to the face or even yawning. Dislocation causes pain at the side of the jaw and makes it impossible to close the mouth.

The bones of the jaw are subject to **fracture,** usually as a result of severe trauma. At the very least, fractures cause pain and joint stiffness; in worse cases, the jaw may be loosened, the teeth misaligned, and nearby nerves damaged. Treatment of a dislocated or fractured jaw usually involves immobilization of the jaw and, in serious cases, surgery to realign the bones.

A variety of jaw-related problems—from sprain (see page 41) to meniscus displacement (see above) and osteoarthritis (see above)—can be found in people with faulty bites, or **malocclusion.** A malocclusion can have any number of causes. It may be a function of how your permanent teeth came in or a result of dental work (crowns, caps, etc.). Or it may be an adjustment to accommodate for tooth pain on one side of the mouth; in this case the problem may become more extreme as you eventually start favoring the "good" side of your mouth to protect the other side. The malocclusion can end up pushing the condyle of the mandible into an improper position, with consequent pressure on the muscles, ligaments, and disk. Orthodontic treatment to correct a congenital malocclusion is often effective, especially if done at an early age.

Although **whiplash** is commonly associated with the neck, it is a condition that affects the jaw as well. Whiplash is a diagnostic term that may be applied to a combination of problems resulting from high-speed back-and-forth movement of the neck and, sometimes, violent opening and closing of the jaw: severe muscle strain or tears, extreme muscle spasm, severe ligament sprain, and/or damaged disks. In such instances pain in the jaw can be produced by injury either to the neck or to the jaw itself. The typical cause of whiplash is an automobile accident in which an automobile is hit from behind, causing the driver's or passenger's neck to snap too far backward (hyperextension), then too far forward (hyperflexion), then sometimes too far backward again. If a car crashes into an immobile object or has a head-on collision, the sequence is reversed. Other traumatic neck injuries from sports accidents can produce trauma similar to whiplash.

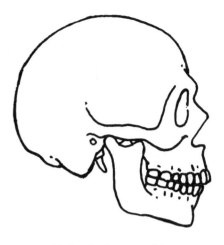

Malocclusion: overbite

Taking Care of Your Jaw

As with many other parts of the body, **proper posture** is an important factor in maintaining a healthy jaw. By preserving the straight vertical alignment of the head and neck, proper posture minimizes stress on the muscles and ligaments of the jaw and helps maintain TMJ alignment. Proper posture should be observed as much as possible while standing, sitting, and lying down; those activities that disrupt proper posture for an extended period, or that do so repeatedly, should be avoided.

Although to some people proper posture seems to come almost naturally, for most of us it takes cultivation (and sometimes even professional guidance). For detailed information on recognizing and developing proper posture, see **Chapter 10—Posture**.

Another important factor in jaw maintenance is **proper body mechanics** in the various activities of daily life. With regard to the jaw, proper body mechanics means using the body and the different parts of the body in ways that are consistent with the smooth functioning of the joints, muscles, ligaments, and disks of the jaw. Among other things, this means avoiding such habits as grinding your teeth or clenching your jaw, resting your chin in the palm of your hand, and chewing ice, hard candy, or pencils. As with proper posture, proper body mechanics can significantly reduce the risk of many jaw problems.

Proper body mechanics are by no means always self-evident; occasionally they may even be counterintuitive. For most of us they need to be learned and adopted. For detailed information on identifying and developing proper body mechanics, see **Chapter 12—Body Mechanics**.

Although they represent somewhat different ways of thinking about the body, posture and body mechanics are closely related phenomena. By

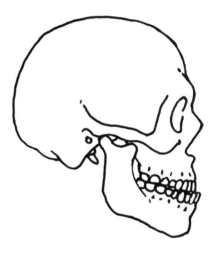

Malocclusion: underbite

Headrests, Airbags, and Your Jaw

One important measure you can take to avoid jaw trauma is to use a car outfitted with headrests and airbags. These features offer the best protection against whiplash caused by auto accidents. Your headrest should be raised so that the middle of the back of your head contacts it and, if possible, adjusted so that it corresponds to the curve of your cervical spine.

definition, proper posture is a prerequisite of proper body mechanics. Indeed, many poor biomechanical habits harmful to the jaw are poor postural habits.

Keeping your jaw healthy also calls for **strength** in the muscles that help to keep the jaw stable, moving, and well aligned—including not just your jaw muscles but the neck and shoulder muscles as well. Well-developed strength prepares the jaw for the demands constantly made on it and provides some protection from injury when our body mechanics are imperfect.

Endurance in the muscles that support the jaw is also essential. Endurance is the ability of the muscles to contract (that is, be in use) over time. The less developed a muscle's endurance, the shorter the amount of time it may be called upon to contract before it tires—forcing other, often more vulnerable parts of the body to do its job and putting itself and those other parts at risk of injury. Because a range of common activities, including talking for any sustained period of time, calls upon our muscles to contract over extended periods, a certain level of endurance is absolutely vital.

Flexibility in the muscles and ligaments is just as critical as muscle strength and endurance. The less flexible your muscles, the more susceptible they are to the natural (and often painful) tightening that comes from everyday activities. And the more susceptible they are to injury from imperfect body mechanics. As with strength, this flexibility must be distributed among all the muscles that support the jaw.

Appropriate strength and flexibility for your jaw (and other parts of your body) may be achieved through a regular program of exercise. For more information, see **Chapter 15—Strength, Endurance, and Flexibility.**

Many lines of **work** carry genuine risks of jaw dysfunction due to strain or overuse. Perhaps the most familiar such jobs are those that demand a considerable amount of talking, such as teaching and lecturing. Other such jobs are those that demand a high degree of concentration, like working at a computer all day, which (among other things) tends to keep the head in a forward, fixed position for hours on end. If you hold a job of this sort—even if your muscle endurance, strength, and flexibility are good—it may be a wise precaution to stretch the jaw (and related) muscles before beginning your workday and several times throughout the day.

It's also important as much as possible to configure your physical work environment so that it does not force you to observe poor body mechanics. If you work at a computer, it is essential that your chair be appropriately supportive and that chair, desk, and monitor be at proper heights.

If your occupation does subject your jaw to strain and overuse, be sure to take a break of at least several minutes every hour. And if you feel any tightness or stiffness *at all*, stretch the muscles a bit (seebelow). In fact, to head off problems, you may want to try this routine even if you don't have tightness or stiffness.

For more information on protecting your jaw and other parts of your body from injury during work activities, see **Chapter 17—Work.**

When Problems Occur

No matter how well you treat your jaw, **occasional temporary tightness or stiffness** may still occur, especially as you age. In these instances, one way to ease your pain is with a few **stretching exercises,** which will bring back some badly needed flexibility and blood flow to your tired or aching muscles. (See the box, "Quick-Relief Jaw Stretches," at right). **Massage,** which may help loosen tight muscles and increase blood flow to constricted areas, may also work nicely. Although electric hand-held massagers and various non-electric massage rollers are available on the market, you're much more likely to get a sensitive massage simply by using your hands.

Sometimes a bout of jaw stiffness or soreness can be traced directly to a particular instance of poor body mechanics. This is often the explanation for pain that occurs during a specific activity—like working at a desk, reading, or even sleeping. If this is the case, double-check your body mechanics; you may find that a simple adjustment will quickly eliminate the problem.

If your jaw discomfort persists for more than a few days, it's a good idea to have it checked out by a dentist. Beyond temporary soreness and stiffness, it is possible that you will experience **more serious jaw problems** of one sort or another at some point in your life.

It is best to see a dentist at the first sign of trouble, no matter how innocent-seeming. This is usually an obvious course of action in the case of a serious traumatic event, such as a car accident or sports injury. In these cases you should seek **immediate professional attention.** In such urgent situations it's also a good idea to know and apply some basics of **first aid.** (See **Appendix A—First Aid Basics.**)

And whether or not it is the result of a traumatic event, any case of severe jaw pain should also get immediate attention (and first aid, if appropriate). **Milder degrees of jaw pain,** if persisting for more than a few days or recurring, should also be evaluated by a physical therapist or dentist. Although minor jaw pain may well be a simple case of muscle tension, it can easily develop into a chronic condition if not addressed (if it isn't chronic already). Of equal concern is the possibility that minor jaw pain is the symptom of an even more involved problem. And, painful or not, any episode of the jaw seeming to "pop out," then "pop in"—or any locking of or clicking in the jaw—is worthy of attention.

Quick-Relief Jaw Stretches

The stretches below may ease (and sometimes even head off) common jaw tightness and stiffness. Feel free to do them as often as you wish. Detailed instructions and appropriate illustrations can be found in Chapter 19—Flexibility Exercises. These exercises are especially valuable if you work long hours at a computer terminal. (These exercises may also help with minor muscle spasm by relaxing the contracted muscles.) If your jaw tightness or stiffness produces more than minor discomfort, consult your dentist or physical therapist before attempting them.

- Jaw Relaxer (p. 241)
- Lateral Jaw Relaxer (p. 242)

Headaches and Your Jaw

Although headaches have a vast range of possible causes—from eating habits to infections to dehydration—they can also have their origin in the TMJ. Muscle tension in the jaw, hyperextension injuries, myofascial pain dysfunction syndrome, and other problems can all refer pain into the head. There is, however, no simple way for you to determine if and when a particular headache has jaw problems as its underlying cause. A severe or persistent headache requires the attention of a physician.

In the meantime, minor jaw pain can be managed by heeding a few simple tips. **Rest** can provide some relief by giving your jaw muscles and other soft tissues a chance to heal. Lie down on a firm supporting surface on your back or side, maintaining the proper alignment of the neck (see **Chapter 10—Posture**). Improper head and neck alignment will negatively affect the position of the jaw and surrounding muscles. Don't stuff too many pillows under your neck, which will only make the problem worse. A contoured cervical pillow is an ideal option.

Because all eating activities, including chewing and swallowing, require constant contraction of the jaw muscles, it is also a good idea to eat softer foods (like yogurt and blended fruit drinks), take smaller bites, and avoid chewing on gum or ice altogether. Also avoid opening your mouth wide to yawn and do less talking to give the muscles a chance to relax.

For a day or two after the appearance of minor jaw pain, you can apply **ice** to the area. The ice numbs the pain and may reduce or prevent any swelling. One good method is to put crushed ice in a sealable plastic bag with a little water, then cover the bag with towels. (A bag of frozen peas or corn works well too; refrigerated towels can be used in a pinch.) To avoid harming the skin or underlying tissues, apply the ice for only 15 to 20 minutes at a time, with 20 to 40 minutes between applications.

After a period of using ice, you may try **moist heat,** applied to the jaw in a 20-minutes-on/20-minutes-off cycle. Moist heat tends to relax tense muscles, offering some relief from pain and stiffness. Warm showers or warm, moist towels work well for this. Heating pads, although not highly recommended, are also acceptable, but take care that the heat is not too intense.

For some people **nonsteroidal anti-inflammatory drugs (NSAIDs)** may help in easing jaw pain. This class of drugs includes aspirin and ibuprofen, both of which are widely available without prescription. Like all drugs, however, NSAIDs have potentially dangerous side effects. Ask your doctor or pharmacist before taking NSAIDs, and follow the directions on the label.

When addressing a jaw problem, your physical therapist has many techniques to draw upon. But—depending on your physical therapist's examination and evaluation—a jaw rehabilitation program will almost certainly incorporate strength, endurance, and flexibility exercises and attention to improved postural alignment and body mechanics. Your dentist or orthodontist may also have some recommendations for addressing a malocclusion if one is present.

CHAPTER FOUR

The Shoulder

The shoulder is capable of a wider and more varied range of motion than any other joint in the human body. This flexibility allows human beings to do everything from paint a ceiling to pitch a baseball. But this flexibility comes at a steep price: The shoulder joint is one of the most unstable in the body—held in place not by the strong bony structure found in other joints but rather by a limited network of muscles, tendons, and ligaments.

"Overhead athletes" (throwers, tennis players, swimmers) are at high risk for shoulder problems, as are people whose occupations require them to reach overhead (such as house painters and construction workers). But all of us are vulnerable to shoulder ailments, especially as we grow older.

How the Shoulder Works

The shoulder region includes four distinct joints: the **acromioclavicular (AC), sternoclavicular (SC), scapulothoracic (ST), and glenohumeral (GH) joints.** The AC joint links a small projection near the outer top of the shoulder blade (**scapula**) to the collarbone (**clavicle**); the SC joint links the breastbone (**sternum**) to the clavicle; and the ST joint links the scapula to the soft tissues of the rib cage (**thorax**). The AC, SC, and ST joints all contribute to the shoulder's functioning, but it is the GH joint that most contributes to the shoulder's remarkable range of motion. Indeed, it is known informally as the "shoulder joint."

The GH joint is a ball-and-socket joint that links the upper arm bone (**humerus**) to the outer border of the shoulder blade, next to the end of the clavicle. (Ball-and-socket joints resemble a golf ball on a tee: the round end of one bone moves freely within the scooped-out hollow of the other bone.) Thus, the large, rounded end of the humerus (the **humeral head**) glides and rotates within the scooped-out socket on the scapula known as the **glenoid fossa**. The glenoid fossa itself is relatively shallow, but it is made deeper by a surrounding ring of cartilage (the **labrum**). The humeral head and the glenoid fossa—like the ends of other bones in the shoulder's joints—are covered with a smooth **articular cartilage** that facilitates movement in the region. The GH joint's unique construction makes it possible for us to move

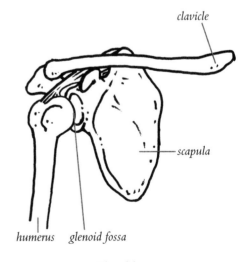

Shoulder

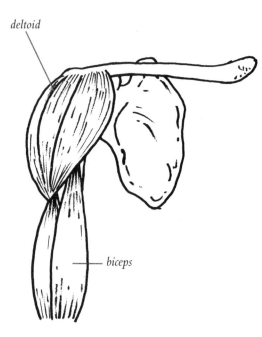

deltoid

biceps

Muscles of shoulder (front view)

the arm forward, backward, and to the side; to rotate it inward and outward; to move it across the body and behind the back; and to circle the arm clockwise and counterclockwise.

Muscles in the back, neck, chest, shoulder, and upper arm all work together to keep the shoulder stable, well aligned, and moving. Among the more important of those muscles is the **deltoid,** which gives the very top of the arm its rounded contour; the **biceps**, which extends from shoulder to elbow; and the **rotator cuff,** formed by four muscles that extend from the scapula to the humerus. Flexible fibrous cords of tissue called **tendons** (technically, extensions of the muscle) attach these and other muscles to the humerus, scapula, and neighboring bones. A number of the tendons—especially rotator cuff tendons and the upper tendon of the biceps muscle—also serve a stabilizing function, keeping the humeral head from popping out of the glenoid fossa during certain activities without interfering with the shoulder's range of motion.

The shoulder mechanism is further reinforced by the **shoulder capsule,** fibrous and connective tissue material that surrounds the joints, and by a range of **ligaments,** tough bands of fibrous tissue that bind together the various joint ends.

Eight **bursa sacs (bursae),** fluid-filled sacs of varying sizes within and around the shoulder, cushion the joints and minimize friction in the region. A **synovial membrane** in the shoulder capsule also provides lubrication for the joints.

The shoulder is part of a kinetic chain that includes the skull, jaw, neck, and upper back at one end and the lower arm, wrist, and hand at the other. The movement and working of all these different areas of the body are interrelated and depend on each other for correct functioning.

What Can Go Wrong

The vast range of motion and flexibility of the shoulder makes it particularly vulnerable to overuse and trauma. The muscles of the rotator cuff and the tendons in the shoulder complex, called upon for so much arm movement, are especially subject to wear and tear. In addition, the shallowness of the GH joint greatly increases the chance that the humeral head will pop out of the glenoid fossa in the event of a traumatic injury. This can cause injury not only to the bones but to the surrounding soft tissue, as well including the rotator cuff.

While shoulder problems may arise as the result of a specific traumatic incident—a fall, work-related accident, or sports injury—they often seem to appear out of nowhere. In cases where there's no obvious cause for pain, the culprit is often the cumulative stress, strain, and abuse from years of poor posture and body mechanics. In young people and active adults, problems tend to be related to overhead sports, which can be punishing to the shoulder.

Shoulder symptoms come in many varieties. Pain can be dull, sharp, constant, intermittent, or like "pins and needles." It is also highly variable, from mild discomfort to extreme pain. It may be site specific or generalized. Only certain motions of the shoulder may cause pain, or the shoulder's range of motion may be limited.

Some shoulder conditions, such as mild strains, sprains, and tendinitis (see below), call for simple home treatments like rest and ice. Others demand more advanced physical therapy techniques: carefully and scientifically tailored exercises to strengthen the shoulder and improve range of motion; adjustments of the posture; mobilization; and perhaps approaches (modalities) like ultrasound and electrical stimulation as well. Still other problems require surgery or other major interventions, although these, too, are usually complemented with an exercise program designed by a physical therapist as part of the rehabilitation stage. In every instance, however, you should look to your physician or physical therapist to make a diagnosis and determine the proper treatment.

The shoulder's muscles are common sites of shoulder dysfunction. Certainly the mildest such dysfunction, if it can even be called that, is the tendency of these muscles—like muscles throughout the body—to become stiff or tight in response to heavy shoulder activity. The result of such **muscle tightness** is usually minor, short-term achiness and may be no cause for concern. (On the other hand, muscle tightness does diminish the shoulder's range of motion, which, unless the muscles are warmed up and stretched, puts the shoulder at risk of injury when called upon to push beyond that range.)

More worrisome is the accumulation of excess lactic acid and other chemicals in the shoulder muscles whenever they are subject to excessive or repetitive stress over prolonged periods of time—for example, when a person does heavy physical labor (especially with an insufficiently warmed-up shoulder). The cellular and chemical responses to excessive stress almost inevitably lead to **muscle inflammation,** the development of hard knots of muscle called **trigger points,** and pain, which only increases if the stress is unrelieved.

The shoulder muscles may also suffer from tearing. This tearing may result from direct trauma, overuse (from engaging in sports or performing a work-related activity), or poor body mechanics. A **muscle strain,** sometimes inaccurately called a "pulled muscle," occurs when the muscle has been overstretched or overexerted and may have microscopic tearing as its cause. When the tearing is more severe, it is called, simply, a **muscle tear,** which may be partial or complete. The symptoms of strains and tears vary only in degree and may include pain, inflammation, bleeding into the surrounding tissues, and muscle spasm (see below). Strains, however, are often mild enough to require little more treatment than rest for a few days.

Strains and tears often trigger **muscle spasm**—the sudden, intense contraction of muscle tissue. Although very painful, a muscle spasm is the body's natural mechanism for protecting injured tissue by acting as a brace. Because it is a protective mechanism, muscle spasm is also present in almost all shoulder disorders.

Injuries to the muscles have much in common, and are often associated, with injuries to their tendons. Like the muscles themselves, the tendons of the muscles can become inflamed when subject to excessive stress. This condition, known as **tendinitis,** is probably the most familiar shoulder ailment. Repeatedly raising the arms overhead, as when pruning a tree, placing items on a shelf, or engaging in overhead sports (like tennis, swimming, or baseball), is one common cause of tendinitis. Another common cause is engaging in sports or similar physical activities without having first warmed up and stretched the tendons. Tendinitis may also strike those who "overdo" a physical activity after an extended period of being sedentary—which is why it is also known as the "weekend athlete syndrome."

Because the tendons lack the same pain nerve endings as other structures, you might not feel any pain due to tendinitis until the surrounding synovial membrane of the joint or the adjacent bursae also become inflamed. Typical symptoms then include a deep generalized ache in the area, an increase in pain when using the shoulder, and localized tenderness. (Tendinitis can be further complicated by the appearance in the tendon of calcium crystals, leading to inflammation and calcification of the bursa and to increased pain that makes moving the shoulder difficult; this condition is called **calcific tendinitis.**)

In some cases a tendon, like a muscle, may **tear** or **rupture** altogether as a result of trauma, leading to significant pain and spasm.

A combination of muscle and tendon problems shows up frequently in the sensitive rotator cuff. The cumulative wear and tear of everyday life alone may be enough to bring muscle strain to the rotator cuff. Inactivity also may lead to problems in the area. And in young and older people alike, the rotator cuff is vulnerable to traumatic injury.

Repetitive overhead stress to the shoulder, furthermore, may lead to **rotator cuff impingement syndrome,** in which not only the rotator cuff muscles and tendons but also sometimes the biceps tendon and even the bursae (see page 52) are involved. In such cases one of the major tendons may become inflamed and can be pinched between the humeral head and the outer end of the scapula when the arm is raised, with painful results. (This condition is also called **painful arc syndrome.**) Other symptoms may include decreased ability to use the arm, and muscle weakness in the shoulder. Physical therapy intervention is important at an early stage to prevent the condition from worsening.

If this problem is allowed to progress untreated, it may lead to muscle strains and tears, including a complete **rotator cuff tear.** In the worst cases this painful injury may be accompanied by a rupturing of the biceps tendon.

When wear and tear on the muscles, tendons, and bursae (see page 52) in the GH joint are accompanied by wear and tear on the shoulder capsule itself, the result can be a tightening of the capsule, causing the shoulder to be fully or partially immobilized. Also a consequence of overuse or trauma—or even the underuse that frequently follows in the wake of an injury to the area—**frozen shoulder (adhesive capsulitis)** is characterized by many of the same symptoms that accompany rotator cuff problems: pain when the arm is raised, muscle weakness, and decreased ability to use the arm. It usually causes pain as well when you lean upon or lie down on the affected shoulder. This condition is more likely to strike women than men, especially women over the age of 50. While a frozen shoulder may heal itself untreated, the whole freezing/frozen/thawing cycle can take years. Physical therapy is essential to managing this condition.

Not unlike the muscles and tendons, the ligaments that support the joints of the shoulder can be overstretched—that is, pushed beyond their normal limits—or microscopically torn. This injury, a **sprain,** can affect any of the shoulder's ligaments and can be produced by trauma (like a fall), overuse (from activities such as gymnastics), the cumulative impact of poor posture, or poor body mechanics (like lifting heavy objects incorrectly). The ligaments of the AC joint, between the collarbone and shoulder blade, may be affected as a result of an impact to the tip of the shoulder. A mild sprain will produce pain and swelling around the joint; in severe cases the collarbone may also be able to slip in and out of the joint or even become separated from the scapula entirely. This phenomenon is sometimes called a **shoulder separation.**

The joints are subject to the degenerative changes associated with **arthritis,** which can lead to both pain and stiffness. This condition can be the result of early trauma to the joints, but there is a wide range of possible causes. The most widespread form of arthritis in the shoulder joints is **osteoarthritis,** the degeneration of the articular cartilage and a wearing down of the joint surfaces. In some cases osteoarthritis may result in the buildup of roughened cartilage or spurs (deposits of bony tissue) on the joint surfaces and the appearance of loose bodies (floating bits of cartilage and bone) within the joint.

Osteoarthritis has a number of possible causes, including trauma, overuse, and inactivity. But by far the most common is simple degeneration of the joint due to age, typical (though not inevitable) among middle-aged individuals. Although it sometimes has no symptoms at all, osteoarthritis may well lead to pain (from mild to severe) and stiffness and decreased movement in the shoulder. Cases of extensive, severe degeneration of the joint may even require surgical replacement of the humeral head.

A rarer but more serious form of arthritis from which the shoulder may suffer is **rheumatoid arthritis,** an inflammatory disease whose origin is not fully understood (but which may be the result of autoimmune mechanisms or viral infections). The disorder is characterized by pain, stiffness, swelling, and warmth in the shoulder joints. Physical therapy is necessary to help maintain mobility and flexibility in the region.

As indicated, the bursae surrounding the GH joint can become irritated by overuse, leading to **bursitis.** When this happens, the bursa sacs thicken and reduce the free movement around the glenohumeral joint, thus limiting the range of motion of the shoulder. Pain, the primary symptom of bursitis, is usually constant and site specific; the pain may worsen, however, when you move your arm out to the side. Bursitis usually occurs in tandem with inflammation or degenerative changes in the rotator cuff (see page 51) or shoulder capsule (see page 51). (The term "bursitis" is often used—incorrectly—to indicate any kind of shoulder pain.)

The GH joint may also suffer **partial dislocation,** in which the humeral head slips (subluxes) partway out of the glenoid fossa. This can result from trauma (such as a fall on an outstretched arm, or a sharp blow to the back or shoulder) or from overuse, often while playing overhead sports. In younger people (roughly ages 14 to 30), a partial dislocation may develop into a recurrent condition, in which the humeral head pops out of place spontaneously and pops back in again by itself. Partial dislocations are not necessarily painful in themselves, but they can become chronic, and repeated popping in and popping out can lead to serious wear and tear on the GH joint, as well as damage to the muscles, ligaments, labrum, nerves, humeral head, and capsule. A **full dislocation,** in which the humeral head comes completely out of the glenoid fossa, has the same causes but is more immediately damaging to the shoulder. Recurring dislocations may require surgical repair to stabilize the joints.

Like all bones, those in the shoulder—especially the upper part of the humerus and the collarbone—are subject to **fracture** as a result of trauma, like a fall or a collision. (Fractures to the shoulder blade are relatively uncommon.) Fractures tend to cause at least pain and joint stiffness. But in some instances fractures in the shoulder region can also damage the radial nerve or the artery leading down the arm—with potentially serious consequences for the wrist and hand. Generally, a shoulder fracture will call for immobilization while the shoulder heals.

The exceptional prominence of the collarbone makes it especially prone to direct trauma, which may result in **bruises**—internal bleeding—in the soft tissue around the bone or even in the bone itself. Although a bruised collarbone is usually not serious in itself, it can lead to **osteolysis,** a painful (if temporary) condition characterized by severe calcium loss in the bone.

Taking Care of Your Shoulder

As with many other parts of the body, **proper posture** is an important factor in maintaining a healthy shoulder. By preserving the straight vertical alignment of the spine, proper posture goes a long way toward ensuring that all the components of the shoulder stay aligned so that it can move without undue stress and strain. Proper posture should be observed as much as possible while standing, sitting, and lying down; those activities that disrupt proper posture for an extended period, or that do so repeatedly, should be avoided. (This admonition should not, however, interfere with normal vigorous activities such as sports, which are in fact much encouraged.)

Although to some people proper posture seems to come almost naturally, for most of us it takes cultivation (and sometimes even professional guidance). For detailed information on recognizing and developing proper posture, see **Chapter 10—Posture.**

Another important factor in shoulder maintenance is **proper body mechanics** in the various activities of daily life. With regard to the shoulder, proper body mechanics means using the body and the different parts of the body in ways that are consistent with the smooth functioning of the

"Double-jointedness"

"Double-jointedness," properly known as **hypermobility**, is a term meant simply to describe a joint that has a much greater range of motion than normal. In and of itself, hypermobility is not a problem. Indeed, for some athletes, like dancers and gymnasts, being hypermobile may be a benefit. But this extreme range of motion can also exact a toll by making the shoulder prone to rotator cuff injuries, subluxations, dislocations, and wear and tear.

region's joints, muscles, tendons, and ligaments. Among other things, this means knowing how to lift and carry heavy objects properly; being careful not to hook your arm over the back of a chair; and not raising your arm repeatedly above shoulder level. As with proper posture, proper body mechanics can significantly reduce the risk of many shoulder problems.

Proper body mechanics are by no means always self-evident; occasionally they may even be counterintuitive. For most of us they need to be learned and consciously adopted. For detailed information on identifying and developing proper body mechanics, see **Chapter 12—Body Mechanics**.

Although they represent somewhat different ways of thinking about the body, posture and body mechanics are closely related. By definition, proper posture is practically a prerequisite of proper body mechanics, because in the absence of proper posture, you are always undermining the smooth functioning of your joints, muscles, tendons, and ligaments. Indeed, quite a few of the poor biomechanical habits harmful to the shoulder are poor postural habits.

Keeping your shoulder healthy also calls for **strength** in the muscles that help to keep the shoulder stable, moving, and well aligned, including not just your shoulder muscles but your lower back, upper back, chest, abdomen, and arm muscles as well. The less developed your muscle strength, the narrower the range of physical activities you are capable of performing—or capable of performing without putting stress on the region. As a result, many common practices of everyday life, from lifting up a child to pushing open a heavy door, become riskier than they should be. A balance of strength in the upper and lower back, chest, abdomen, and arm muscles is important too so that one area need not compensate for weakness in another.

Endurance in the muscles that support the shoulder is also essential. Endurance is the ability of the muscles to contract (that is, be in use) over time. The less developed a muscle's endurance, the shorter the amount of time it can be called upon to contract before it tires—forcing other, often more vulnerable parts of the body to do its job and putting itself and those other parts at risk of injury. On the other hand, well-conditioned muscles are less susceptible to strain and thus provide some protection from injury and trauma when our body mechanics are less than perfect. Because a range of common activities, including many sports and work activities, calls upon our muscles to contract over extended periods, a certain level of endurance is absolutely vital. If you're going to be involved in an overhead sport or work-related activity, you need to be especially diligent about conditioning your shoulder.

Flexibility in the muscles, tendons, and ligaments is just as critical as muscle endurance and strength. The less flexible your muscles and ligaments, the more susceptible they are to the natural (and sometimes painful) tightening that comes from everyday activities. And the more susceptible they are to injury when called upon to perform many common practices, like closing a garage door or putting away groceries. As with endurance and strength, this flexibility must be distributed among all the muscles that support the shoulder.

Appropriate endurance, strength, and flexibility for your shoulder (and other parts of your body) may be achieved through a regular program of exercise. For more information, see **Chapter 15—Strength, Endurance, and Flexibility.**

Although all parts of the body are at greater risk of injury when you are engaged in **sports** or other vigorous activities, the structure and function of the shoulder and its wide range of motion make it especially vulnerable, even for those who generally have good endurance, strength, and flexibility. Sudden strain on the shoulder or the repeated lifting of the arm overhead—common in many sports and activities, from tennis to tree pruning to weight training—make the shoulder vulnerable to tendinitis, rotator cuff tears, and other problems. While the risks tend to increase the older you are and the more intense your workout is, it is nevertheless a good idea for anyone to fully prepare the shoulder for such a workout: warm up through gentle aerobic activity (such as walking for 5 or 10 minutes, being sure to move the arms) and then stretch the shoulder muscles.

It should be noted that sports-related repetitive-motion injuries to the shoulder may often be prevented by taking care to use proper form. If you engage in racquet sports, sports that require throwing (like baseball), or swimming (especially freestyle and butterfly), you should have an expert evaluate your form.

Still, common sense is the best line of defense against injury. If you don't play sports or engage in similar physical activities regularly, it is important not to push yourself too much when you do. And if you do experience any pain in the shoulder, stop what you're doing at once. To try to "play through it" is to risk injury.

For more information on protecting your shoulder and other parts of your body from injury during particular sports and activities, see **Chapter 16—Sports.**

Like sports, many lines of **work** carry considerable risks of shoulder injury due to repetitive strain or overuse. Just about any sort of heavy labor

Shoulder Inactivity

In one form or another, stress on the shoulder is certainly the most familiar cause of injury to the muscles and joints. Another cause, however, is only slightly less threatening: simple inactivity. Failure regularly to use the muscles of the shoulder and to bring the joints to the limits of their range of motion through moderately vigorous activity makes the region particularly susceptible to sudden overuse and other kinds of stress. The joints stiffen; ligaments and muscles may contract; good blood flow is inhibited. Even more noteworthy, inactivity may make the shoulder more susceptible to general joint degeneration.

The effects of inactivity tend to be magnified with age. And it is inactivity, more than aging itself, that leads to the conditions generally associated with growing older, like osteoarthritis. Regular exercise—power walking with good shoulder movement, swimming, or golf, for example— may well keep these problems at bay.

Quick-Relief Shoulder Stretches

The stretches below may ease (and sometimes even head off) common shoulder tightness and stiffness, especially tightness and stiffness brought on by repetitive stress. Feel free to do them as often as you wish. Detailed instructions and appropriate illustrations can be found in Chapter 19—Flexibility Exercises. (These exercises may also help with muscle spasm.) If your shoulder tightness and stiffness produce more than minor discomfort, consult your physical therapist before attempting them. Be sure to warm up your muscles prior to doing these exercises by, for instance, getting up and walking around your office while moving your arms.

• Upper Back/Shoulder Stretch (p. 243)
• Shoulder Roll (p. 243)
• Arm Circles (p. 251)
• Shoulder Release (p. 252)
• Shoulder Dip (p. 252)
• Corner Stretch (p. 236)

that involves lifting and carrying, especially lifting and carrying overhead, falls into this category: construction work, furniture moving, and baggage handling, for example. If your occupation requires this sort of activity—even if your muscle endurance, strength, and flexibility are good—it is a wise precaution to first warm up and then stretch the shoulder muscles before beginning your workday and several times throughout the day.

It's also important as much as possible to configure your physical work environment so that it does not force you to use poor body mechanics. Using step ladders or lowering work shelves, for example, can reduce the need for overhead lifting.

Finally, if your occupation does subject your shoulder to repetitive stress, reduce the stress by varying your movements slightly and, if possible, alternating hands. Also be sure to take a short break every hour, and if you feel any tightness or stiffness *at all*, stretch the muscles a bit (see below). In fact, to head off problems, you may want to try this routine even if you don't have tightness or stiffness.

For more information on protecting your shoulder and other parts of your body from injury during workplace activities, see **Chapter 17—Work.**

When Problems Occur

No matter how well you treat your shoulder, **occasional temporary tightness and stiffness** may occur, especially as you grow older. After all, even the simple activities of everyday life, from putting on a sweater to carrying luggage, can be tough on the shoulder. One way to ease your discomfort is with a few focused **stretching exercises,** which will bring back some badly needed flexibility and blood flow to your tired or aching muscles. (See the box, **"Quick-Relief Shoulder Stretches,"** at left.)

Massage, which increases blood flow to the region while warming and stretching the shoulder muscles and soft tissue, may also work nicely. Although electric hand-held massagers and various nonelectric massage rollers are available on the market, you're much more likely to get a sensitive massage from someone just using the hands.

Sometimes a bout of shoulder stiffness or soreness can be traced directly to a particular instance of poor posture or poor body mechanics. This is often the explanation for pain that occurs during a specific activity—like sitting in a movie theater with your arm up on the seat beside you. If this is the case, double-check your body mechanics; you may discover that a simple adjustment will quickly eliminate the problem.

If your shoulder discomfort persists for more than a few days, it's a good idea to have your shoulder checked by a physical therapist or physician.

Beyond temporary soreness and stiffness, it is possible that you will experience **more serious shoulder problems** of one sort or another at some point in your life, even if you have generally healthy shoulders. The normal wear and tear of everyday living may stress the region. Age, too, takes its toll, and with it may come osteoarthritis and general joint degeneration. Falls and accidents may result in sprains, muscle tears, or even fractures. Anyway, few of us can claim perfect shoulder maintenance, which makes us especially vulnerable to a whole range of shoulder problems.

Especially because shoulder problems can have repercussions for your neck, elbow, wrist, and hand, it is best to see a physical therapist or physician at the first sign of trouble, no matter how innocent-seeming. This is usually an obvious course of action in the case of a traumatic event, like a dislocation caused by a fall or collision. In these cases you should seek **immediate professional attention.** In such urgent situations it's also a good idea to know some basics of **first aid.** (See Appendix A—First Aid Basics.)

Even if it's not the result of a traumatic event, any case of severe shoulder pain should also get immediate professional attention (and, if appropriate, first aid).

Milder degrees of shoulder pain, if persisting for more than a few days or recurring, should also be evaluated by a physical therapist or physician. This includes the familiar achiness and stiffness that characterize tendinitis, often brought on by overuse and often associated with sports and other physical activities. If not addressed, minor shoulder pain can easily develop into a chronic condition (if it isn't chronic already). Of equal concern is the possibility that minor shoulder pain may be the symptom of an even more involved problem. Any grinding or clicking, muscle weakness, loss of range of motion, or episode of the shoulder seeming to "pop out" and then "pop in," painful or not, should also be cause for concern.

In the meantime, minor shoulder pain can be managed by heeding a few simple tips. **Rest** can provide some relief by giving the tissue some time to heal and regenerate: no sports, no repetitive motion of the arm, no reaching or lifting. Prolonged immobilization, however, is not recommended; gentle movement and stretching and a gradual return to normal activity are best.

For the first day or two after the appearance of minor shoulder pain, you may apply **ice** to the affected area. The ice numbs the pain temporarily and may reduce or prevent swelling. One good method for applying ice is to put crushed ice in a sealable plastic bag with a little water, then cover the bag with towels. (A bag of frozen peas or corn works well too; refrigerated towels can be used in a pinch.) To avoid harming the skin or underlying tissues, apply the ice for only 15 to 20 minutes at a time, with 20 to 40 minutes between applications.

After a period of using ice, you may try **moist heat,** applied to the shoulder in a 20-minutes-on/20-minutes-off cycle. Moist heat tends to relax tense, strained muscle fibers, offering some relief from pain and stiffness. Warm showers or warm, moist towels work well for this; whirlpools and hot tubs are fine too. Heating pads, although not highly recommended, are also acceptable, but take care that the heat is not too intense.

For some people **nonsteroidal anti-inflammatory drugs (NSAIDs)** can be very effective in easing shoulder pain. This class of drugs includes aspirin and ibuprofen, both of which are widely available without prescription. Like all drugs, however, NSAIDs have potentially dangerous side effects. Ask your doctor or pharmacist before taking NSAIDs, and follow the directions on the label.

When addressing a particular shoulder problem, your physical therapist has a wide range of techniques to draw upon. But—depending on the physical therapist's examination and evaluation—a shoulder rehabilitation program will almost certainly incorporate strength, endurance, and flexibility exercises and attention to improved postural alignment and body mechanics.

CHAPTER FIVE

The Elbow

Activities as diverse as pounding a hammer, lifting a fork, and swinging a tennis racquet would be impossible without the elbow. Yet we tend to overlook this crucial link in the arm's kinetic chain…at least until something goes wrong.

The elbow, after all, is subjected to punishing day-in and day-out use—especially in people who carry heavy briefcases, who play sports such as golf and tennis, or whose jobs (carpentry, assembly-line work, etc.) involve repetitive-motion stress on the elbow. In addition, the normal wear and tear of the aging process makes us all vulnerable to elbow pain.

The elbow can be deceptive in its apparent simplicity. This is all the more reason to learn a little about how it functions and how you can head off pain and dysfunction before they require professional intervention.

How the Elbow Works

The elbow is the point at which the single bone of the upper arm (the **humerus**) meets the two bones of the lower arm (the **radius** and the **ulna**). (If you hold your arm out in the "thumbs up" position, the radius is the upper bone, and the ulna is the lower.) The bony tip of the elbow, the **olecranon,** is part of the ulna. The two bony knobs on the inside and the outside of the elbow, the **epicondyles,** are part of the lower humerus.

The elbow is actually composed of three joints. One, the **radiohumeral joint,** links the humerus to the radius; another, the **ulnohumeral joint,** links the humerus to the ulna. A third joint, the **superior radioulnar joint,** connects the upper portions of the radius and the ulna to each other. The joint surfaces are covered with a smooth **articular cartilage** that facilitates movement in the region. These joints together allow the elbow to bend and straighten like a hinge and also permit the forearm to rotate without moving the upper arm.

Muscles in the upper and lower arm all work together to keep the elbow stable, well aligned, and moving. Among the more important of these muscles are the **biceps** and the **brachials** in the front of the upper arm, and the **triceps** and **aconeus** in the back of the upper arm. Flexible fibrous

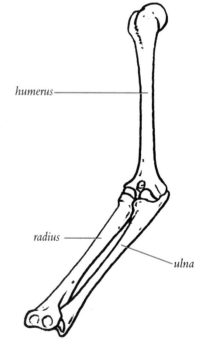

humerus

radius

ulna

Elbow (right)

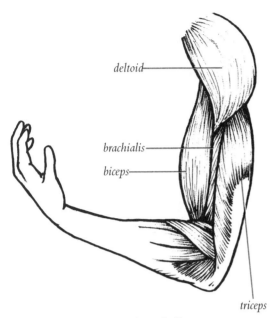

deltoid

brachialis

biceps

triceps

Muscles of elbow

cords of tissue called **tendons** (technically extensions of the muscle) attach the muscles to the humerus, radius, and ulna.

The elbow mechanism is further reinforced by the **joint capsule,** fibrous and connective tissue material that surrounds the joints, and by a range of **ligaments,** tough bands of fibrous tissue that bind together the various joint ends. Major ligaments run from the two epicondyles to the upper ulna and to the upper radius (the **medial collateral ligament,** or **MCL,** and the **lateral collateral ligament,** or **LCL**). Another important ligament (the **annual ligament**) encircles the upper radius.

Three major nerves—the **median, ulnar,** and **radial nerves**—run the length of the arm, crossing the elbow at various points. Each of these nerves allows us to contract specific muscles in the arm and hand and to perceive sensations such as touch, temperature, and pain. (Because these nerves run the length of the arm, pain in the hand or fingers is sometimes a symptom of a problem in the elbow.)

The **olecranon bursa,** a fluid-filled sac at the elbow tip, cushions the joints and minimizes friction in the region. A **synovial membrane** in the elbow capsule also provides lubrication for the elbow unit.

The elbow functions as part of a kinetic chain that includes the neck, shoulder, and upper arm at one end and the forearm, wrist, and hand at the other. All these different areas of the body are interrelated and depend on each other for correct functioning and movement.

What Can Go Wrong

The construction of the elbow is relatively simple; consequently, it is somewhat more durable than many of the body's other joints. Still, it is by no means free from risk. Repetitive-motion injuries are especially common in the elbow. Furthermore, elbow injuries take on an added degree of seriousness because they sometimes translate into wrist and hand problems.

While elbow problems may arise as the result of a specific traumatic incident—a fall, work-related accident, or sports injury—they often seem to appear out of nowhere. In cases where there's no obvious cause for pain, the culprit is often the cumulative stress, strain, and abuse from years of poor body mechanics. In young people and active adults, problems tend to be related to sports, which can be punishing on the elbow.

Elbow symptoms come in many varieties. Pain can be dull, sharp, constant, intermittent, or like "pins and needles." It is also variable, from mild discomfort to intense pain. It may be site specific or generalized. It may appear only with certain motions of the arm, or the elbow's range of motion may be limited.

Some elbow conditions, such as mild strains, sprains, and tendinitis (see below), call for simple home treatments like rest and ice. Others demand more advanced physical therapy techniques: carefully and scientifically tailored exercises to strengthen the elbow and improve range of motion; mobilization; and perhaps approaches (modalities) like ultrasound and electrical stimulation as well. Still other problems require surgery or other major interventions, although these, too, are usually complemented with an exercise program designed by a physical therapist as part of the rehabilitation stage. In every instance, however, you should look to your physician or physical therapist to make a diagnosis and determine treatment.

The elbow's muscles are common sites of elbow dysfunction. Certainly the mildest such dysfunction, if it can even be called that, is the tendency of these muscles—like muscles throughout the body—to become stiff or tight in response to heavy elbow activity. The result of such **muscle tightness** is usually minor, short-term achiness and may be no cause for concern. (On the other hand, muscle tightness does diminish the elbow's range of motion, which, unless the muscles are warmed up and stretched, puts the elbow at risk of injury when called upon to push beyond that range.)

More worrisome is the accumulation of excess lactic acid and other chemicals in the elbow muscles whenever they are subject to excessive stress over prolonged periods—for example, when a person does heavy physical labor (especially with an insufficiently warmed-up elbow). The cellular and chemical responses to excessive stress almost inevitably lead to **muscle inflammation** and pain, which only increases if the stress is unrelieved.

The elbow muscles may also suffer from tearing. This tearing may result from direct trauma, overuse of the muscle (from engaging in sports or a work-related activity), or poor body mechanics. A **muscle strain,** sometimes inaccurately called a "pulled muscle," occurs when the muscle has been overstretched or overexerted and may have microscopic tearing as its cause. When the tearing is more severe, it is called, simply, a **muscle tear,** which may be partial or complete. The symptoms of strains and tears vary only in degree and may include pain, inflammation, bleeding into the surrounding tissues, and muscle spasm (see below). Strains, however, are often mild enough to require little more treatment than rest for a few days.

Strains and tears often trigger **muscle spasm**—the sudden, intense contraction of muscle tissue. Although very painful, a muscle spasm is the body's natural mechanism for protecting injured tissue by acting as a brace. Because it is a protective mechanism, spasm is present in a wide range of elbow disorders.

Injuries to the muscles have much in common, and are often associated, with injuries to their tendons. Like the muscles themselves, the tendons of the muscles can become inflamed when subject to excessive stress. This condition, known as **tendinitis,** is probably the most familiar elbow ailment. Any activity that stretches the tendons beyond their usual range of motion can cause tendinitis. Another common cause is engaging in sports or similar vigorous activities without having first warmed up and stretched the tendons. Tendinitis may also strike those who "overdo" a physical activity after an extended period of being sedentary—which is why it is also known as the "weekend athlete syndrome."

Because the tendons lack the same pain nerve endings as other structures, you might not feel any pain due to tendinitis until the surrounding synovial membrane of the joint or the adjacent bursa also become inflamed. Typical symptoms then include a deep generalized ache in the area, an increase in pain when using the elbow, and localized tenderness.

In some cases a tendon, like a muscle, may **tear** or **rupture** altogether as a result of trauma, leading to significant pain and spasm.

A combination of muscle and tendon problems characterizes a number of elbow injuries. With **tennis elbow (lateral epicondylitis),** the muscles and tendons along the outside of the forearm, particularly where they attach to the outer (lateral) epicondyle, become inflamed. This condition, caused by any motion involving the repetitive criss-crossing of the radius and ulna (as in a faulty backhand tennis stroke), can bring nagging or sporadic soreness to the area. **Pitcher's** or **golfer's elbow (medial epicondylitis)** displays a similar inflammation of the muscles and tendons along the inside of the forearm, particularly where they attach to the inner (medial) epicondyle. This condition, similar in its symptoms to tennis elbow, is caused by any motions involving the repetitive bending of the forearm in toward the body with the wrist flexed (as in a golf swing or baseball pitch).

Not unlike the muscles and tendons, the ligaments that support the joints of the elbow can be overstretched—that is, pushed beyond their normal limits—or microscopically torn. This injury, a **sprain,** can affect any of the elbow's ligaments and can be produced by trauma (like a fall), overuse (from activities such as racquetball), or poor body mechanics (like lifting heavy objects incorrectly). But it most commonly strikes the medial collateral ligament or, less commonly, the lateral collateral ligament. Because MCL sprains are often the result of repetitive throwing motions, this condition is sometimes called "Little League elbow." A mild sprain will produce pain and swelling around the joint and possibly weakness in the muscles; over time the joint may become stiff and restricted. In more severe cases there may be a feeling of slippage in the joint.

The joints are subject to the degenerative changes associated with **arthritis,** which can lead to both pain and stiffness. This condition can be the result of early trauma to the joints, but there is a wide range of possible causes. The most widespread form of arthritis in the elbow joints is **osteoarthritis,** the degeneration of the articular cartilage and a wearing down of the joint surfaces. In some cases osteoarthritis may result in the buildup of roughened cartilage or spurs (deposits of bony tissue) on the joint surfaces and the appearance of loose bodies (floating bits of cartilage and bone) within the joint.

Osteoarthritis has a number of possible causes, including trauma, overuse, and inactivity. But by far the most common is simple degeneration of the joint due to age, typical (though not inevitable) among middle-aged individuals. Although it sometimes has no symptoms at all, osteoarthritis may well lead to pain (from mild to severe) and stiffness and decreased movement in the elbow.

A rarer but more serious form of arthritis from which the elbow may suffer is **rheumatoid arthritis,** an inflammatory disease whose origin is not fully understood (but which may be the result of autoimmune mechanisms or viral infections). The disorder is characterized by pain, stiffness, swelling, and warmth in the elbow joints. Physical therapy is necessary to help maintain mobility and flexibility in the region.

The experience of hitting the "funny bone," with its brief sensation of numbness and tingling, is in fact a case of hitting the ulnar nerve where it passes between the medial epicondyle and the olecranon. While this is harmless in itself, repeated trauma may cause scar tissue to form, leading to nerve entrapment or compression. This condition, known as **cubital tunnel syndrome** (named after the narrow channel through which the ulnar nerve runs), causes continuous pain, as well as tingling or numbness in the fourth and fifth fingers of the hand and weakness in those muscles controlled by the ulnar nerve.

The bursae in the elbow are subject to **bursitis**—an inflammation brought on by trauma or overuse—but none more so than the olecranon bursa at the elbow tip. Continually leaning on the elbow, a familiar practice among students poring over their books, is one common cause of bursitis in the olecranon bursa (hence the nickname "student's elbow"). Repeatedly bumping the elbow tip, as plumbers and others who perform manual labor in tight spaces often do, is another cause. When this happens, the bursa sac may thicken and reduce the free movement around the joint, thus limiting the elbow's range of motion. Pain, the primary symptom of bursitis, is usually constant and site specific; it may worsen when the arm is bent or straightened.

Like all bones, those in the elbow are subject to **fractures, dislocations,** and related injuries as a result of trauma, particularly because of our instinct to break a fall with our outstretched arms. Fractures, cracks, and chips of the olecranon; hairline fractures of the radial head; and fractures to the lower portion of the humerus are the most frequent such injuries. Fractures tend to cause at least pain and joint stiffness. But in some instances fractures or dislocations in the elbow can also damage the nerves or arteries in the region—with potentially serious consequences for the wrist and hand. The complicated structure of the elbow can often make fractures difficult to treat; in most cases surgical intervention is called for.

Taking Care of Your Elbow

As with many other parts of the body, an essential factor in elbow maintenance is **proper body mechanics** in the various activities of daily life. With regard to the elbow, proper body mechanics means using the body and the different parts of the body in ways that are consistent with the smooth functioning of the region's joints, muscles, tendons, and ligaments. Among other things, this means knowing how to lift and carry heavy objects properly, being careful not to lean on or bump the elbow tip, and not repeatedly bending and straightening the arm. Proper body mechanics can significantly reduce the risk of many elbow problems.

Proper body mechanics are by no means always self-evident; occasionally they may even be counterintuitive. For most of us they need to be learned and adopted. For detailed information on identifying and developing proper body mechanics, see **Chapter 12—Body Mechanics.**

Keeping your elbow healthy also calls for **strength** in the muscles that help to keep the elbow stable, moving, and well aligned, including not just the elbow muscles but the neck, shoulder, forearm, wrist, and hand muscles as well. The less developed your muscle strength, the narrower the range of physical activities you are capable of performing—or capable of performing without putting stress on the region. As a result, many common practices of everyday life, like lifting up a child, become riskier than they should be. A balance of strength in the upper and lower arm muscles is important too, so that one area need not compensate for weakness in another.

Endurance in the muscles that support the elbow is also essential. Endurance is the ability of the muscles to contract (that is, be in use) over time. The less developed a muscle's endurance, the shorter the amount of time it can be called upon to contract before it tires—forcing other, often more vulnerable parts of the body to do its job and putting itself and those other parts at risk of injury. On the other hand, well-conditioned muscles are less susceptible to strain and thus provide some protection from injury and trauma when our body mechanics are less than perfect. Because a range of common activities, including many sports and work activities, calls upon our muscles to contract over extended periods, a certain level of endurance is absolutely vital. If you're going to be involved in racquet sports, golf, bowling, or sports that require throwing, you need to be especially diligent about conditioning your elbow.

Flexibility in the muscles, tendons, and ligaments is just as critical as muscle endurance and strength. The less flexible your muscles and ligaments, the more susceptible they are to the natural (and sometimes painful) tightening that comes from everyday activities. And the more susceptible they are to injury when called upon to perform many common practices, like carrying a heavy briefcase. As with endurance and strength, this flexibility must be distributed among all the muscles that support the elbow.

Appropriate endurance, strength, and flexibility for your elbow (and other parts of your body) may be achieved through a regular program of exercise. For more information, see **Chapter 15—Strength, Endurance, and Flexibility**.

Although all parts of the body are at greater risk of injury when you are engaged in **sports** or similar vigorous activities, the structure and function of the elbow make it especially vulnerable, even for those who generally have good endurance, strength, and flexibility. Sudden strain on the elbow or the repeated bending and straightening of the arm—common occurrences in many sports and activities, from swimming to tennis—make the elbow vulnerable to tendinitis and other minor and major problems. While the risks tend to increase the older you are and the more intense your workout is, it is nevertheless a good idea for anyone to fully prepare the elbow for such a workout: warm up through gentle aerobic activity (such as walking for 5 or 10 minutes, being sure to move the arms), and then stretch the elbow muscles.

It should be noted that sports-related repetitive-motion injuries to the elbow may often be prevented by using proper form. If you engage in racquet sports, sports that require throwing, or golf, you should have an expert evaluate your form. Also make sure your racquet and golf clubs fit your grip properly; the wrong equipment can contribute to elbow problems.

Still, common sense is the best line of defense against injury. If you don't

Elbow Inactivity

In one form or another, excessive stress on the elbow is certainly the most familiar cause of injury to the muscles and joints. Another cause, however, is only slightly less threatening: simple inactivity. Failure regularly to use the muscles of the elbow and to bring the joints to the limits of their range of motion through moderately vigorous activity makes the region particularly susceptible to sudden overuse and other kinds of stress. The joints stiffen; ligaments and muscles may contract; good blood flow is inhibited. Even more noteworthy, inactivity may make the elbow more susceptible to general joint degeneration.

The effects of inactivity tend to be magnified with age. And it is inactivity, more than aging itself, that leads to the conditions generally associated with growing older, like osteoarthritis. Regular exercise—swimming or golf, for example—may well keep these problems at bay.

play sports or engage in similar physical activities regularly, it is important not to push yourself too much when you do. And if you do experience any pain in the elbow, stop what you're doing at once. To try to "play through it" is to risk serious injury.

Sports in particular also make the elbow susceptible to traumatic injuries from falls. (Cycling and in-line skating are two of the more familiar culprits.) And though such injuries are by nature unpredictable, often you can avoid them simply by wearing elbow protectors.

For more information on protecting your elbow and other parts of your body from injury while participating in particular sports, see **Chapter 16—Sports.**

Like sports, many lines of **work** carry considerable risks of elbow injury due to strain or overuse. Meat cutting, baggage handling, shelf stacking, and assembly-line work, which often require repetitive and even awkward elbow motion, are just a few of the jobs that fall into this category. If you hold an occupation of this sort—even if your muscle endurance, strength, and flexibility are good—it is a wise precaution first to warm up and then to stretch the elbow muscles before beginning your workday and several times throughout the day.

It's also important as much as possible to configure your physical work environment so that it does not force you to use poor body mechanics. Something as simple as raising or lowering your work surface can minimize stress on the elbow.

Finally, if your occupation does subject your elbow to repetitive stress, you can reduce the stress by varying your movements slightly, keeping your elbows in close to the body, and, if possible, alternating hands. Also be sure to take a break of at least several minutes every hour, and if you feel any tightness or stiffness *at all*, shake out your hands to get the blood circulating and stretch your elbow muscles a bit (see below). In fact, to head off problems, you may want to try this routine even if you don't have tightness or stiffness.

For more information on protecting your elbow and other parts of your body from injury during workplace activities, see **Chapter 17—Work**.

When Problems Occur

No matter how well you treat your elbow, **occasional temporary tightness and stiffness** may occur, especially as you grow older. After all, with such a wide range of common activities demanding the use of the elbow, everyday life can be tough on the joint. One way to ease your discomfort is with a few focused **stretching exercises,** which will bring back some badly needed flexibility and blood flow to your tired or aching muscles. (See the box, **"Quick-Relief Elbow Stretches,"** at right.)

Massage, which increases blood flow to the region while warming and stretching the elbow muscles and soft tissue, may also work nicely. Although electric hand-held massagers and various nonelectric massage rollers are available on the market, you're much more likely to get a sensitive massage by using your hands. Simply **shaking out** the hands and arms is another alternative.

Sometimes a bout of elbow stiffness or soreness can be traced directly to a particular instance of poor body mechanics. This is often the explanation for pain that occurs during a specific activity—leaning on your elbow when you read the paper, for example. If this is the case, double-check your body mechanics; you might find that a simple adjustment will quickly eliminate the problem.

If your discomfort, however mild, persists for more than a few days, it's a good idea to have your elbow checked by a physical therapist or physician.

Beyond temporary soreness and stiffness, it's possible that you will experience **more serious elbow problems** of one sort or another at some point in your life, even if you have a generally healthy elbow. The normal wear and tear of everyday living may stress the region. Age, too, takes its toll, and with it may come osteoarthritis and general joint degeneration. Falls or accidents may result in strains, sprains, muscle tears, or even fractures. Anyway, few of us can claim perfect elbow maintenance, which makes us especially vulnerable to a whole range of elbow problems.

Because elbow problems can have repercussions for your hand and wrist, it's best to see a physical therapist or physician at the first sign of trouble, no matter how innocent-seeming. This is usually an obvious course of action in the case of a traumatic event, like a fall on the elbow that leaves it too painful to move. In these cases you should seek **immediate professional attention.** In such urgent situations it's also a good idea to know some basics of **first aid.** (See Appendix A—First Aid Basics.)

Even if it's not the result of a traumatic event, any case of severe elbow pain or serious swelling should also get immediate professional attention (and, if appropriate, first aid).

Milder degrees of elbow pain, if persisting for more than a few days or recurring, should be evaluated by a physical therapist or physician. This includes the familiar achiness and stiffness that characterize tendinitis, often brought on by overuse and often associated with sports and other physical activities. If not addressed, minor elbow pain can easily develop into a

Quick-Relief Elbow Stretches

The stretches below may ease (and sometimes head off) common elbow tightness and stiffness, especially tightness and stiffness brought on by repetitive stress. Feel free to do them as often as you wish. Detailed instructions and appropriate illustrations can be found in Chapter 19—Flexibility Exercises. (These exercises may also help with muscle spasm.) If your elbow tightness and stiffness produce more than minor discomfort, consult your physical therapist before attempting them. Be sure to warm up your muscles prior to doing these exercises by, for instance, getting up and walking around your office while moving your arms.

- Elbow Stretch (p. 253)
- Triceps Stretch (p. 253)

chronic condition (if it isn't chronic already). Of equal concern is the possibility that minor elbow pain is the symptom of an even more involved problem. Any grinding or clicking in the elbow should also be cause for concern.

In the meantime, minor elbow pain can be managed by heeding a few simple tips. **Rest** can provide some relief by giving the tissue some time to heal and regenerate: no sports and no repetitive motion of the arm. Prolonged immobilization, however, is not recommended; gentle movement and stretching and a gradual return to normal activity are best.

For the first day or two after the appearance of minor elbow pain, you may apply **ice** to the affected area. The ice numbs the pain temporarily and may reduce or prevent swelling. One good method for applying ice is to put crushed ice in a sealable plastic bag with a little water, then cover the bag with towels. (A bag of frozen peas or corn works well too; refrigerated towels can be used in a pinch.) To avoid harming the skin or underlying tissues, apply the ice for only 15 to 20 minutes at a time, with 20 to 40 minutes between applications.

After a period of using ice, you may try **moist heat,** applied to the elbow in a 20-minutes-on/20-minutes-off cycle. Moist heat tends to relax tense, strained muscle fibers, offering some relief from pain and stiffness. Warm showers or warm, moist towels work well for this; whirlpools and hot tubs are fine too. Heating pads, although not highly recommended, are also acceptable, but take care that the heat is not too intense.

For some people **nonsteroidal anti-inflammatory drugs (NSAIDs)** can be very effective in easing elbow pain. This class of drugs includes aspirin and ibuprofen, both of which are widely available without prescription. Like all drugs, however, NSAIDs have potentially dangerous side effects. Ask your doctor or pharmacist before taking NSAIDs, and follow the directions on the label.

When addressing a particular elbow problem, your physical therapist has a wide range of techniques to draw upon. But—depending on the physical therapist's examination and evaluation—an elbow rehabilitation program will almost certainly incorporate strength, endurance, and flexibility exercises and attention to improved postural alignment and body mechanics.

The Wrist & Hand

Much of what human beings have achieved can be ascribed not just to intelligence but also to the unique structure of the wrist and hand unit. The human hand's combination of fine motor movement, dexterity, grasping power, and opposability (ability to pick up an object between the thumb and another finger) is practically unmatched in nature.

In combination with the flexibility and leverage provided by the wrist and the elbow, the hand has allowed human beings to create everything from stone arrowheads to computers. The multiple types of grips of which the hand is capable enable us to pick up a glass, hold an egg without breaking it, carry a suitcase, turn the key in a lock, even pick up a grain of rice. And the fingers and hands, so richly supplied with nerve endings, are sensory organs nearly as important as our eyes and ears.

Injuries and dysfunctions in the hand and wrist should never be taken lightly: for many people even a partial loss of function can have grave consequences. You owe it to yourself to treat your wrist and hand with kid gloves.

How the Wrist and Hand Work

The wrist, which links the hand with the arm, is a complex mechanism constructed of 8 small bones known collectively as the **carpal bones,** arrayed in two interrelated rows. One row connects with the ends of the two forearm bones, the **radius** and the **ulna.** (If you hold out your arm in the "thumbs up" position, the radius is the upper bone, and the ulna is the lower.) The other row connects with the bones of the palm of the hand. The joint surfaces are covered with a smooth **articular cartilage** that facilitates movement in the region. The wrist's bony structure permits it to bend up and down and from side to side and to move in a circular path both clockwise and counterclockwise.

The hand itself contains 19 bones: 5 elongated **metacarpal bones,** which extend from the wrist and make up the palm, and 14 **phalanges,**

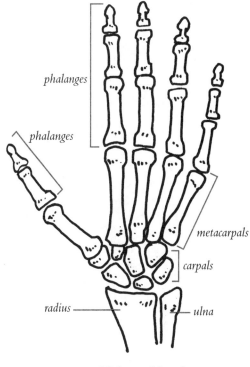

phalanges

phalanges

metacarpals

carpals

radius

ulna

Wrist and hand

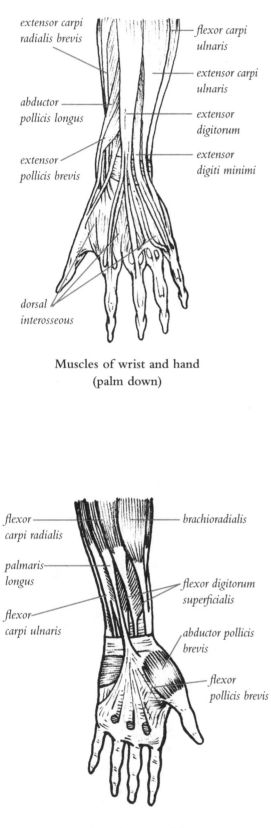

extensor carpi
radialis brevis

flexor carpi
ulnaris

extensor carpi
ulnaris

abductor
pollicis longus

extensor
digitorum

extensor
pollicis brevis

extensor
digiti minimi

dorsal
interosseous

Muscles of wrist and hand
(palm down)

flexor
carpi radialis

brachioradialis

palmaris
longus

flexor digitorum
superficialis

flexor
carpi ulnaris

abductor pollicis
brevis

flexor
pollicis brevis

Muscles of wrist and hand
(palm up)

which collectively make up the fingers. (Each finger consists of 3 phalanges, except for the thumb, which consists of 2 phalanges.) Among them, these 19 bones make for 14 separate joints. The knuckle joints, or **metacarpophalangeal (MCP) joints,** join the fingers with the palm. The finger joints are called the **interphalangeal (IP) joints.** All these elements are packed into an exceptionally tight space.

The hand's construction allows the fingers to flex into a fist and open back up again, spread apart from one another and come back together, and move independently. But the most remarkable feature of the hand is the thumb's opposability, which allows the thumb to touch all the other fingers and to grasp objects. Like all joints, those of the hand feature articular cartilage on the bone surfaces.

Muscles in the forearm and the palm all work together to keep the wrist and hand stable, aligned, and moving. Flexible fibrous cords of tissue called **tendons**—technically, extensions of the muscle—attach these muscles to the radius, ulna, carpals, metacarpals, and phalanges. A number of the tendons also serve a stabilizing function.

The wrist and hand are further reinforced by a range of **ligaments,** tough bands of fibrous tissue that bind together the various joint ends. Six major ligaments provide stability for the wrist, joining the lower radius to various carpal bones and binding the two rows of carpal bones together. These ligaments are joined by others that link the bones of the hand.

Other stabilizers in the wrist and hand include the **joint capsules,** fibrous and connective tissue material that surrounds the joints, and for the hand only, **volar plates,** small shields of cartilage and membranes on the palm side of the knuckles. A **synovial membrane** in the joint capsules provides lubrication for all the joints.

Three major nerves—the **median, radial,** and **ulnar nerves**—run the length of the arm, crossing the wrist en route to the hand. Each of these three nerves allows us to contract specific muscles in the wrist and hand and to perceive sensations such as touch, temperature, and pain.

The hand is the terminus of a kinetic chain that includes the neck, shoulder, upper arm, elbow, forearm, and wrist. All these different areas of the body are interrelated and depend on each other for correct movement and functioning.

What Can Go Wrong

The wrist and hand are subject to a number of problems because of the complexity and compactness of their design. Repetitive-motion injuries are especially common and are often work related. Assembly-line workers, computer operators, construction workers, and meat cutters are among those at risk. Similar injuries to the wrist and hand are common in sports, particularly among tennis players, pitchers, swimmers, and golfers.

The intricate construction of the wrist and hand, the sensitive nerve endings in the fingers, and our heavy dependence on the hand and wrist in our everyday lives tend to magnify the seriousness of any injury. Even seemingly minor injuries or problems can have major implications.

For example, simple **inflammation** is far more serious in the wrist and hand than it is just about anywhere else in the body (except, perhaps, the ankle and foot). When inflammation occurs, fluids can become trapped in the compact hand and wrist area. If the inflammation is not relieved, these fluids may change from a thin liquid into a fibrous, glue-like substance. At the least, recovery is delayed; at the worst, permanent changes or dysfunction in the hand may result. (To get an idea of how easy it is for fluid to accumulate in the hand area, gently squeeze the skin on the top of your hand and lift it up. Notice how loose that skin is; when swelling occurs, there's a lot of space for fluid to fill.)

Some wrist and hand conditions, such as mild sprains and tendinitis (see page 72), call for simple home treatments like rest and ice. Others demand more advanced physical therapy techniques: carefully and scientifically tailored exercises to strengthen the wrist and hand and improve range of motion; mobilization; and perhaps approaches (modalities) like ultrasound and electrical stimulation as well. Still other problems require surgery or other major interventions, although these, too, are usually complemented with an exercise program designed by a physical therapist as part of the rehabilitation stage. In every instance, however, you should look to your physician or physical therapist to make a diagnosis and determine the proper treatment.

Probably the mildest wrist and hand dysfunction, if it can even be called that, is the tendency of the region's muscles—like muscles throughout the body—to become stiff or tight in response to heavy wrist and hand activity. The result of such **muscle tightness** is usually minor, short-term achiness and may be no cause for concern. (On the other hand, muscle tightness does diminish the wrist/hand unit's range of motion; unless the muscles are warmed up and stretched, the region is at risk of injury when called upon to move beyond the usual range.)

More worrisome is the accumulation of excess lactic acid and other chemicals in the hand and wrist muscles whenever they are subject to excessive stress over prolonged periods of time, like engaging in heavy physical labor (especially with an insufficiently warmed-up hand/wrist). The cellular and chemical responses to excessive stress almost inevitably lead to **muscle inflammation** and pain, which only increases if the stress is unrelieved. So-called **"writer's cramp,"** caused by tightly gripping a pen or pencil for long periods, is a common example of this condition.

The wrist and hand muscles may also suffer from tearing. This tearing may result from direct trauma or overuse of the muscle (from engaging in sports or other activities, such as repeated grasping). A **muscle strain,** sometimes inaccurately called a "pulled muscle," occurs when the muscle has been over-stretched or overexerted and may have microscopic tearing as its cause. When the tearing is more severe, it is called, simply, a **muscle tear**, which may be partial or complete. Tears rarely strike the small intrinsic muscles of the hand, but they may occur in those of the forearm, which control much wrist and hand movement. The symptoms of strains and tears vary only in degree and may include pain, inflammation, bleeding into the surrounding tissues, and muscle spasm (see below). Strains, however, are often mild enough to require little more treatment than rest for a few days.

Strains and tears often trigger **muscle spasm**—the sudden, intense contraction of muscle tissue. Although very painful, a muscle spasm is the body's natural mechanism for protecting injured tissue by acting as a brace. Because it is a protective mechanism, muscle spasm is present in many other wrist and hand disorders.

Injuries to the muscles have much in common, and are often associated, with injuries to their tendons. Like the muscles, the tendons may become inflamed when subject to excessive stress, which can considerably impede their normal gliding motions. This relatively familiar condition is known as **tendinitis.**

Because the tendons lack pain nerve endings, you might not feel any pain due to tendinitis until the surrounding synovial membrane of the joint also becomes inflamed. Typical symptoms then include a deep generalized ache in the area, an increase in pain when using the hand and wrist, and localized tenderness.

In the wrist tendinitis may strike the tendons that stretch from the radius to the thumb. Pain in the area may also radiate into the hand or forearm and be accompanied by a catching sensation when you bend your thumb. This condition is called **de Quervain's disease.** In the hand tendinitis generally affects tendons of the fingers or thumb; a nodule may even develop on the covering of the tendon in the palm. As a result, there may be a popping or clicking sensation when you bend the finger. In extreme cases this may develop into a **trigger finger,** in which the finger locks in a flexed position. A trigger finger is sometimes a consequence of repeatedly grasping objects—as when working on an assembly line—or of sustaining trauma to the palm.

Many of the causes of tendinitis may also lead to tendon **strain,** especially in the tendons of the hand itself, leading to pain and usually spasm as well. A tendon may even **tear** or **rupture** altogether as a result of trauma.

Not unlike the muscles and tendons, the ligaments of the wrist and hand can be overstretched—that is, pushed beyond their normal limits—or microscopically torn. This injury, a **sprain,** can range from the minor to the severe. A mild sprain will produce pain and swelling around the joint, a loss of motion, and possibly weakness in the hand; in more severe cases there may also be a feeling of slippage in the joints involved.

Sprains most commonly occur in the wrist as the result of a fall on an open hand or repetitive stress at the workplace. Any of the wrist's ligaments can be sprained. In the hand, sprains tend to occur in the fingers and thumb. Although these sprains, too, may be work related, more often they are the result of trauma, especially sports-related trauma. One such sprain is a **jammed finger,** an injury caused by the head-on collision of a finger and a hard object (like a baseball). With a jammed finger, the finger bone itself may temporarily become dislocated (see page 75), damaging not only the ligaments but possibly the volar plates, tendons, and cartilage as well. Despite its innocuous-sounding name, this is a serious condition that may cause permanent harm to the affected finger if not treated promptly. At the very least, temporary immobilization of the finger is required.

The joints of the wrist and hand are subject to the degenerative changes associated with **arthritis,** which can lead to both pain and stiffness. In the hand arthritis may also be accompanied by muscle weakness and an inability to pick up or hold objects. Arthritis can be the result of early trauma to the joints, but there is a wide range of possible causes. One form of arthritis in the wrist and hand joints is **osteoarthritis,** the degeneration of the articular cartilage and a wearing down of the joint surfaces. In some cases osteoarthritis may result in the buildup of roughened cartilage or spurs (deposits of bony tissue) on the joint surfaces and the appearance of loose bodies (floating bits of cartilage and bone) within the joint.

Osteoarthritis has a number of possible causes, including trauma, overuse, and inactivity. But by far the most common is simple degeneration of the joint due to age, typical (although not inevitable) among middle-aged individuals. Although it sometimes has no symptoms at all, osteoarthritis may

Knuckle-cracking

The distinctive popping sound that frequently occurs when you pull on, bend, or twist the fingers is actually a product of the change in air pressure caused by the abrupt disruption of the alignment of the joint's bones. But as satisfying as it may be to crack the knuckles, it does not in fact serve any sort of beneficial purpose, like freeing up excessively tight joints. Indeed, knuckle-cracking may be quite harmful to the fingers—stretching the joint capsules and ligaments and possibly leading to an unhealthy joint laxity. A word to the wise, then, on knuckle-cracking: don't do it.

well lead to pain (from mild to severe) and stiffness and decreased movement in the region. In the hand it can affect many of the 14 joints, but it may be most troublesome when it strikes the joint at the base of the thumb.

Perhaps the more serious form of arthritis from which the wrist and hand may suffer is **rheumatoid arthritis,** an inflammatory disease whose origin is not fully understood (but which may be the result of autoimmune mechanisms or viral infections). The disorder is characterized, at the very least, by pain, stiffness, swelling, and warmth in the joints of the wrist, hand, and thumb. In more advanced forms rheumatoid arthritis may lead to deformity of the hand, the destruction of the MCP and IP joints, dislocation, and tendon rupture. Physical therapy is necessary to help maintain mobility and flexibility in the region; in advanced cases surgical replacement of the joints may even be required.

The nerves that run through the wrist and into the hand are vulnerable to injury. One of the most familiar of these injuries involves the compression of the median nerve, that is, swelling and pressure on the nerve as it passes thorugh the wrist. This condition, known as **carpal tunnel syndrome** (named after the narrow channel through which the nerve passes), can result when ligaments in the wrist become thickened with scar tissue or when the sheaths surrounding the tendons become swollen as a result of overuse. Although carpal tunnel syndrome can be triggered by fractures of the wrist bones or even fluid retention during pregnancy, it is more commonly the result of repetitive motion and overuse—for example, from typing at a keyboard all day long. Carpal tunnel syndrome is perhaps the most familiar of all workplace injuries.

Because the median nerve serves all the fingers except the little finger, gripping an object may be painful or impossible. There may also be a sensation of tingling or numbness. Symptoms of carpal tunnel syndrome may appear abruptly and then worsen progressively. (Symptoms may present themselves in the middle of the night.) This condition can be addressed through a wide variety of sophisticated physical therapy techniques—including approaches (modalities) like electric stimulation and ultrasound—as well as more straightforward means, such as the use of a custom wrist support or splint to calm the inflamed tissue around the nerve and the use of strengthening and flexibility exercises; in severe cases, however, surgery may be required.

Compression or entrapment of the ulnar nerve has similar symptoms, leading to continuous pain and tingling or numbness in the fourth and fifth fingers (the ring and little fingers) and weakness in some of the finger muscles. This may be caused by the pressure on the nerve either where it crosses the wrist en route to the hand or where it crosses the elbow—a part of the anatomy known informally as the "funny bone." This condition, **cubital tunnel syndrome** (named after the narrow channel in the elbow through which the nerve passes), occurs as a result of repeated trauma to the "funny bone"—such as continually leaning on the elbow.

Wristdrop, a condition in which the wrist cannot be straightened, is yet another nerve-related disorder—in this case one that involves the radial nerve. It is often associated with fracture of the upper arm bone (humerus), which in turn damages the radial nerve. Because the radial nerve controls the muscles on the back of the hand, opening the hand is considerably impaired.

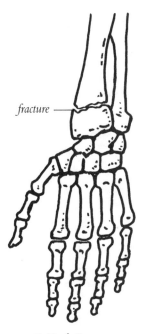

fracture

Colles' fracture

Like all bones, those in the wrist are subject to **fractures** and **dislocations** as a result of trauma, particularly because of our instinct to break a fall with an open hand. The most common such injury, a **Colles' fracture,** is a fracture at the base of the radius. Although technically it is the forearm that is broken, this fracture is generally referred to as a "broken wrist." The scaphoid bone, one of the carpals adjacent to the radius, can also be fractured in a fall; this injury is often mistaken for a less serious one, such as a sprain or simple bruise, but it may take months to heal. Wrist fractures and dislocations almost always cause swelling and pain, especially when the wrist is moved. A fracture at the wrist needs to be immobilized in a cast to heal.

Fingers, too, can become dislocated at one or more of the joints, usually as a result of violent impact due to falls, industrial accidents, sports activities, or automobile accidents. Sometimes, as in the case of a jammed finger (see page 73), a dislocated finger is accompanied by severe ligament sprain. A **broken finger** is an especially common sports injury but is rarely serious if treated promptly.

The worst sort of hand fracture involves **multiple broken bones** in the palm of the hand and is usually caused by the hand smashing into or being smashed by a solid object—again, often during sports or in automobile accidents. Because of the potential for swelling and nerve and soft tissue damage, with consequent permanent effects on the hand, this kind of fracture is always a medical emergency.

Taking Care of Your Wrist and Hand

As with many other parts of the body, **proper body mechanics** in the various activities of daily life are an essential factor in maintaining a healthy wrist and hand. For the wrist/hand unit, proper body mechanics means using the body and the different parts of the body in ways that are consistent with the smooth functioning of the region's joints, muscles, tendons,

Wrist and Hand Inactivity

In one form or another, excessive stress on the wrist/hand unit is certainly the most familiar cause of injury to the muscles and joints. Another cause, however, is only slightly less threatening: simple inactivity. Failure regularly to use the muscles of the wrist and hand and to bring the joints to the limits of their range of motion through moderately vigorous activity makes the region particularly susceptible to sudden overuse and other kinds of stress. The joints stiffen; ligaments and muscles may contract; good blood flow is inhibited. Even more noteworthy, inactivity may make the wrist and hand more susceptible to general joint degeneration.

The effects of inactivity tend to be magnified with age. And it is inactivity, more than aging itself, that leads to the conditions generally associated with growing older, like osteoarthritis. Regular exercise—gardening, swimming, or golf, for example—may well keep these problems at bay.

and ligaments. Among other things, this means knowing how to lift and carry heavy objects properly, being sure to use wrist and elbow supports when working at a computer, and not holding the hands in a contorted position for prolonged periods, as when knitting. Proper body mechanics can significantly reduce the risk of many wrist and hand problems.

Proper body mechanics are by no means always self-evident; occasionally they may even be counterintuitive. For most of us they need to be learned and consciously adopted. For detailed information on identifying and developing proper body mechanics, see **Chapter 12—Body Mechanics.**

Keeping your wrist and hand healthy also calls for **strength** in the muscles that help to keep the wrist and hand stable, moving, and well aligned—specifically those of the palm and forearm. The less developed your muscle strength, the narrower the range of physical activities you are capable of performing—or capable of performing without putting stress on the region. As a result, many common practices of everyday life, from lifting up a child to opening a tight jar, become riskier than they should be. A balance of strength in the forearm and hand muscles is important too so that one area need not compensate for weakness in another.

Endurance in the muscles that support the wrist and hand is also essential. Endurance is the ability of the muscles to contract (that is, be in use) over time. The less developed a muscle's endurance, the shorter the amount of time it can be called upon to contract before it tires—forcing other, often more vulnerable parts of the body to do its job and putting itself and those other parts at risk of injury. Since a range of common activities, including many sports and work activities (like typing and writing), calls upon our muscles to contract over extended periods, a certain level of endurance is absolutely vital.

Flexibility in the muscles, tendons, and ligaments is just as critical as muscle endurance and strength. The less flexible your muscles and ligaments, the more susceptible they are to the natural (and sometimes painful) tightening that comes from everyday activities. And the more susceptible they are to injury when called upon to perform many common practices, including many grasping activities. As with endurance and strength, this flexibility must be distributed among all the muscles that support the wrist and hand.

Appropriate endurance, strength, and flexibility for your wrist and hand (and other parts of your body) may be achieved through a regular program of exercise. For more information, see **Chapter 15—Strength, Endurance, and Flexibility.**

Although all parts of the body are at greater risk of injury when you are engaged in **sports** or other vigorous activities, the structure and function of the wrist and hand make it especially vulnerable, even for those who generally have good strength, endurance, and flexibility. First of all, the hand and wrist are usually exposed and unprotected, making them vulnerable to trauma. Second, strain or repetitive motion, such as from playing golf or playing piano, can increase the likelihood of problems. While the risks tend to increase the older you are and the more intense your workout is, it is nevertheless a good idea for anyone to fully prepare the wrist and hand for such a workout: warm up through gentle aerobic activity (such as walking for 5 or 10 minutes, being sure to move the arms) and then stretch the wrist and hand muscles.

It should be noted that sports-related repetitive-motion injuries to the wrist may often be prevented by taking care to use proper form. If you engage in racquet sports, sports that require throwing, or golf, you should have an expert evaluate your form. Also make sure your racquet and golf clubs fit your grip properly; the wrong equipment can contribute to wrist and finger problems.

Still, common sense is the best line of defense against injury when you play sports. If you don't play sports or engage in similar physical activities regularly, it is important not to push yourself too much when you do. And if you do experience any pain in the wrist or hand, stop what you're doing at once. To try to "play through it" is to risk injury.

Sports in particular also make the wrist and hand susceptible to traumatic injuries from falls (as in in-line skating) and collisions (as in football). And though such injuries are by nature unpredictable, often you can avoid or minimize them simply by wearing wrist protectors.

For more information on protecting your wrist, hand, and other parts of your body from injury during particular sports, see **Chapter 16—Sports**.

Like sports, many lines of **work** carry considerable risks of wrist and hand injury due to strain or overuse. Assembly-line workers, meat cutters, textile workers, and construction workers—among others—all face a higher risk of hand and wrist dysfunction due to repetitive motion. (They're also at a higher risk for serious trauma.) And since virtually every office worker now works at a computer, formerly obscure repetitive-motion ailments such as carpal tunnel syndrome have become household words. If you hold an occupation of this sort—even if your muscle endurance, strength, and flexibility are good—it is a wise precaution first to warm up and then to stretch the wrist and hand muscles before beginning your workday and several times throughout the day.

It's also important as much as possible to configure your physical work environment so that it does not force you to use poor body mechanics. Drafters, for example, who work at too-high tables that force them to flex their wrists excessively might try standing on a platform or adjusting the height of their work surface. If you work at a computer, it's essential that your chair, desk, and monitor be at proper heights, that your chair have armrests, and that your keyboard have a wrist rest.

Finally, if your occupation does subject your wrist and hand to stress, try varying your movements slightly and, if possible, alternating hands. And if you feel any tightness or stiffness *at all*, stretch the muscles a bit (see below). In fact, to head off problems, you may want to try this routine even if you don't have tightness or stiffness.

For more information on protecting your wrist, hand, and other parts of your body from injury during workplace activities, see **Chapter 17 — Work**.

When Problems Occur

No matter how well you treat your wrist and hand, **occasional temporary tightness and stiffness** may occur, especially as you grow older. After all, with such a wide range of common activities demanding the use of the wrist and hand, everyday life can be hard on the region. One way to ease your discomfort is with a few focused **stretching exercises,** which will bring back some badly needed flexibility and blood flow to your tired or aching muscles. (See the box, **"Quick-Relief Wrist and Hand Stretches,"** on page 79.)

Massage, which increases blood flow to the region while warming and stretching the wrist and hand muscles and soft tissue, may also work nicely. Although electric hand-held massagers and various nonelectric massage rollers are available on the market, you're much more likely to get a sensitive massage by using your hands. Simply **shaking out** the arms and hands is another alternative.

Sometimes a bout of wrist and hand stiffness or soreness can be traced directly to a particular instance of poor body mechanics. This is often the explanation for pain that occurs during a specific activity, like computer keyboarding without wrist support. If this is the case, double-check your body mechanics to make sure they're correct; you might find that a simple adjustment will eliminate the problem.

If your wrist and hand discomfort, however mild, persists for more than a few days, it's a good idea to have the region checked by a physical therapist or physician.

Beyond temporary soreness and stiffness, it's possible you will experience **more serious wrist and hand problems** at some point in your life, even if you have a generally healthy wrist and hand. The normal wear and tear of everyday living may stress the region—especially if you work at a computer, as increasing numbers of people do. Age, too, takes its toll, and with it may come osteoarthritis and other degenerative disorders. Falls or accidents may result in strains, sprains, or even fractures. Anyway, few of us can claim perfect wrist and hand maintenance, which makes us especially vulnerable to a whole range of problems.

Because wrist and hand problems can have major repercussions for the use of your hands, it's necessary to see a physical therapist or physician at the first sign of trouble. This is an obvious course of action in the case of a traumatic event, like a hard fall on the hand that leaves it too painful to move. In these cases you should seek **immediate professional attention.** In such urgent situations it's also a good idea to know some basics of **first aid.** (See Appendix A—First Aid Basics.)

Even if it's not the result of a traumatic event, any case of severe wrist and hand pain—or any swelling of the wrist or hand—requires immediate professional attention (and, if appropriate, first aid).

Milder degrees of wrist and hand pain, whether recurring or persisting for more than a few days, also should be evaluated by a physical therapist or physician.

In the meantime, minor wrist and hand pain can be managed by heeding a few simple tips. **Rest** from strenuous or repetitive tasks can provide some relief by giving the tissue some time to heal and regenerate. Prolonged immobilization, however, is not recommended; gentle movement and stretching and a gradual return to normal activity are best.

For the first day or two after the appearance of minor wrist or hand pain, you may apply **ice** to the affected area. The ice numbs the pain temporarily and may reduce or prevent swelling. One good method for applying ice is to put crushed ice in a sealable plastic bag with a little water, then cover the bag with towels. (A bag of frozen peas or corn works well too; refrigerated towels can be used in a pinch.) To avoid harming the skin or underlying tissues, apply the ice for only 15 to 20 minutes at a time, with 20 to 40 minutes between applications.

After a period of using ice, you may try **moist heat,** applied to the

Quick-Relief Wrist and Hand Stretches

The stretches below may ease (and sometimes head off) common wrist and hand tightness and stiffness, especially tightness and stiffness brought on by repetitive stress. Feel free to do them as often as you wish. Detailed instructions and appropriate illustrations can be found in Chapter 19—Flexibility Exercises. If your wrist and hand tightness and stiffness are persistent or produce more than just mild discomfort, consult your physical therapist before attempting them. Be sure to warm up your muscles prior to doing these exercises by, for instance, getting up and walking around your office and shaking out your wrists and hands.

- Palm-Up Wrist/Finger Extension (p. 255)
- Palm-Down Wrist/Finger Flexion (p. 255)
- Wrist Abduction/Adduction (p. 256)
- Fist Flex (p. 257)
- Thumb Circles (p. 260)

wrist/hand in a 20-minutes-on/20-minutes-off cycle. Moist heat tends to relax tense muscles, offering some relief from pain and stiffness. Warm showers or warm, moist towels work well for this. Heating pads or gloves, although not highly recommended, are also acceptable, but take care that the heat is not too intense.

For some people **nonsteroidal anti-inflammatory drugs (NSAIDs)** can be effective in easing wrist and hand pain. This class of drugs includes aspirin and ibuprofen, both of which are widely available without prescription. Like all drugs, however, NSAIDs have potentially dangerous side effects. Ask your doctor or pharmacist before taking NSAIDs, and follow the directions on the label.

When addressing a particular wrist or hand problem, your physical therapist has a wide range of techniques to draw upon. But—depending on the physical therapist's examination and evaluation—a wrist/hand rehabilitation program will almost certainly incorporate strength, endurance, and flexibility exercises and attention to improved postural alignment and body mechanics.

CHAPTER SEVEN

The Hip

Compared with such complex areas of the body as the back and the knee, the hip region is a model of straightforward sturdiness. It takes great force to seriously damage a healthy hip, and the large, strong muscles of the thighs (which help support and move the hips) are usually able to withstand more than their share of abuse.

Injuries and problems still occur, however, particularly in runners and in older individuals. Osteoarthritis in the hip afflicts many in the general population. And elderly people are subject to life-threatening hip fractures due to osteoporosis, the disease that causes brittle bones.

How the Hip Works

The hip is the point at which the thigh bone (**femur**) meets the three bones that make up each side of the pelvis: the **ilium,** the **pubis** (or **pubic bone**), and the **ischium.** The ilium, known informally as the hipbone, is a prominent arching bone on either side of the pelvis that can be felt by touching the waist. The pubis attaches to the lower part of the ilium and curves forward. The ischium loops below and slightly behind the pubis. The three bones converge to form a deep socket, the **acetabulum,** at the bottom outer edge of the basin-shaped pelvis, where it connects with the femur. The femur is the longest bone in the body, and the bump found on the outer side of the upper leg just below the hip joint is a part of the femur known as the **greater trochanter.**

The hip is a ball-and-socket joint. (Ball-and-socket joints resemble a golf ball on a tee: the round end of one bone moves freely within the scooped-out hollow of the other bone.) Thus, the large, rounded end of the femur (the **femoral head**) glides and rotates within the acetabulum. The femoral head and the acetabulum are covered with a smooth **articular cartilage** that facilitates movement within the joint. This arrangement allows the leg to move forward and backward, away from and across the body, and to pivot inward and outward—a combination essential to the activities of daily life.

Muscles in the thigh and lower back work together to keep the hip stable, well aligned, and moving. Among the more important of these

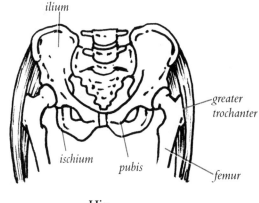

ilium

greater trochanter

ischium

pubis

femur

Hip

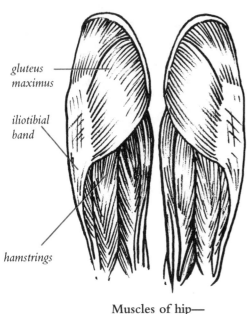

gluteus
maximus

iliotibial
band

hamstrings

Muscles of hip—
superficial muscles (back view)

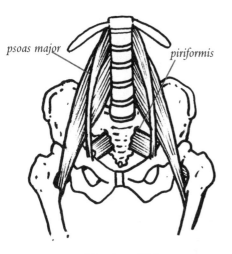

psoas major

piriformis

Muscles of hip—
deep muscles (front view)

muscles are the **gluteus maximus,** the large buttock muscle; the **hamstrings,** a trio of muscles in the back of the leg from the pelvis to just below the knee; and the **iliopsoas,** a pair of muscles running from the lower back and pelvis to the front of the upper leg—although a number of other muscles make essential contributions as well. Flexible fibrous cords of tissue called **tendons** (technically, extensions of the muscle) attach the muscles to the pelvis, lumbar vertebrae, and femur. These tendons also serve a stabilizing function.

The hip mechanism is further reinforced by the **joint capsule,** fibrous and connective tissue material that surrounds the joint, and by a range of **ligaments,** tough bands of fibrous tissue that bind together the bones of the hip joint. Three major ligaments in particular link the femur to the ilium, the pubis, and the ischium. Yet another stabilizer of the hip is the **iliotibial band (ITB),** a belt of fascia that runs along the outside of the thigh from the hip down to the knee.

Several nerves branching off from the **sciatic nerve,** which originates in the back, cross through the hip and down the leg. Each of these nerves allows us to contract specific muscles in the thigh, lower leg, and foot and to perceive sensations such as touch, temperature, and pain.

Three **bursa sacs (bursae),** fluid-filled sacs of varying sizes within and around the hip, cushion the joints and minimize friction in the region; perhaps the most significant of these is the **trochanteric bursa,** which lies over the greater trochanter of the femur. A **synovial membrane** in the joint capsule also facilitates smooth movement for the hip.

The hip is part of a kinetic chain that includes the back on one end and the knee, ankle, and foot on the other. All these areas of the body are interrelated and depend on each other for correct functioning and movement.

What Can Go Wrong

The tightly constructed hip joint is exceptionally stable. It is the "workhorse" joint of the human body, built solidly to support the weight of our bodies and keep us moving. As a result, what hip problems people do experience tend to be associated with inactivity, aging (including hip fractures among the elderly), and disease.

Young people are not immune from hip trouble, however. Trauma, most often from automobile accidents or rough sports, can also produce injuries. And while not as common as in other areas of the body, wear-and-tear and overuse injuries to the hip region, especially among runners and other athletes, are possible.

Hip symptoms come in many varieties. Pain can be dull, sharp, constant, or intermittent. It is also highly variable, from mild discomfort to extreme pain. There may be grinding or clicking in the joint or muscle weakness around it. The hip's range of motion may be limited.

Some hip conditions, such as mild strains, sprains, and tendinitis (see page 84), call for simple treatments like rest and ice. Others demand more advanced physical therapy techniques: carefully and scientifically tailored exercises to strengthen the hip and improve range of motion; adjustments of the gait; mobilization; and perhaps approaches (modalities) like ultrasound and electrical stimulation as well. Still other problems require surgery or other major interventions, although these, too, are usually complemented with an exercise program designed by a physical therapist as part of the rehabilitation stage. In every instance, however, you should look to your physician or physical therapist to make a diagnosis and determine treatment.

The hip's muscles are occasional sites of hip dysfunction. Certainly the mildest such dysfunction, if it can even be called that, is the tendency of these muscles—like muscles throughout the body—to become stiff or tight in response to heavy hip activity. The result of such **muscle tightness** is usually minor, short-term achiness and may be no cause for concern. (On the other hand, muscle tightness does diminish the hip's range of motion, which, unless the muscles are warmed up and stretched, puts the hip at risk of injury when called upon to push beyond that range.)

More worrisome is the accumulation of excess lactic acid and other chemicals in the hip muscles whenever they are subject to excessive or repetitive stress over prolonged periods of time—for example, when a person engages in heavy running or jumping (especially with an insufficient warmup period). The cellular and chemical responses to excessive stress almost inevitably lead to **muscle inflammation** and pain, which only increases if the stress is unrelieved.

When inflammation or tightening strikes the piriformis muscle, which is located (in most people) over the sciatic nerve, the symptoms can resemble those of a low back disorder: pain radiating into the leg, loss of hip motion, and difficulty with daily activities, especially those performed while standing or seated. This condition is sometimes called **piriformis syndrome.**

The hip muscles may also suffer from tearing. This tearing may result from direct trauma, overuse (from engaging in sports or some other activity), or poor body mechanics (such as improper lifting or an improper gait). A **muscle strain,** sometimes inaccurately called a "pulled muscle," occurs when the muscle has been overstretched or overexerted and may have microscopic tearing as its cause. When the tearing is more severe, it is called, simply, a **muscle tear,** which may be partial or complete. The two most frequently strained or torn muscles around the hip are the hamstrings, which run down the back of the upper leg, and the rectus femoris, which runs from the pelvis to just below the knee in the front of the leg. The symptoms of strains and tears vary only in degree and may include pain, inflammation, bleeding into the surrounding tissues, and muscle spasm (see below). Strains, however, are often mild enough to require little more treatment than rest for a few days.

Strains and tears often trigger **muscle spasm**—the sudden, intense contraction of muscle tissue. Although very painful, a muscle spasm is the body's natural mechanism for protecting injured tissue by acting as a brace. Because it is a protective mechanism, muscle spasm is also present in many other hip disorders.

Injuries to the muscles have much in common, and are often associated, with injuries to their tendons. Like the muscles themselves, the tendons of the muscles can become inflamed when subject to excessive stress. This condition is known as **tendinitis.** Any activity that stretches the tendons beyond their usual range of motion can cause tendinitis. But certainly the most common cause is engaging in running or similar vigorous activities without having first warmed up and stretched the tendons. Tendinitis may also strike those who "overdo" a physical activity after an extended period of being sedentary.

Because the tendons lack the same pain nerve endings as other structures, you might not feel any pain due to tendinitis until the surrounding synovial membrane of the joint or the bursa also become inflamed. Typical symptoms then include a generalized ache in the area, an increase in pain when using the hip, and localized tenderness where the tendon meets the bone.

In some cases a tendon, like a muscle, may even **tear** or **rupture** altogether as a result of trauma, leading to significant pain and spasm.

Not unlike the muscles and tendons, the ligaments of the hip can be overstretched—that is, pushed beyond their normal limits—or even torn. This injury, a **sprain,** can affect any of the hip's ligaments and can be produced by trauma, overuse, or poor body mechanics. A mild sprain will produce pain and swelling around the joint and possibly weakness in the muscles. Because of the great anatomical stability of this joint, however, sprains in the hip are relatively rare.

Like the muscles, the iliotibial band is prone to tightening in response to heavy activity, such as running and cycling. While this is harmless in itself, the ITB does become vulnerable to **iliotibial band syndrome (ITBS),** a condition caused by the repeated rubbing of the tightened ITB against the bony edges on the outer side of the femur. This can cause pain and irritation around the hip (and, more severely, along the outer side of the knee).

The hip joint is subject to the degenerative changes associated with **arthritis,** which can lead to both pain and stiffness. This condition can be the result of early trauma to the joints, but there is a wide range of possible causes. The most widespread form of arthritis in the hip joint is **osteoarthritis,** the degeneration of the articular cartilage and a wearing down of the joint surfaces. In some cases osteoarthritis may result in the buildup of roughened cartilage or spurs (deposits of bony tissue) on the joint surfaces and the appearance of loose bodies (floating bits of cartilage and bone) within the joint.

Osteoarthritis has a number of possible causes, including trauma, overuse, and inactivity. But by far the most common is simple degeneration of the joints due to age, typical (though not inevitable) among middle-aged individuals. Although it sometimes has no symptoms at all, osteoarthritis may well lead to pain (from mild to severe) and stiffness in the hip. In some cases it may be completely debilitating and require surgical replacement of the hip.

A rarer but more serious form of arthritis from which the hip may suffer is **rheumatoid arthritis,** an inflammatory disease whose origin is not fully understood (but which may be the result of autoimmune mechanisms or viral infections). The disorder is characterized by pain, stiffness, swelling, and warmth in the joints and can be debilitating. Like severe osteoarthritis, rheumatoid arthritis may call for surgical hip replacement.

All the bursae in the hip are subject to **bursitis,** an inflammation usually brought on by trauma or overuse, but none more so than the trochanteric bursa. An improper gait is one common cause of bursitis in the hip, a problem whose effects are greatly magnified by the relentless, repetitive force put on the hips by runners and other athletes. Pain, the primary symptom of bursitis, is usually constant and site specific. Bursitis can become a chronic disorder in which the bursa sacs thicken and reduce free movement around the joint, thus limiting the hip's range of motion.

Although extremely rare, the hip joint may suffer **dislocation,** in which the femoral head comes partway or completely out of the acetabulum. This results almost exclusively from the force of major trauma and must be treated as a medical emergency. Such an injury may not only damage the sciatic nerve but, more significantly, interrupt the blood supply to the femur, causing the bone to die.

Like all bones, those in the hip—especially at or just below the femoral head where it fits into the hip socket—are subject to **fracture.** Hairline cracks in the femur are possible among runners or others who engage in demanding activities; such an injury is known as a **stress fracture.** Mildly painful, it is easy to confuse with muscle strain (see page 83), tendinitis (see page 84), or bursitis (see page 85); an early, accurate diagnosis is critical because, without treatment, healing of the fracture may be compromised.

More serious fractures to the femur may result from trauma, especially falls and automobile or motorcycle accidents. These fractures are characterized by acute pain and an inability to walk. Like dislocations, they risk interrupting the supply of blood to the femur and must be treated as medical emergencies. Surgery is generally necessary to stabilize the fracture or to replace the hip altogether.

Such fractures can, of course, happen to anyone, but they are more likely among people who suffer from **osteoporosis**—a disease, most commonly found in older women, that causes bones to become weak and brittle. Hip fractures associated with osteoporosis are among the most familiar and threatening of injuries to the elderly.

The prominence of the hip makes it especially prone to **bruises**—internal bleeding—in the soft tissue around the bone or in the bone itself as a result of trauma, such as a fall or a collision. Such injuries are characterized by a black, blue, purple, and green appearance of the skin at the point of contact, the result of broken blood vessels under the skin or in the muscle. In many cases body fluids seep into the damaged tissue and cause swelling. Football players in particular are vulnerable to contusions along the rim of the pelvis, near the waist. This injury, a **hip pointer,** is very painful.

Taking Care of Your Hip

One of the most important factors in maintaining a healthy hip is a **proper gait.** The term "gait" refers to your particular manner of walking or running, and a proper gait is a manner of walking or running that displays symmetry, rhythm, and even leg and foot alignment. And while there is no one proper gait, gaits that do not meet these criteria may increase stress on the hip and on other parts of the body (like the knee, ankle, and foot) as well. This is particularly true for serious athletes and anyone else who does a lot of running.

Like good posture, a proper gait comes naturally to many people, while others may need to cultivate it. In some instances a proper gait is not even attainable without the right tools, like corrective footwear. For more information on identifying and developing a proper gait, see **Chapter 11—Gait.**

Another important factor in hip maintenance is **proper body mechanics** in the various activities of daily life. With regard to the hip, proper body mechanics means using the body and the different parts of the body in ways that are consistent with the smooth functioning of the region's joints, muscles, tendons, and ligaments. Among other things, this means not squatting down or climbing stairs for a prolonged period. Like proper gait, proper body mechanics can significantly reduce the risk of many hip problems.

Proper body mechanics are by no means always self-evident; sometimes they are even counterintuitive. They need to be learned and consciously adopted. For detailed information on identifying and developing proper body mechanics, see **Chapter 12—Body Mechanics**.

Although they represent slightly different ways of thinking about the body, gait and body mechanics are closely related phenomena. A proper gait is practically a prerequisite of proper body mechanics, because in the absence of a proper gait, you are always undermining the smooth functioning of your joints, muscles, tendons, and ligaments. In fact, some of the poor biomechanical habits most harmful to the hip are poor gait habits.

Weight control is a factor that's easily overlooked when it comes to keeping your hip healthy. But, in fact, excess weight can significantly magnify the stress on the hip joints. To avoid this burden on your hip, it's important to remain within your appropriate weight range. (Your weight also has implications for other parts of your body, including your back, knees, ankles, and feet.) For more information, see **Chapter 13—Body Weight**.

Keeping your hip healthy also calls for **strength** in the muscles that help to keep the hip stable, moving, and well aligned, including not just your hip muscles, but your thigh, buttock, back, and abdomen muscles as well. The less developed your muscle strength, the narrower the range of physical activities you are capable of performing—or capable of performing without putting stress on your hip. As a result, many common practices of everyday life, like squatting down to lift a child off the ground, become riskier than they should be. Furthermore, a certain amount of strength is necessary simply to hold the body upright and keep it moving. A balance of strength in the thighs, buttocks, back, and abdomen is important too so that one area need not compensate for weakness in another.

Endurance in the muscles that support the hip is also essential. Endurance is the ability of the muscles to contract (that is, be in use) over time. The less developed a muscle's endurance, the shorter the amount of time it can be called upon to contract before it tires—forcing other, often more vulnerable parts of the body to do its job and putting itself and those other parts at risk of injury. Because practically any upright activity calls upon the muscles in the hip region to contract over extended periods, a cer-

Hip Inactivity

In one form or another, excessive stress on the hip is certainly the most familiar cause of injury to the muscles and joints. Another cause, however, is only slightly less threatening: simple inactivity. Failure regularly to use the muscles of the hip and to bring the joints to the limits of their range of motion through moderately vigorous activity makes the region particularly susceptible to sudden overuse, an improper gait, and other kinds of stress. The joints stiffen; ligaments and muscles may contract; good blood flow is inhibited. Even more noteworthy, inactivity may make the hip more susceptible to general joint degeneration.

The effects of inactivity tend to be magnified with age. And it is inactivity, more than aging itself, that leads to the conditions generally associated with growing older, like osteoarthritis. Regular exercise—walking, swimming, or golf, for example—may well keep these problems at bay.

tain level of endurance is absolutely vital. And this is even more true for anyone involved in an activity that requires a great deal of running or other repetitive hip movement.

Flexibility in the muscles, tendons, and ligaments is just as critical as muscle endurance and strength. The less flexible your muscles, the more susceptible they are to the natural (and often painful) tightening that comes from everyday activities. And the more susceptible they are to injury when called upon to perform many common practices—from hopping over a puddle to getting into a taxi. As with endurance and strength, this flexibility must be distributed among all the muscles that support the hip.

Appropriate endurance, strength, and flexibility for your hip (and other parts of your body) may be achieved through a regular program of exercise. For more information, see **Chapter 15—Strength, Endurance, and Flexibility**.

Although **sports** and other vigorous activities are highly recommended, they do put the hip at greater risk of injury, even for those who generally have good endurance, strength, and flexibility in the muscles. Sudden or, more significantly, repetitive stress on the hip makes the joint vulnerable to muscle strain, tendinitis, and other minor and major problems. While the risks tend to increase the older you are and the more intense your workout is, it is nevertheless a good idea for anyone to fully prepare the hip for such a workout: warm up through gentle aerobic activity (such as walking for 5 or 10 minutes) and then stretch the hip muscles.

It should be noted that sports-related repetitive-motion injuries to the hip—generally, those associated with running or jumping—may often be prevented by taking care to use proper form. If you are a serious runner, you may want to consider having a physical therapist perform a gait analysis, a detailed study of your particular gait. This may help pinpoint idiosyncracies in your form that could represent poor body mechanics; your physical therapist may then be able to suggest biomechanical adjustments or corrective footwear to improve your gait before problems arise. But, with or without a gait analysis, you should make sure you have sufficiently supportive shoes for the activity; the wrong shoes can increase the stresses to the hip associated with sports and magnify any preexisting biomechanical or anatomical defects.

Still, common sense is the best line of defense against injury. If you don't engage in sports regularly, it's important not to push yourself too much when you do. And if you do experience any pain in the hip, stop what you're doing at once. To try to "run through it" is to risk injury.

Some sports (especially rough sports such as tackle football or rugby) make the hip susceptible to traumatic injuries, including hip pointers and even fractures. Fractures, fortunately, are fairly rare; hip pointers can be prevented simply by wearing hip pads.

For more information on protecting your hip and other parts of your body from injury during particular sports, see **Chapter 16—Sports.**

When Problems Occur

No matter how well you treat your hip, **occasional temporary tightness and stiffness** may occur, especially as you grow older. After all, between walking, climbing stairs, and playing sports, everyday life can be tough on the hip, resilient as it may be. One way to ease the discomfort is with a few focused **stretching exercises,** which will bring back some badly needed flexibility and blood flow to your tired or aching muscles. (See the box, "Quick-Relief Hip Stretches," on page 90.)

Massage, which increases blood flow to the region while warming and stretching the hip's muscle and soft tissue, may also work nicely. Although electric hand-held massagers and various nonelectric massage rollers are available on the market, you're much more likely to get a sensitive massage from someone just using the hands.

If your hip discomfort, however mild, persists for more than a few days, it's a good idea to have your hip checked by a physical therapist or physician.

Beyond temporary soreness and stiffness, it's possible that you will experience **more serious hip problems** at some point in your life, even if you have a generally healthy hip. The normal wear and tear of everyday life may stress the joint. Age, too, takes its toll, and with it may come osteoarthritis and possibly osteoporosis or other problems. Falls or accidents may result in sprains, muscle tears, or even fractures. Anyway, few of us can claim perfect hip maintenance, which makes us more vulnerable to a range of hip problems.

It's best to see a physical therapist or physician at the first sign of trouble, no matter how innocent-seeming. This is usually an obvious course of action in the case of a traumatic event, such as a hard fall on your hip or a collision that leaves you unable to walk. In these cases you should seek **immediate professional attention.** In such urgent situations it's also a good idea to know some basics of **first aid.** (See Appendix A—First Aid Basics.)

Even if it's not the result of a traumatic event, any case of severe hip pain should also get immediate medical attention (and, if appropriate, first aid).

Milder degrees of hip pain, if recurring or persisting for more than a few days, should also be evaluated by a physical therapist or physician. This

A Hip-Safe Home

Not enough can be said about the importance of avoiding trauma to the hip for those with osteoporosis. Because this disease, common among the elderly, leaves the bones so fragile, even a gentle fall can lead to a life-threatening fracture. At the very least, practical changes should be made to the household to minimize the possibility of tumbles: no loose electrical cords, no slippery throw rugs, etc. You should also be sure to mop up any spills right away and always turn on the lights when you enter a room. It is also highly recommended that those with osteoporosis consult a physical therapist to develop an exercise program to increase strength, balance, and coordination to make a fall less likely—and to try to enhance bone density as well.

Quick-Relief Hip Stretches

The stretches below may ease common hip tightness and stiffness. Feel free to do them as often as you wish. Detailed instructions and appropriate illustrations can be found in Chapter 19—Flexibility Exercises. (These exercises can also help with muscle spasm.) If your hip tightness and stiffness produce more than minor discomfort, consult your physical therapist before attempting them.
Be sure to warm up your muscles prior to doing these exercises by, for instance, getting up and walking around your office.

- Lunge Stretch (p. 262)
- Butterfly Stretch (p. 263)
- Hip Abductor Stretch (p. 265)
- V-Sit Stretch (p. 263)
- Buttocks Stretch (p.265)

includes the familiar achiness and stiffness that characterize osteoarthritis or tendinitis, the latter often brought on by overuse and often associated with sports and other physical activities. Of equal concern is the possibility that minor hip pain may be the symptom of bursitis or a more serious problem, such as a stress fracture. Any grinding or clicking in the joint should also be cause for concern.

In the meantime, minor hip pain can be managed by heeding a few simple tips. **Rest** may provide some relief by giving the tissue some time to heal and regenerate: no running, climbing, squatting, or similarly demanding activities. Prolonged bed rest, however, is not recommended and may result in debilitation; a gradual return to normal activities is best. Continuing to walk, even in the initial stages, may be helpful.

For the first day or two after the appearance of minor hip pain, you may apply **ice** to the affected area. The ice numbs the pain temporarily and may reduce or prevent swelling. One method for applying ice is to put crushed ice in a sealable plastic bag with a little water, then cover the bag with towels. (A bag of frozen peas or corn works well too; refrigerated towels can be used in a pinch.) To avoid harming the skin or underlying tissues, apply the ice for 15 to 20 minutes at a time, with 20 to 40 minutes between applications.

After a period of using ice, you may try **moist heat,** applied to the hip in a 20-minutes-on/20-minutes-off cycle. Moist heat tends to relax tense, strained muscle fibers, offering some relief from pain and stiffness. Warm showers or warm, moist packs or towels work well for this; whirlpools and hot tubs are fine too. Heating pads, although not highly recommended, are also acceptable, but take care that the heat is not too intense.

For some people **nonsteroidal anti-inflammatory drugs (NSAIDs)** can be very effective in easing hip pain. This class of drugs includes aspirin and ibuprofen, both of which are widely available without prescription. Like all drugs, however, NSAIDs have potentially dangerous side effects. Ask your doctor or pharmacist before taking NSAIDs, and follow the directions on the label.

When addressing a particular hip problem, the physical therapist has a wide range of techniques to draw upon. But—depending on your physical therapist's examination and evaluation—a hip rehabilitation program will almost certainly incorporate strength, endurance, and flexibility exercises and attention to improved body mechanics and gait. Your physical therapist may also recommend corrective footwear.

The Knee

There's a paradox about knee ailments: while problems in other joints can make you feel like you're over the hill, knee ailments are sometimes a point of pride, especially among athletes. A "trick knee" is sometimes seen as proof that you've paid your dues for being active. Unfortunately, the causes of knee pain—including overuse injuries and wear and tear over a long period of time—aren't always glamorous, and the results are often bothersome, painful, and debilitating.

The knee is the largest and most complicated joint in the body. It is also one of the most vulnerable. Like the spine, another region that's particularly susceptible to injury, the knee bears enormous loads while providing flexible movement. When walking, for example, each knee supports up to one-and-a-half times your body weight. Climbing stairs typically magnifies that ratio to three to four times, and squatting to seven to eight times. Just the normal activities of daily life place enormous stresses on the joint.

Physical therapists know that it's crucial to prevent knee injuries and to intervene as early as possible to keep minor problems from becoming major ones. If you take your knees seriously and work hard to prevent or overcome problems, you can avoid years of chronic pain and dysfunction.

How the Knee Works

The knee is the point at which the thigh bone (**femur**) meets the shin bone (**tibia**). It is actually made up of two separate joints: the **tibiofemoral joint** and the **patellofemoral joint.** The tibiofemoral joint links the femur to the tibia. The top of the tibia is made up of two **plateaus** and a knuckle-like protuberance in between known as the **tibial tubercle.** Between the femur and tibia and attached to the top of the tibia, on each side of the tibial plateaus, lie two crescent-shaped pads of shock-absorbing, stabilizing cartilage called **menisci.**

The patellofemoral joint links the femur to the kneecap (**patella**), which lies over the front of the knee; the patella glides along the bottom front surface of the femur in a groove between two protuberances called **femoral condyles.**

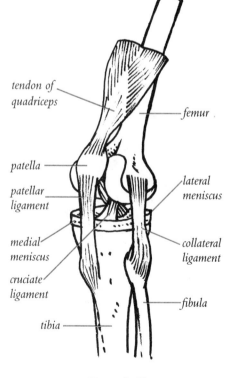

Knee (left)

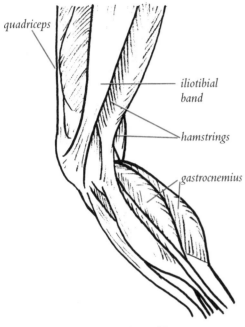

quadriceps

iliotibial band

hamstrings

gastrocnemius

Muscles of knee

The surfaces of the tubercle and condyle and the underside of the patella are covered with a smooth **articular cartilage** that facilitates movement in the region. Together, the two joints create a modified hinge joint, not only allowing the knee to bend and straighten but also to rotate slightly in a semicircular motion and from side to side.

Muscles in the leg all work together to keep the knee stable, well aligned, and moving. Among the more important of these muscles are the **hamstrings,** actually a group of three muscles running down the back of the thigh, and the **quadriceps,** a group of four muscles running down the front of the thigh. Other muscles in the lower leg also play a role in the knee's function. Flexible fibrous cords of tissue called **tendons** (technically, extensions of the muscle) attach the muscles to various parts of the pelvis, femur, kneecap, tibia, and **fibula** (the second bone in the lower leg). A number of tendons also serve a stabilizing function.

The knee mechanism is further reinforced by a **joint capsule,** fibrous and connective tissue material that surrounds the joints, and by a range of **ligaments,** tough bands of fibrous tissue that bind together the bones of the knee joint. A pair of major ligaments (the **collateral ligaments**) run from the femoral condyle to the upper tibia along the inside of the knee and from the femoral condyle to the fibula on the outside of the knee. Two others (the **cruciate ligaments**) run diagonally and crisscross each other within the center of the knee unit. Yet another important ligament connects the patella with the tibia. A belt of fascia known as the **iliotibial band (ITB)** runs along the outside of the leg from the hip down to the knee and helps keep the lateral movement of the knee in check.

Up to 13 **bursa sacs (bursae),** fluid-filled sacs of varying sizes within and around the knee, cushion the joints and minimize friction in the region; among the most significant of these is the **prepatellar bursa,** located at the front of the knee. A **synovial membrane** in the joint capsule also provides lubrication for the knee.

The knee is part of a kinetic chain that includes the pelvis, hip, and upper leg on one end and the lower leg, ankle, and foot on the other. All these different areas of the body are interrelated and depend on each other for correct functioning and movement.

What Can Go Wrong

The knee is a little like an expensive sports car: remarkably engineered, capable of great bursts of power, but not the most durable of mechanisms. The way the bones of the knee are put together—with the patella "floating" in front of the joint and with a relatively large space between the femur and the tibia—makes the knee dependent on the muscles, tendons, ligaments, and fascia to keep the joint stable. Thus the particular structure of the knee makes it unusually vulnerable to injury due to overuse, repetitive motion, or trauma.

While knee pain may arise as the result of a specific traumatic incident—an accident, fall, work-related injury, or sports injury—it sometimes seems to appear out of nowhere. In cases where there's no obvious cause for pain, the culprit is often the cumulative stress, strain, and overuse from years of poor body mechanics. In young people and active adults, problems tend to be related to playing sports, which can often be punishing on the knee. After all, the familiar overuse and repetitive-motion injuries with athletic-sounding names ("jumper's knee," "runner's knee") are not the sole domain of professional athletes.

Knee symptoms come in many varieties. Pain can be dull, sharp, constant, or intermittent. It is also highly variable, from mild discomfort to agonizing pain. The knee's range of motion may become restricted—or excessive. There may be grinding or clicking in the joint; the joint may lock; or the muscles may feel weak.

Some knee conditions, such as mild strains, sprains, and tendinitis (see below), call for simple home treatments like rest and ice. Others demand more advanced physical therapy techniques: carefully and scientifically tailored exercises to strengthen the knee and improve range of motion; adjustments of the gait; mobilization; and perhaps approaches (modalities) like ultrasound and electrical stimulation as well. Still other problems require surgery or other major interventions, although these, too, are usually complemented with an exercise program designed by a physical therapist as part of the rehabilitation stage. In every instance, however, you should look to your physician or physical therapist to make a diagnosis and determine treatment.

The knee's muscles are occasional sites of knee dysfunction. Certainly the mildest such dysfunction, if it can even be called that, is the tendency of these muscles—like muscles throughout the body—to become stiff or tight in response to heavy knee activity. The result of such **muscle tightness** is usually minor, short-term achiness and may be no cause for concern. (On the other hand, muscle tightness does diminish the knee's range of motion, which, unless the muscles are warmed up and stretched, puts the knee at risk of injury when called upon to push beyond that range.)

More worrisome is the accumulation of excess lactic acid and other chemicals in the knee muscles whenever they are subject to excessive or repetitive stress over prolonged periods of time—for example, when a person engages in heavy running or jumping (especially with an insufficient warm-up period). The cellular and chemical responses to excessive stress almost inevitably lead to **muscle inflammation** and pain, which only increases if the stress is unrelieved.

The knee muscles may also suffer from tearing. This tearing may result from direct trauma, overuse (from engaging in sports or some other activity), or poor body mechanics (such as an improper gait). A **muscle strain,** sometimes inaccurately called a "pulled muscle," occurs when the muscle has been overstretched or overexerted and may have microscopic tearing as its cause. When the tearing is more severe, it is called, simply, a **muscle tear,** which may be partial or complete. The symptoms of strains and tears vary only in degree and may include pain, inflammation, bleeding into the surrounding tissues, and muscle spasm (see below). Strains, however, are often mild enough to require little more treatment than rest for a few days.

Strains and tears often trigger **muscle spasm**—the sudden, intense contraction of muscle tissue. Although very painful, a muscle spasm is the body's natural mechanism for protecting injured tissue by acting as a brace. Because it is a protective mechanism, muscle spasm is also present in many other knee disorders.

Injuries to the muscles have much in common, and are often associated, with injuries to their tendons. Like the muscles themselves, the tendons of the muscles can become inflamed or microscopically torn (strained) when subject to excessive stress. This condition, known as **tendinitis,** is probably the most familiar knee ailment. Any activity that stretches the tendons beyond their usual range of motion can cause tendinitis. But certainly the most common cause is engaging in running or similar vigorous activities without having first warmed up and stretched the tendons. Tendinitis may also strike those who "overdo" a physical activity after an extended period of being sedentary.

Because the tendons lack the same pain nerve endings as other structures, you might not feel any pain due to tendinitis until the surrounding synovial membrane of the joints or the adjacent bursa also become inflamed. Typical symptoms then include a deep generalized ache in the area, an increase in pain when using the knee, and localized tenderness.

In some cases a tendon, like a muscle, may even **tear** or **rupture** altogether as a result of trauma, leading to significant pain and spasm.

One of the more common varieties of tendinitis is so-called **jumper's**

knee, which afflicts the tendon attached to the patella (specifically, the quadriceps tendon). This tendon, which is involved in straightening the leg, experiences a great deal of stress whenever your foot hits the ground forcefully, as in running or repetitive jumping—especially if the quadriceps muscle isn't sufficiently strong and flexible.

The two menisci are vulnerable to tears, often as a result of a direct blow to the knee—during sports, for example—in which they are pinched between the femur and the tibia. Depending on which one is injured, a **meniscus tear** causes pain to the inside or the outside of the knee, which can become quite intense when a person is walking or climbing stairs. The knee may even lock. Surgery is generally used only as a last resort in the treatment of this condition, and then it tends to be aimed at repairing the tear rather than removing the meniscus altogether.

Occasionally the back of the knee's joint capsule may become weakened, leading to a rupture through which the synovial membrane emerges. The result is a painful swelling behind the knee known as a **Baker's cyst.** This injury shows up in runners and tennis players as a consequence of overuse. Sometimes a Baker's cyst will go away by itself; in other cases it may become a chronic condition.

Not unlike the muscles and tendons, the ligaments of the knee can suffer microtrauma or be overstretched—that is, pushed beyond their normal limits—or even sometimes torn. This injury, a **sprain,** can affect any of the knee's ligaments and can be produced by trauma, overuse, or poor body mechanics (like an improper gait). Skiing, running, football, soccer, and other contact sports are some of the principal sprain producers. The most common sprain results from a violent blow to the outer side of the knee, stretching the medial collateral ligament (MCL), which runs along the inside of the knee. In rarer cases the knee is struck on the inner side, causing stretching or tearing of the lateral collateral ligament (LCL), which runs along the outside of the knee. A sprain to one of the crisscrossing ligaments, the anterior cruciate ligament (ACL), may occur when the tibia is pushed sharply forward of the femur—an occurrence frequently associated with skiing accidents. If the ACL is completely torn, you may hear a pop or feel a snapping sensation at the time of the injury. Surgery is required to repair a torn ligament.

A mild sprain will produce pain and swelling around the joint and possibly weakness in the muscles. In more severe cases there may be a feeling of slippage in the joint; severe sprains may make it too painful to walk.

Simultaneous tears of the medial collateral ligament, the anterior cruciate ligament, and another ligament called the medial capsular ligament—and often one of the menisci (specifically, the medial meniscus, to the inside of the joint)—are all components of an injury sometimes called the **"clipping injury."** This exceptionally acute traumatic injury is associated largely with contact sports. It, too, must be addressed surgically.

Like the muscles, the iliotibial band is prone to tightening in response to heavy activity, such as running and cycling. While this is harmless in itself, the ITB does become vulnerable to **iliotibial band syndrome (ITBS),** a condition caused by the repeated rubbing of the tightened ITB against the bony edges on the outer side of the femoral condyle. This can cause pain and irritation along the outer side of the knee.

The knee joint is subject to the degenerative changes associated with **arthritis,** which can lead to both pain and stiffness. This condition can be the result of early trauma to the joints, but there is a wide range of possible causes. The most widespread form of arthritis in the knee joint is **osteoarthritis,** the degeneration of the articular cartilage and a wearing down of the joint surfaces. In some cases osteoarthritis may result in the buildup of roughened cartilage or spurs (deposits of bony tissue) on the joint surfaces and the appearance of loose bodies (floating bits of cartilage and bone) within the joint.

Osteoarthritis has a number of possible causes, including trauma, overuse, and inactivity. But by far the most common is simple degeneration of the joints due to age, typical (though not inevitable) among middle-aged individuals. Although it sometimes has no symptoms at all, osteoarthritis may well lead to pain (from mild to severe) and stiffness in the knee. In some cases it may be completely debilitating and requires surgical knee replacement.

A loose body can only further complicate matters, sometimes floating into places where it causes pain or even causes the knee to lock. The presence of one or several loose bodies—or "mice in the knee," as the condition is often called—characterizes the loosely defined condition known as a **"trick knee."**

A rarer but more serious form of arthritis is **rheumatoid arthritis,** an inflammatory disease whose origin is not fully understood (but which may be the result of autoimmune mechanisms or viral infections). The disorder is characterized by pain, stiffness, swelling, and warmth in the knee joints. Physical therapy is necessary to help maintain mobility and flexibility in the region.

Patellofemoral pain syndrome is a generic term used to refer to a number of dysfunctions of the patella and the patellofemoral joint—

including misalignment of the patella and laxity of the joint. It is caused by improper movement of the patella during bending and straightening of the knee and by mechanical imbalances at the patellofemoral joint over long periods of time. Symptoms include pain around the patella while moving, swelling, creaking in the knee, and muscle weakness. This condition may cause pain upon standing up after sitting for an extended period of time and is sometimes called the "moviegoer's sign." Patellofemoral pain syndrome may also involve partial dislocation of the patella (see below).

Another joint disorder from which the knee may suffer is **chondroma-lacia patellae,** a degeneration in the cartilage on the underside of the patella, ranging from minor roughness to major cracks and fissures. It may feel like there's sand or gravel under the kneecap, and the area around the kneecap may fill with fluid. Sometimes the pain is so severe that it is difficult to sit with the knees bent for more than a few minutes at a time. Severe chondromalacia may require surgical treatment of the patellofemoral joint. Chondromalacia patellae is often incorrectly diagnosed as patellofemoral pain syndrome (see page 96).

All the bursae in the knee are subject to **bursitis,** an inflammation brought on by trauma or overuse, but none more so than the prepatellar bursa. Continually kneeling down—a familiar practice among roofers, electricians, plumbers, carpet layers, and others—is one common cause of bursitis in the prepatellar bursa. (This condition sometimes goes by the old-fashioned name of **"housemaid's knee."**) Pain, the primary symptom of bursitis, is usually constant and site specific. Bursitis can become a chronic disorder in which the bursa sacs thicken and reduce free movement around the joint, thus limiting the knee's range of motion.

During adolescence (ages 12 to 16), the tibia enters a period of growth that makes it very sensitive to constant tugging of the patellar tendon, which is part of just about all vigorous activities: running, jumping, and cycling, for example. As a result, the tibial tubercle may become enlarged and irritated, causing a dull pain in the knee and the appearance of a larger than usual bony knob below the kneecap. This condition, known as **Osgood-Schlatter's disease,** is more likely to affect boys, who are especially active at that age, than girls.

The knee may also suffer **partial dislocation,** in which the patella slips (subluxes) partway out of the shallow groove between the femoral condyles. It may become positioned too high or too low; it may become excessively rotated or tilted. This usually results from a traumatic accident. A subluxed patella stretches and strains the ligaments, tendons, and other elements

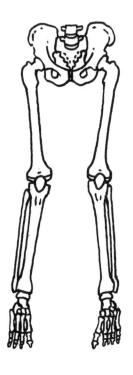

Valgus deformity

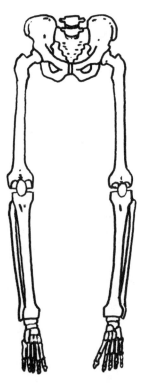

Varus deformity

within the knee, which may in turn cause sharp pain and a feeling of buckling or giving way. Often partial dislocation becomes noticeable when a person is climbing stairs or rising after being seated for a long time. Women are more susceptible to this disorder for several reasons, such as the groove between the femoral condyles being more shallow in females. Indeed, once a woman's patella has become subluxed, it may become a recurring problem. Realignment of the patella, exercises, and even surgery may be required to resolve the problem. A **full dislocation,** in which the patella comes completely out of the groove, has the same causes but is more immediately damaging to the knee and requires medical attention.

Like all bones, those in the knee—especially the patella, the femoral condyles, and the upper end of the tibia—are subject to **fractures** as a result of trauma. Fractures are serious not only because they damage the bone itself but because of possible secondary damage to the soft tissue around the bone. They may also result in the appearance of loose bodies in the area, leading to a so-called "trick knee" (see page 96). Knee fractures cause pain and joint stiffness and usually need to be immobilized in a cast to heal; in severe cases a fracture may require surgical intervention.

A variety of knee problems—including muscle strain, muscle inflammation, tendinitis, and ligament sprains—may also be found in people with a **valgus deformity** or a **varus deformity**. A valgus deformity, or **"knock knee,"** is a condition in which the knees lean slightly inward; a varus deformity, or **"bow leg,"** is a condition in which the knees lean slightly outward. The possible causes (both direct and indirect) of a valgus or varus deformity are many and include, among others, arthritis (see page 96), flat-footedness, and bone disorders such as rickets; in many cases these disorders may be congenital. The cumulative impact of years of walking and running with valgus or varus deformities, with the stress it places on the structures in and around the joint, may have serious long-term implications for the knee. In some instances there may even be a narrowing of the joint space on the inner or outer side of the knee and a general degeneration of the joint.

Taking Care of Your Knee

One of the most important factors in maintaining a healthy knee is a **proper gait.** The term "gait" refers to your particular manner of walking or running; and a proper gait is a manner of walking or running that displays symmetry, rhythm, and even leg and foot alignment. And while there is no one proper gait, gaits that do not meet these criteria may increase stress on the knee and on other parts of the body (like the hip, ankle, and foot) as well. This is particularly true for serious athletes and anyone else who does a lot of running.

Like good posture, a proper gait comes naturally to many people, while others may need to cultivate it. In some instances a proper gait is not even attainable without the right tools, like corrective footwear. For more information on identifying and developing a proper gait, see **Chapter 11 — Gait**.

Another important factor in knee maintenance is **proper body mechanics** in the various activities of daily life. With regard to the knee, proper body mechanics means using the body and the different parts of the body in ways that are consistent with the smooth functioning of the region's joint, muscles, tendons, and ligaments. Among other things, this means not squatting down or climbing stairs for prolonged periods; never sitting on the floor with the knees turned in and the feet splayed out to the side; and being sure to wear knee pads when kneeling, as when cleaning or gardening. Like proper gait, proper body mechanics can significantly reduce the risk of many knee problems.

Proper body mechanics are by no means always self-evident; sometimes they are even counterintuitive. They need to be learned and consciously adopted. For detailed information on identifying and developing proper body mechanics, see **Chapter 12 — Body Mechanics**.

Although they represent slightly different ways of thinking about the body, gait and body mechanics are closely related phenomena. A proper gait is practically a prerequisite of proper body mechanics, because in the absence of a proper gait, you are always undermining the smooth functioning of your joints, muscles, tendons, and ligaments. In fact, some of the poor biomechanical habits most harmful to the knee are poor gait habits.

Weight control is a factor that's easily overlooked when it comes to keeping your knee healthy. But, in fact, excess weight can significantly magnify any stress on the knee joints. To avoid this burden on your knee, it's important to remain within your appropriate weight range. (Your weight also has implications for other parts of your body, including your back, hips, ankles, and feet.) For more information on healthy body weight, see **Chapter 13 — Body Weight**.

Keeping your knee healthy also calls for **strength** in the muscles that help to keep the knee stable, moving, and well aligned, including not just your knee muscles but your thigh and lower leg muscles as well. The less developed your muscle strength, the narrower the range of physical activities you are capable of performing—or capable of performing without putting stress on your knee. As a result, many common practices of everyday

Knee Inactivity

In one form or another, excessive stress on the knee is certainly the most familiar cause of injury to the muscles and joints. Another cause, however, is only slightly less threatening: simple inactivity. Failure regularly to use the muscles of the knee and to bring the joints to the limits of their range of motion through moderately vigorous activity makes the region particularly susceptible to sudden overuse, an improper gait, and other kinds of stress. The joints stiffen; ligaments and muscles may contract; good blood flow is inhibited. Even more noteworthy, inactivity may make the knee more susceptible to general joint degeneration.

The effects of inactivity tend to be magnified with age. And it is inactivity, more than aging itself, that leads to the conditions generally associated with growing older, like osteoarthritis. Regular exercise—walking, swimming, or golf, for example—may well keep these problems at bay.

life, like squatting or climbing stairs or lifting heavy objects, become riskier than they should be. Furthermore, a certain amount of strength is necessary simply to hold the body upright and keep it moving. A balance of strength in the thighs, buttocks, and lower legs is important too so that one area need not compensate for weakness in another.

Endurance in the muscles that support the knee is also essential. Endurance is the ability of the muscles to contract (that is, be in use) over time. The less developed a muscle's endurance, the shorter the amount of time it can be called upon to contract before it tires—forcing other, often more vulnerable parts of the body to do its job and putting itself and those other parts at risk of injury. Because practically any upright activity calls upon the muscles in the knee region to contract over extended periods, a certain level of endurance is absolutely vital. And this is even more true for anyone involved in an activity that requires a great deal of running or any repetitive knee movement.

Flexibility in the muscles, tendons, and ligaments is just as critical as muscle endurance and strength. The less flexible your muscles, the more susceptible they are to the natural (and often painful) tightening that comes from everyday activities. And the more susceptible they are to injury when called upon to perform many common practices—from rising from a chair to getting out of bed. As with endurance and strength, this flexibility must be distributed among all the muscles that support the knee.

Appropriate strength, endurance, and flexibility for your knee (and other parts of your body) may be achieved through a program of exercise. For more information, see **Chapter 15—Strength, Endurance, and Flexibility**.

Although **sports** and other such activities are highly recommended, they do put the knee at greater risk of injury, even for those who generally have good endurance, strength, and flexibility in the muscles. Sudden, intense, or, more significantly, repetitive stress on the knee makes the joint vulnerable to muscle strain, tendinitis, and other minor and major problems. While the risks tend to increase the older you are and the more intense your workout is, it is nevertheless a good idea for anyone to fully prepare the knee for such a workout: warm up through gentle aerobic activity (such as walking for 5 or 10 minutes), and then stretch the knee muscles.

It should be noted that sports-related repetitive-motion injuries to the knee—generally, those associated with running—may often be prevented by taking care to use proper form. If you are a serious runner, you may want to consider having a physical therapist perform a gait analysis, a detailed study of your particular gait. This may help pinpoint idiosyncracies in your form that could represent poor body mechanics; your physical therapist may then be able to suggest biomechanical adjustments or corrective footwear to improve your gait before problems arise. But, with or without a gait analysis, you should make sure you have sufficiently supportive shoes for the activity; the wrong shoes can cause stresses to the knee associated with sports and magnify any preexisting biomechanical or anatomical defects.

Still, common sense is the best line of defense against injury. If you don't engage in sports regularly, it's important not to push yourself too much when you do. And if you do experience any pain in the knee, stop what you're doing at once. To try to "run through it" is to risk serious injury.

Sports in particular make the knee susceptible to traumatic injuries from falls and collisions. Cycling, skateboarding, and in-line skating are some of the more familiar culprits, as are tennis, soccer, basketball, and football, which require considerable movement and abrupt changes of direction. Although such injuries are by nature unpredictable, often they can be avoided simply by wearing knee pads. It is not a good idea, however, to rely on neoprene braces for stabilization or protection; these may create a false sense of security, setting you up for serious knee problems.

For more information on protecting your knee and other parts of your body from injury during particular sports, see **Chapter 16—Sports**.

Like sports, many lines of **work** carry considerable risks of knee injury due to strain or overuse. Needless to say, just about any sort of labor that involves repetitive or sharp bending of the knees (like carpet laying) falls into this category. If you hold an occupation of this sort—even if your muscle endurance, strength, and flexibility are good—it is a wise precaution first to warm up and then stretch the knee muscles before beginning your workday and several times throughout the day.

Also, if your occupation does subject your knee to strain and overuse, be sure to take a break of at least several minutes every hour, and if you feel any tightness or stiffness *at all*, stretch the muscles a bit (see below). In fact, to head off problems, you may want to try this routine even if you don't have tightness or stiffness.

For more information on protecting your knee and other parts of your body from injury during work activities, see **Chapter 17—Work**.

When Problems Occur

No matter how well you treat your knee, **occasional temporary tightness and stiffness** may occur, especially as you grow older. After all, between climbing stairs and sitting for hours with your knees bent, everyday

Quick-Relief Knee Stretches

The stretches below may ease (and sometimes head off) common knee tightness and stiffness, especially tightness and stiffness brought on by repetitive stress. Feel free to do them as often as you wish. Detailed instructions and appropriate illustrations can be found in Chapter 19—Flexibility Exercises. If your knee tightness and stiffness produce more than minor discomfort, consult your physical therapist before attempting them. Be sure to warm up your muscles prior to doing these exercises by, for instance, getting up and walking around your office.

- Standing Hamstring Stretch (p. 271)
- Standing Quad Stretch (p. 272)

life can be tough on the knees. One way to ease your discomfort is with a few focused **stretching exercises,** which will bring back some badly needed flexibility and blood flow to your tired or aching muscles. (See the box, **"Quick-Relief Knee Stretches,"** at left.)

Massage, which increases blood flow to the region while warming and stretching the elbow muscles and soft tissue, may also work nicely. Although electric hand-held massagers and various nonelectric massage rollers are available on the market, you're much more likely to get a sensitive massage by using your hands.

Sometimes a bout of knee stiffness or soreness can be traced directly to a particular instance of poor body mechanics. This is often the explanation for pain that occurs during a specific activity—like resting on your knees to wash the floor. If this is the case, double-check your body mechanics to make sure they are correct; you might find that a simple adjustment will quickly eliminate the problem.

If your knee discomfort, however mild, persists for more than a few days, it's a good idea to have your knee checked by a physical therapist or physician for proper diagnosis.

Beyond temporary soreness and stiffness, it is possible that you will experience **more serious knee problems** of one sort or another at some point in your life, even if you have a generally healthy knee. The normal wear and tear of everyday living can stress the joint. Age, too, takes its toll, and with it may come osteoarthritis and other dysfunctions. Falls or accidents may bring sprains, muscle tears, or even fractures. Anyway, few of us can claim perfect knee maintenance, which makes us especially vulnerable to a whole range of knee problems.

It is best to see a physical therapist or physician at the first sign of trouble, no matter how innocent-seeming. This is usually an obvious course of action in the case of a traumatic event, like a severe twist or a fall that pops the knee out of place. In these cases you should seek **immediate professional attention.** In such urgent situations it's also a good idea to know some basics of **first aid.** (See Appendix A—First Aid Basics.)

Even if it's not the result of a traumatic event, any case of severe knee pain—or of the knee's locking—should also get immediate medical attention (and, if appropriate, first aid).

Milder degrees of knee pain, if persisting for more than a few days or recurring, should be evaluated by a physical therapist or physician, even though they do not demand such urgency. This includes the familiar achiness and stiffness that characterize tendinitis, often brought on by overuse and often associated with sports and other physical activities. If not addressed, minor knee pain can easily develop into a chronic condition (if it isn't chronic already). Of equal concern is the possibility that minor knee pain is the symptom of an even more involved problem—one that will lead to major impairments or disability. Any grinding or clicking in the knee, muscle weakness, loss of range of motion, or episode of the patella seeming to pop out of place, painful or not, should also be cause for concern and should be evaluated immediately.

In the meantime, minor knee pain can be managed by heeding a few simple tips. **Rest** can provide some relief by giving the tissue some time to heal and regenerate: no sports, running, or similarly demanding activities. Prolonged bed rest, however, is not recommended and may result in debilitation; a gradual return to normal activities is best. Continuing to walk, even in the initial stages, may be helpful.

For the first day or two after the appearance of minor knee pain, you may apply **ice** to the affected area. The ice numbs the pain temporarily and may reduce or prevent swelling. One good method for applying ice is to put crushed ice in a sealable plastic bag with a little water, then cover the bag with towels. (A bag of frozen peas or corn works well too; refrigerated towels can be used in a pinch.) To avoid harming the skin or underlying tissues, apply the ice for 15 to 20 minutes at a time, with 20 to 40 minutes between applications.

After a period of using ice, you may try **moist heat,** applied to the knee in a 20-minutes-on/20-minutes-off cycle. Moist heat tends to relax tense, strained muscle fibers, offering some relief from pain and stiffness. Warm showers or warm, moist towels work well for this; whirlpools and hot tubs are fine too. Heating pads, although not highly recommended, are also acceptable, but take care that the heat is not too intense.

For some people, **nonsteroidal anti-inflammatory drugs (NSAIDs)** can be very effective in easing knee pain. This class of drugs includes aspirin and ibuprofen, both of which are widely available without prescription. Like all drugs, however, NSAIDs have potentially dangerous side effects. Ask your doctor or pharmacist before taking NSAIDs, and follow the directions on the label.

When addressing a particular knee problem, your physical therapist has a wide range of techniques to draw upon. But—depending on the physical therapist's examination and evaluation—a knee rehabilitation program will almost certainly incorporate strength, endurance, and flexibility exercises. In addition, your knee rehabilitation program may include attention to improved body mechanics and gait. Your physical therapist may also recommend corrective footwear.

The Ankle & Foot

Your ankle and foot take more direct punishment than almost any other part of the body. They not only bear enormous weight with each step but undergo even greater stress when you run, climb stairs, participate in sports, or walk uphill. Add poorly fitting shoes or an improper gait to the mix and you can almost guarantee yourself problems.

Trauma to the ankle and foot must always be taken particularly seriously. The intricate construction of the region, the sensitive nerve endings in the foot, and our heavy dependence on the ankle and foot in our everyday lives tend to magnify the seriousness of any injury.

Many of these problems can easily be prevented or at least minimized. Others, such as sports and running injuries, can be avoided through appropriate exercise, wearing the right shoes, and consulting with a physical therapist *before* problems occur.

How the Ankle and Foot Work

The ankle is the point at which the uppermost bone in the foot, the **talus,** meets the bones of the lower leg, the **tibia** and **fibula.** (The tibia, or "shinbone," is the bone at the front of the lower leg, and the fibula is along the outer side of the lower leg.) The bottommost portions of these two bones, with their familiar projections to the inner and outer sides of the ankles, form a box-like structure known as the **ankle mortise,** in which the talus rests. The joint surfaces are covered with a smooth **articular cartilage** that facilitates movement in the region. The ankle's bony structure permits the foot to move up and down.

The foot itself contains 28 bones: 7 interconnected **tarsal bones**—including the talus and the heel bone (**calcaneus**), the foot's largest bone—arrayed below the ankle toward the back of the foot; 5 elongated **metatarsal bones,** which make up the front half of the foot; 2 small **sesamoid bones,** set at the base of the great (or big) toe; and 14

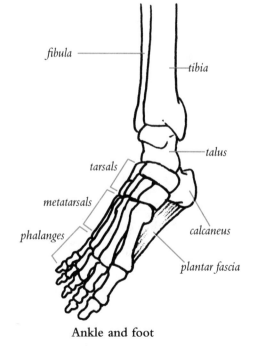

fibula

tibia

talus

tarsals

metatarsals

calcaneus

phalanges

plantar fascia

Ankle and foot

phalanges, which collectively make up the toes. (Each toe consists of 3 phalanges, except for the big toe, which consists of 2.) Between them, these 28 bones make for 32 separate joints. The **metatarsophalangeal (MTP) joints** join the toes with the body of the foot. The toe joints are called the **interphalangeal (IP) joints.**

The arrangement of bones forms a gentle arch running lengthwise along the instep at the base of the foot (the **longitudinal arch**), and another arch running crosswise (the **transverse arch**). This arched arrangement considerably enhances the foot's flexibility, stability, and ability to adapt to uneven surfaces, allowing the foot to absorb shock and still be rigid enough to propel the body forward.

Like the hand, the bones of the foot are packed into an exceptionally tight space. They are, however, considerably stronger and larger than those of the hand, built to bear the body's full weight. Its structure allows the foot to move up and down and from side to side, to rotate, and to turn inward and outward; it also allows the toes to move up and down, spread apart from one another and come back together again, and (to some degree) to move independently. Like all joints, those of the foot, too, feature articular cartilage on the bone surfaces.

All the bones of the ankle and foot work together to provide a stable base of support and to adjust our feet to different and uneven surfaces when we walk, run, or play sports.

Muscles in the lower leg and the foot all work together to keep the ankle and foot stable, aligned, and moving. Among the more important of these are the **gastrocnemius,** the large rounded muscle at the back of the lower leg; the **soleus,** a flat muscle lying just below the gastrocnemius (not pictured); and the **anterior tibialis,** in the front of the lower leg. Flexible fibrous cords of tissue called **tendons** (technically, extensions of the muscle) extend from the ends of these muscles and attach them to the tibia, fibula, calcaneus, tarsals, metatarsals, and other neighboring bones. A number of the tendons—most notably, the **Achilles tendon,** an extension of the gastrocnemius and soleus muscles, located at the back of the ankle—also serve a stabilizing function.

The ankle and foot mechanism is further reinforced by a range of **ligaments,** tough bands of fibrous tissue that bind together the various bone ends. Several major ligaments provide stability for the ankle, joining the lower tibia and lower fibula to the talus and calcaneus. These ligaments are joined by a range of others linking the various bones of the foot.

Other stabilizers in the ankle and foot include the **joint capsules,**

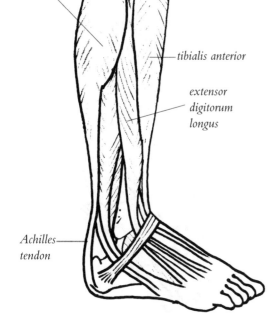

gastrocnemius (soleus invisible beneath)

tibialis anterior

extensor digitorum longus

Achilles tendon

Muscles of ankle and foot

fibrous and connective tissue material that surrounds the joints. In addition, a long, strong sheet of **plantar fascia** runs the length of the longitudinal arch. A **synovial membrane** in the joint capsules provides lubrication for the ankle/foot joints.

Several major **nerves**—most notably the **tibial nerve** and **common peroneal nerve**—run from the lower leg, crossing the ankle en route to the foot, then further subdividing. Each of these nerves allows us to contract specific muscles in the ankle and foot and to perceive sensations such as touch, temperature, and pain.

Four major **bursa sacs (bursae),** fluid-filled sacs of varying sizes within and around the ankle and foot, cushion the joints and minimize friction in the region. One is located at the back of the heel, another between the Achilles tendon and the bone, yet another between the Achilles tendon and the skin, and the fourth outside the metatarsal head of the big toe. A fifth, smaller bursa is also found outside the metatarsal head of the little toe. The heel and the ball of the foot are each also protected by a thick pad of fatty tissue.

The ankle and foot are the terminus of a kinetic chain that includes the pelvis, hip, upper leg, knee, and lower leg. All these different areas of the body are interrelated and depend on each other for correct functioning and movement.

What Can Go Wrong

The ankle and foot region is subject to constant stresses and hazards—from the effects of ill-fitting shoes and traumatic sports injuries to the degenerative changes that occur with the aging process. And because they may affect our posture and gait, abnormalities in feet can have repercussions for the knee, the hip, and even the lower back.

The intricate construction of the ankle and foot, the sensitive nerve endings in the toes, and our heavy dependence on the ankle and foot in our everyday lives tend to magnify the seriousness of any injury. And this is true not only with traumatic injuries. Even seemingly minor injuries or problems in the ankle and foot can have major implications.

For example, **inflammation** is far more serious in the ankle and foot than it is anywhere else in the body other than the wrist and hand. When inflammation occurs, fluids can become trapped in the compact ankle and foot area. If the inflammation is not addressed, these fluids may change from a soft substance into a fibrous, glue-like substance. At the least, recovery is delayed; at the worst, permanent dysfunction in the foot may result.

Some ankle and foot conditions, such as mild sprains and shin splints (see below), call for simple home treatments like rest and ice. Others demand more advanced physical therapy techniques: carefully and scientifically tailored exercises to strengthen the ankle and foot and improve range of motion; adjustments of the gait; mobilization; and perhaps approaches (modalities) like ultrasound and electrical stimulation as well. Still other problems require surgery or other major interventions, although these, too, are usually complemented with an exercise program designed by a physical therapist as part of the rehabilitation stage. In every instance, however, you should look to your physician or physical therapist to make a diagnosis and determine the treatment that is best for you.

Certainly the mildest ankle and foot dysfunction, if it can even be called that, is the tendency of the region's muscles—like muscles throughout the body—to become stiff or tight in response to heavy ankle and foot activity. The result of such **muscle tightness** is usually minor, short-term achiness and may be no cause for concern. (On the other hand, muscle tightness does diminish the ankle/foot unit's range of motion, which, unless the muscles are warmed up and stretched, puts the ankle and foot at risk of injury when called upon to push beyond that range.)

More worrisome is the accumulation of excess lactic acid and other chemicals in the ankle and foot muscles whenever they are subject to excessive or repetitive stress over prolonged periods of time—for example, when a person engages in heavy running or jumping (especially with an insufficient warmup period). The cellular and chemical responses to excessive stress almost inevitably lead to **muscle inflammation** and pain, which only increases if the stress is unrelieved.

The ankle and foot muscles may also suffer from tearing. This tearing may result from direct trauma, overuse (from engaging in sports or some other physical activity), or poor body mechanics (such as an improper gait). A **muscle strain,** sometimes inaccurately called a "pulled muscle," occurs when the muscle has been overstretched or overexerted and may have microscopic tearing as its cause. When the tearing is more severe, it is called, simply, a **muscle tear,** which may be partial or complete. The symptoms of strains and tears vary only in degree and may include pain, inflammation, bleeding into the surrounding tissues, and muscle spasm (see page 109).

Strains and tears can strike any of the region's muscles, but strains, at least, are more frequently seen in the muscles at the front of the ankle and up the shin. This disorder, called **shin splints,** is usually the result of running on hard surfaces, although inappropriate footwear and an improper gait may also be contributing factors.

Strains and tears often trigger **muscle spasm**—the sudden, intense contraction of muscle. Although very painful, a muscle spasm is the body's natural mechanism for protecting injured tissue by acting as a brace. Because it is a protective mechanism, muscle spasm is also present in many other ankle and foot disorders.

Injuries to the muscles have much in common, and are often associated, with injuries to their tendons. Like the muscles themselves, the tendons of the muscles become inflamed when subject to excessive stress or overuse, considerably impeding their normal gliding motions. This relatively familiar condition is known as **tendinitis.** While any activity that stretches the tendons beyond their usual range of motion can cause tendinitis, certainly the most common cause is engaging in running or similar vigorous activities without having first warmed up and stretched the tendons. Tendinitis may also strike those who "overdo" a physical activity after an extended period of being sedentary.

Because the tendons lack the same pain nerve endings as other structures, you might not feel any pain due to tendinitis until the surrounding synovial membrane of the joint or the adjacent bursa also becomes inflamed. Typical symptoms then include a deep generalized ache in the area, an increase in pain when using the ankle or foot, and localized tenderness in the area.

In the ankle tendinitis most frequently strikes the Achilles tendon. This condition, for obvious reasons called **Achilles tendinitis,** usually results in pain and swelling around the tendon and difficulty putting weight on the area.

In some rare cases a tendon may even **tear** or **rupture** altogether as a result of trauma, leading to sudden and intense pain. If the tendon in question is the Achilles tendon, pushing off or rising up on the toes of that foot will also be impossible. An Achilles tendon rupture is a medical emergency and will often require surgery to repair.

Not unlike the tendons, the ligaments of the ankle and foot can suffer microtrauma or be overstretched—that is, pushed beyond their normal limits—or even torn. This injury, a **sprain,** can range from the minor to the severe. A mild sprain will produce pain and swelling around the joint, a loss of motion, and possibly weakness in the muscles; in more severe cases there may also be a feeling of slippage in the joints involved.

The most common sort of ankle sprain is an **inversion sprain,** in which

Calluses and Corns

A callus is a thickening of the skin where it rubs against your shoe or against another part of the foot. A corn is a small callus located between the toes, on the side of the feet, or on the top of the toes. Calluses and corns represent the skin's effort to protect itself from friction by adding extra layers and becoming tougher. They grow over time, actually increasing the friction in the area and often becoming inflamed and extremely painful. The bone beneath a callus, especially on the bottom of the foot, may even come to exert pressure on nerves, with painful consequences.

Calluses and corns are common symptoms of the range of disorders involving minor deformities of the foot or improper gait. They may also arise independently, as a result of wearing ill-fitting shoes.

Resist the temptation to perform "bathroom surgery" on your calluses and corns; don't use chemicals and don't try to cut or trim them. It's a good idea to have calluses and corns checked by a podiatrist. For temporary relief, you may try soaking your feet in warm water and (for corns) separating the toes with cotton or a foam rubber or gel protector or using self-adhesive pads to minimize friction.

But you will still need to address the cause of the problem. Simply switching to better-fitting shoes might be solution enough. (See Chapter 14—Footwear.) If the friction or any other symptoms remain after a few days, you should consult your physical therapist or podiatrist.

the ligaments on the outside of the ankle are overstretched. This is caused by a sudden turning over onto the outside of the ankle, the result of stumbling into a hole, landing awkwardly on the foot during sports activities, taking a bad fall, or similar mishaps. Inversion sprains are particularly dangerous because they can damage muscles, blood vessels, and even nerves in addition to ligaments. They should be examined by a physician to rule out fracture (see page 112).

In people whose gait leads them to roll the foot too far inward (over-pronate) while walking or running, the plantar fascia may be subject to repetitive stress—with unpleasant consequences. Under the arch of the foot near the heel, the fascia may become inflamed or suffer microscopic tearing (strain); a bony growth (or heel spur) may appear on the bottom of the heel at the point where the fascia connects to and pulls on the calcaneus. Over time, the fascia may even tear away from the heel bone. This condition, **plantar fasciitis,** generally leads to intermittent pain on the inner side of the heel; perhaps its most common symptom is severe pain upon taking the first step out of bed in the morning. Athletes, especially runners, who over-pronate (roll the feet excessively inward) are at greatest risk of developing plantar fasciitis. This also tends to afflict people with flat feet (see page 114).

The joints of the ankle and foot are also subject to the degenerative changes associated with **arthritis,** which can lead to both pain and stiffness. This condition can be the result of early trauma to the joints, but there is a wide range of possible causes. The most widespread form of arthritis in the ankle and foot joints is **osteoarthritis,** the degeneration of the articular cartilage and a wearing down of the joint surfaces. In some cases osteoarthritis may result in the buildup of roughened cartilage or spurs (deposits of bony tissue) on the joint surfaces and the appearance of loose bodies (floating bits of cartilage and bone) within the joint.

Osteoarthritis has a number of possible causes, including trauma, overuse, and inactivity. But by far the most common is simple degeneration of the joints due to age, typical (though not inevitable) among middle-aged individuals. Although it sometimes has no symptoms at all, osteoarthritis may well lead to pain (from mild to severe) and stiffness and decreased movement in the ankle and foot.

In some instances osteoarthritis may even lead to **hallux rigidus,** in which the joint at the base of the big toe loses its movement. Pushing off from the toe becomes painful; this, in turn, may alter the way you put your weight on other parts of the foot, enhancing their risk of injury.

A rarer but more serious form of arthritis from which the ankle and foot may suffer is **rheumatoid arthritis,** an inflammatory disease whose origin is not fully understood (but which may be the result of autoimmune mechanisms or viral infections). The disorder is characterized by pain, stiffness, swelling, and warmth in the joints of the ankle and foot. Physical therapy is necessary to help maintain mobility and flexibility in the region once rheumatoid arthritis has set in.

The big toe in particular is susceptible to yet another form of arthritis called **gout.** Characterized by pain, swelling, and warmth in the MTP joint, gout is triggered by deposits of the salts of uric acid in the surrounding tissues, the result of an increase in uric acid in the blood. Physicians often prescribe medications and dietary changes to manage acute attacks of this ailment.

The nerves that run through the ankle and into the foot are vulnerable to injury. One such injury involves the compression of one branch of the tibial nerve (namely, the posterior tibial nerve), a condition caused by the ligaments in the ankle becoming thickened with scar tissue. This condition, known as **tarsal tunnel syndrome** (named after the narrow channel through which the nerve passes), can be triggered by trauma to the ankle or foot. But it is more commonly the result of repetitive motion and overuse, such as running or prolonged periods of standing; wearing shoes that allow the foot to overpronate only increases the likelihood of this sort of injury. People with flat feet (see page 114) are also more likely to experience tarsal tunnel syndrome. The symptoms of this disorder are burning, cramping, and tingling sensations in the ankle or foot, which can occur at any time, but are usually worse at night.

Compression or entrapment of a nerve at the heel may lead to **"jogger's foot"**: a burning sensation in the heel and sometimes a lack of feeling in the sole of the foot near the big toe. Jogger's foot—an injury associated, appropriately enough, with running—is usually caused by trauma to the heel pad when landing on the foot or by insufficiently protective shoes. The resulting inflammation of the area leads to compression of the medial plantar nerve, which branches off the tibial nerve.

Smaller nerves in the foot may be pinched between the heads of adjacent metatarsal bones, leading to inflammation, sharp pain, and numbness in the ball of the foot—and, in some instances, in the two toes of the affected metatarsals as well. This condition is known as **Morton's neuroma** or interdigital neuroma. Although it seems to run in families, the precise cause of the nerve compression is frequently difficult to pinpoint in any particular case. Wearing high heels or other tight, pointy shoes; overpronation;

osteoarthritis (see page 110); rheumatoid arthritis (see page 111); bunions (see page 113); and diabetes are a few of the many possible suspects.

The general term to describe pain and tenderness in the foot resulting from irritation of or pressure on nerve roots in the region is **metatarsalgia.** Metatarsalgia is often a symptom of other foot problems, but it is a genuine dysfunction in its own right. Metatarsalgia is often accompanied by corns and calluses resulting from changes in your gait. Women are more prone to developing metatarsalgia than men, largely because of high-heeled shoes.

Footdrop, a condition in which the foot cannot be actively pulled up toward the shin, is yet another disorder related to the nerves—frequently to one of the branches of the common peroneal nerve. It has a number of causes, ranging from diabetes, which can lead to significant nerve damage in the lower extremities, to a herniated disk in the spine, which can have implications all the way down the leg. Damage to muscles in the front of the lower leg may also be characterized by footdrop.

The bursae around the heel and at the base of the big and little toes are subject to **bursitis,** an inflammation brought on by trauma or overuse. One of the most common causes is the constant pressure of ill-fitting shoes. Pain, the primary symptom of bursitis, is usually constant and site specific. But bursitis can become a chronic disorder in which the bursa sacs thicken and reduce free movement around the joint, thus limiting the ankle/foot unit's range of motion. Inflammation of the bursae is also a component of bunions and bunionettes (see page 113).

Like all bones, those in the ankle are subject to **fractures** and **dislocations** as a result of trauma, particulary awkward falls and severe twists during sports activities. One of the more common such injuries, a **Pott's fracture,** involves fractures at the base of the fibula and tibia (and damage to the ligaments as well). Although technically it is the lower leg that is broken, this may be referred to as a "broken ankle." Ankle fractures and dislocations almost always cause swelling and pain, especially when a person tries to move the ankle.

Fractures in the foot occur most often when it is crushed with a heavy object or stepped on. (The toes are especially vulnerable to this sort of injury.) A fracture to the heel bone, or **calcaneal fracture,** can also occur, as a result of landing on your feet after jumping or falling from a height. And the toes may become dislocated at one or more of the joints, usually the result of violent impact during sports activities.

The intense, ongoing pressure put on the bones of the feet by such activities as ballet dancing, marathon running, and long-distance hiking may result

fracture

Pott's fracture

in **stress fractures.** These injuries, which are sometimes only hairline cracks in the bone, often go undetected, even when x-rays are taken. The pain caused by stress fractures is often quite minimal, although nagging, and will subside with proper rest and treatment.

Because of the risk of swelling, all fractures to the ankle or foot should be treated as medical emergencies.

A variety of foot problems is associated with the minor bone deformities known as **bunion** (or **hallux valgus**) in the big toe and **bunionette** in the little toe. A bunion is a condition—inherited or acquired through over-stressing the joint during such activities as ballet dancing—in which the metatarsal bone at the base of the big toe bulges outward and the phalanges of the toe itself point inward; a bunionette is a similar misalignment of the little toe. In both cases the deformity causes stretching of the muscles, ligaments, and joint capsule of the affected toe; the bursa that covers the joint becomes inflamed and thickens. Once one of these misalignments makes its appearance, often triggered by tight shoes, it grows progressively worse, particularly as the metatarsal head strains against the side of the shoe. Bunions and, to a lesser degree, bunionettes can be quite painful. And if they lead to compensatory distortions of your posture or gait, they may have repercussions along the entire kinetic chain. Surgical removal of the bunion or bunionnette and realignment of the bones may be required.

Similar, if less severe, pains are associated with such other minor deformities as **mallet toe,** in which the end joint of a toe curls under, and **hammer toe,** in which the middle joint curls under. (A toe featuring both deformities has the distinctive name of **claw toe.**) Mallet toe and hammer toe (and claw toe) may be congenital but are more likely to be the result of an improper gait, ill-fitting shoes, or crowding caused by a hallux valgus (see above). Their most unpleasant symptom is the consequent development of corns or calluses on top of or on the tip of the toe. These disorders, too, can have adverse effects on your posture or gait. Although corrective surgery may occasionally be required to address these conditions, often an orthotic device—a buildup inside the shoe—is enough to reposition the toe and relieve pain or pressure in the area.

Women suffer disproportionately from such foot ailments, largely because of shoes that sacrifice fit to fashion. High heels and pointed-toe shoes are responsible for countless cases of bunions, bunionettes, mallet toes, hammer toes, claw toes, and other disorders. Men, too, suffer foot problems from pointed cowboy boots and tight, nonsupportive loafers.

Feet whose natural bone structure makes for unusually low arches

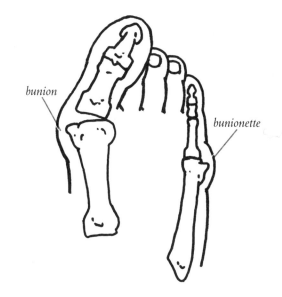

bunion

bunionette

Bunion and bunionette

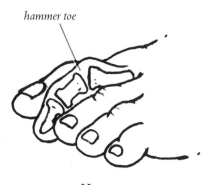

hammer toe

Hammer toe

are known as **flat feet** (or pancake feet). There are many degrees of flat feet, and they are rarely a problem in themselves. Flat feet may, however, contribute to more serious conditions, including plantar fasciitis (see page 110) and tarsal tunnel syndrome (see page 111). An orthotic device may be necessary to prevent strain on the foot.

Another congenital disruption of the foot's bone structure is **Morton's syndrome,** a condition in which an excessively short first metatarsal bone results in the second metatarsal being forced to bear excessive weight. This puts considerable stress on the ligaments, muscles, and joint capsule at the base of the second metatarsal, with consequent metatarsalgia (see page 112).

Taking Care of Your Ankle and Foot

As with many other parts of the body, **proper posture** while standing is an important factor in maintaining a healthy foot. By preserving the straight vertical alignment of the body, proper posture provides an even distribution of weight on the base of the foot. As a rule, activities that disrupt good standing posture for an extended period, or that do so repeatedly, should be avoided. (This admonition should not, however, interfere with normal vigorous activities such as sports, which are, in fact, much encouraged.)

Although to some people, proper posture seems to come almost naturally, for most of us it takes cultivation (and sometimes even professional guidance). For detailed information on recognizing and developing proper posture, see **Chapter 10—Posture.**

Another important factor in ankle and foot maintenance is a **proper gait.** The term "gait" refers to your particular manner of walking or running, and a proper gait is a manner of walking or running that displays symmetry, rhythm, and even leg and foot alignment. And while there is no one proper gait, gaits that do not meet these criteria may increase stress on the ankle and foot and on other parts of the body (like the hip and knee) as well. This is particularly true for serious athletes and anyone else who does a lot of running.

Like proper posture, a proper gait comes naturally to many people, while others may need to cultivate it. In some instances a proper gait is not even attainable without the right tools, like corrective footwear. For more information on identifying and developing a proper gait, see **Chapter 11—Gait.**

Yet another essential ingredient in maintaining a healthy ankle and foot is **proper body mechanics** in the various activities of daily life. With regard to the ankle and foot, proper body mechanics means using the body and the different parts of the body in ways that are consistent with the smooth functioning of the region's joints, muscles, tendons, and ligaments. Among other things, this means not standing on the feet or walking or running (especially on uneven surfaces) for prolonged periods. Like proper posture and proper gait, proper body mechanics can significantly reduce the risk of many ankle and foot problems.

Proper body mechanics are by no means always self-evident; sometimes they are even counterintuitive. They need to be learned and consciously adopted. For detailed information on identifying and developing proper body mechanics, see **Chapter 12—Body Mechanics**.

Although posture, gait, and body mechanics represent slightly different ways of thinking about the body, they are closely related phenomena. Indeed, proper posture and a proper gait are practically prerequisites of proper body mechanics, because in their absence, you are always undermining the smooth functioning of your joints, muscles, tendons, and ligaments. In fact, some of the poor biomechanical habits most harmful to the ankle and foot are poor postural and gait habits.

Weight control is a factor that's easily overlooked when it comes to keeping your ankle and foot healthy. But, in fact, excess weight can significantly magnify the stress on the joints. To avoid this burden on your ankle and foot, it's important to remain within your appropriate weight range. (Your weight also has implications for other parts of your body, including your back, hips, and knees.) For more information, see **Chapter 13—Body Weight.**

Many ankle and foot problems may be prevented simply by choosing **appropriate footwear.** Everyday shoes that fit properly and maintain the foot's natural shape and balance may ward off bunions, various deformities of the toes, and some seemingly cosmetic ills (like calluses and corns) that can put pressure on the nerves. When you run or engage in sports, shoes that provide support and shock absorption can help ward off repetitive-motion injuries. High heels and narrow toes should be avoided as much as possible. For more information, see **Chapter 14—Footwear.**

Keeping your ankle and foot healthy also calls for **strength** in the muscles that help to keep the ankle and foot stable, moving, and well aligned—including those in the lower leg and in the foot itself. The less developed your muscle strength, the narrower the range of physical activities you are capable of performing—or capable of performing without putting stress on your ankle and foot. As a result, many common practices of everyday life, such as standing up on your toes or jumping in the air, become riskier than they should be. Furthermore, a certain amount of strength is necessary

Ankle and Foot Inactivity

In one form or another, excessive stress on the ankle/foot unit is certainly the most familiar cause of injury to the muscles and joints. Another cause, however, is only slightly less threatening: simple inactivity. Failure regularly to use the muscles of the ankle and foot and to bring the joints to the limits of their range of motion through moderately vigorous activity makes the region particularly susceptible to sudden overuse, an improper gait, and other kinds of stress. The joints stiffen; ligaments and muscles may contract; good blood flow is inhibited. Even more noteworthy, inactivity may make the ankle and foot more susceptible to general joint degeneration.

The effects of inactivity tend to be magnified with age. And it is inactivity, more than aging itself, that leads to the conditions generally associated with growing older, like osteoarthritis. Regular exercise—walking, swimming, or golf, for example—may well keep these problems at bay.

simply to hold the body upright and keep it moving. A balance of strength in the muscles of the lower leg and foot is important too so that one area need not compensate for weakness in another.

Endurance in the muscles that support the ankle and foot is also essential. Endurance is the ability of the muscles to contract (that is, be in use) over time. The less developed a muscle's endurance, the shorter the amount of time it can be called upon to contract before it tires—forcing other, often more vulnerable parts of the body to do its job and putting itself and those other parts at risk of injury. Because practically any upright activity calls upon the muscles in the ankle and foot region to contract over extended periods, a certain level of endurance is absolutely vital. And this is even more true for anyone involved in an activity that requires a great deal of running or similar movement.

Flexibility in the muscles, tendons, and ligaments is just as critical as muscle endurance and strength. The less flexible your muscles, the more susceptible they are to the natural (and often painful) tightening that comes from everyday activities. And the more susceptible they are to injury when called upon to perform many common practices—like walking on uneven terrain. As with endurance and strength, this flexibility must be distributed among all the muscles that support the ankle and foot.

Appropriate endurance, strength, and flexibility for your ankle and foot (and other parts of your body) may be achieved through a regular program of exercise. For more information, see **Chapter 15—Strength, Endurance, and Flexibility**.

Although all parts of the body are at greater risk of injury when you are engaged in **sports** or similar vigorous activities, the structure and function of the ankle and foot make them especially so, even for those who generally have good endurance, strength, and flexibility in the muscles. Sudden strain on the ankle and foot and repetitive stress on the joints—common occurrences in many sports and other activities, from soccer to running to skating—make the ankle and foot vulnerable to tendinitis and other minor and major problems. While the risks tend to increase the older you are and the more intense your workout is, it is nevertheless a good idea for anyone to fully prepare the ankle and foot for such a workout: warm up through gentle aerobic activity (such as walking for 5 or 10 minutes), and then stretch the ankle and foot muscles.

It should be noted that sports-related repetitive-motion injuries to the ankle and foot—generally, those associated with running—may often be prevented by taking care to use proper form. If you are a serious runner, you may want to consider having a physical therapist perform a gait analysis, a detailed study of your particular gait. This may help pinpoint idiosyncracies in your form that could represent poor body mechanics; your physical therapist may then be able to suggest biomechanical adjustments or corrective footwear to improve your gait before problems arise.

With or without a gait analysis, you should make sure you have comfortable, good-quality, supportive shoes that absorb shock and don't constrict the bones and joints of the foot. Air-soled sneakers and cushioned or gel inserts in your shoes may also help alleviate some of the impact of the ankle and foot joint during physical activity. The wrong shoes can increase the stresses to the ankle and foot associated with sports and magnify any preexisting biomechanical or anatomical defects.

Still, common sense is the best line of defense against injury. If you don't usually run or play sports, it's important not to push yourself too much when you do. And if you do experience any pain in the ankle and foot, stop what you're doing at once. To try to "run through it" is to risk seriously injuring yourself.

Sports in particular make the ankle and foot susceptible to traumatic injuries from falls, twists, and collisions. You can protect your ankle to some degree by wearing ankle supports or high-top sneakers.

For more information on protecting your ankle and foot and other parts of your body from injury during particular sports and activities, see **Chapter 16—Sports**.

Like sports, many lines of **work** carry considerable risks of ankle and foot injury due to strain or overuse. Assembly-line workers, teachers, textile workers, salespersons, trial lawyers, nurses, food servers, and others who are on their feet for prolonged periods should wear proper footwear. If you hold an occupation of this sort—even if your muscle endurance, conditioning, strength, and flexibility are good—it is a wise precaution first to warm up and then stretch the ankle and foot muscles before beginning your workday.

It's also important as much as possible to configure your physical work environment so that it does not force you to use poor body mechanics or otherwise stress the ankles or feet. If you work at a counter or on an assembly line, for example, a padded floor mat can take some pressure off your feet. And for those who work at a desk or a computer station, a foot rest can have a similar effect.

Finally, if your occupation does place your ankle and foot under continual or repetitive stress, try to take a break of at least several minutes every

Quick-Relief Ankle and Foot Stretches

The stretches below may ease (and sometimes even head off) common ankle and foot tightness and stiffness, especially tightness and stiffness brought on by repetitive stress. Feel free to do them as often as you wish. Detailed instructions and appropriate illustrations can be found in Chapter 19—Flexibility Exercises. (These exercises can also help with muscle spasm.) Remember to stretch the foot slowly at first because the foot muscles are often ones that we do not stretch out and may therefore feel a little stiff. If your ankle and foot tightness and stiffness produce more than minor discomfort, consult your physical therapist before attempting these exercises. Be sure to warm up your muscles before you begin by, for instance, getting up and walking around your office.

- Runner's Stretch (p. 274)
- Calf Stretch with Flexed Knee (p. 275)
- Lower Leg Lengthener (p. 277)
- Toe Flexor (p. 279)
- Toe Extension and Spread (p. 279)

hour, and if you feel any tightness or stiffness *at all*, stretch and flex the ankle and foot muscles a bit (see below). In fact, to head off problems, you may want to try this routine even if you don't have tightness or stiffness.

For more information on protecting your ankle and foot and other parts of your body from injury during workplace activities, see **Chapter 17—Work**.

When Problems Occur

No matter how well you treat your ankle and foot, **occasional temporary tightness and stiffness** may occur, especially as you grow older. After all, everyday life can be punishing on the ankle and foot; they take more than their share of stress as they move us around, often confined to tight, ill-fitting shoes. One way to ease your discomfort is with a few focused **stretching exercises,** which will bring back some badly needed flexibility and blood flow to your tired or aching muscles. (See the box, **"Quick-Relief Ankle and Foot Stretches,"** at left.)

Simply **shaking out** the ankles and feet can also work nicely. Even better for the foot is a basic **massage.** To do this yourself, sit on the floor with legs outstretched and knees soft; bend one foot toward you, and gently massage the entire bottom of your foot using circular movements of your thumbs. **Soaking** the feet in warm water for 15 to 20 minutes may also provide some relief.

Sometimes a bout of ankle or foot stiffness or soreness can be traced directly to a particular instance of poor body mechanics. This is often the explanation for pain that occurs during a specific activity—standing on an uneven surface, for example. If this is the case, double-check your body mechanics; you might find that a simple adjustment will quickly eliminate the problem. Pain in the foot, especially at points where it makes contact with your shoe, may be resolved simply by switching to more comfortable, supportive footwear.

If your ankle or foot discomfort, however mild, persists for more than a few days, it's a good idea to have your ankle and foot checked by a physical therapist, primary-care physician, or podiatrist.

Beyond temporary soreness and stiffness, it is possible that you will experience **more serious ankle and foot problems** of one sort or another at some point in your life, even if you have a generally healthy ankle and foot. The normal wear and tear of everyday living can stress the joints. Age, too, takes its toll, and with it comes the possibility of osteoarthritis and other dysfunctions. (In addition, problems such as bunions tend only to get worse with time.) Falls and accidents may bring strains, sprains, or even fractures.

Anyway, few of us can claim perfect ankle and foot maintenance, which makes us especially vulnerable to a whole range of ankle and foot problems.

Because ankle and foot problems can have major repercussions for the use of your feet, it's necessary to see a physical therapist, primary care physician, or podiatrist at the first sign of trouble. This is an obvious course of action in the case of a traumatic event, such as a ruptured Achilles tendon. In these cases you should seek **immediate professional attention.** In such urgent situations it's also a good idea to know some basics of **first aid.** (See **Appendix A—First Aid Basics.**)

Even if it's not the result of a traumatic event, any case of severe ankle or foot pain—or any swelling of the ankle or foot—requires immediate professional attention (and, if appropriate, first aid).

Milder degrees of ankle and foot pain, if recurring or persisting for more than a few days, also should be evaluated by a physical therapist or physician. In the meantime, minor ankle and foot pain can be managed by heeding a few simple tips. **Rest** can provide some relief by giving the tissue some time to heal and regenerate; keep the weight off the foot, and avoid running, stair climbing, and excessive walking.

For the first day or two after the appearance of minor ankle or foot pain, you may apply **ice** to the affected area. The ice numbs the pain temporarily and may prevent swelling. One good method for applying ice is to put crushed ice in a sealable plastic bag with a little water, then cover the bag with towels. (A bag of frozen peas or corn works well too; refrigerated towels may be used in a pinch.) To avoid harming the skin or underlying tissues, apply the ice for 15 to 20 minutes at a time, with 20 to 40 minutes between applications.

After a period of using ice, you may try **moist heat,** applied to the ankle or foot in a 20-minutes-on/20-minutes-off cycle. Moist heat tends to relax tense muscles, offering some relief from pain and stiffness. Warm showers or warm, moist towels work well for this. Heating pads, although not highly recommended, are also acceptable, but take care that the heat is not too intense.

For some people **nonsteroidal anti-inflammatory drugs (NSAIDs)** can be effective in easing ankle and foot pain. This class of drugs includes aspirin and ibuprofen, both of which are widely available without prescription. Like all drugs, however, NSAIDs have potentially dangerous side effects. Ask your doctor or pharmacist before taking NSAIDs, and follow the directions on the label.

When addressing a particular ankle or foot problem, your physical therapist has a wide range of techniques to draw upon. But—depending on the physical therapist's examination and evaluation—an ankle/foot rehabilitation program will almost certainly incorporate strength, endurance, and flexibility exercises. In addition, your ankle/foot rehabilitation program may include attention to improved body mechanics and gait. Your physical therapist may also recommend corrective footwear.

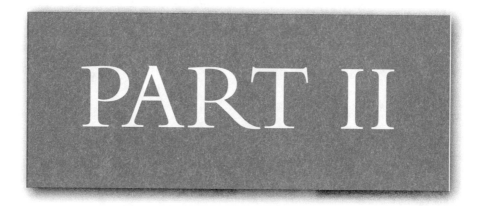

PART II

CHAPTER TEN

Posture

Although for some people the word "posture" conjures up images of being pestered by parents and grandparents to "stand up straight!" the term actually has a much broader meaning. Posture refers generally to *the position of your body in space*—not only when standing up but also when walking, running, sitting, squatting, kneeling, or lying down. Posture is not a fixed phenomenon. In the course of performing a single activity, like playing tennis or preparing a meal, your posture may change dozens of times.

Posture has significant implications for the general health and well-being of much of the body. This is because, by and large, it determines the amount and distribution of stress on the body's various bones, muscles, tendons, ligaments, and disks. "Proper posture" keeps the total stress to a minimum and distributes the stress to those structures most capable of bearing it. "Poor posture" has the opposite effect, increasing the total stress and distributing it to those structures less able to bear it.

All varieties of proper posture are characterized, first and foremost, by one essential feature: a properly aligned spine. A properly aligned spine runs straight down the center of the body, from the back of your head to your tailbone. From the side it displays three natural curves, with the neck at the top forming a gentle "C" curve, the upper back a gentle backward "C" curve, and the lower back another gentle "C" curve. Generally speaking, any posture that fails to maintain this position is poor posture.

The back, and the lower back in particular, is especially sensitive to proper or poor posture. Poor posture of practically any sort puts the back and neck at risk of strains and other disorders. Some varieties of poor posture may also displace the scapula and interfere with the free movement of the shoulder joint. When standing or squatting, poor posture may distribute excess body weight to vulnerable parts of the feet. Poor posture may even affect your gait—that is, your particular way of walking or running—increasing the stress on your hips, knees, ankles, and feet. (See **Chapter 11— Gait** for further information.) Poor posture is almost certain to lead to short-term pain in one or more of these areas, especially the low back; it is also likely to exacerbate any existing problems. Continuous or repeated poor

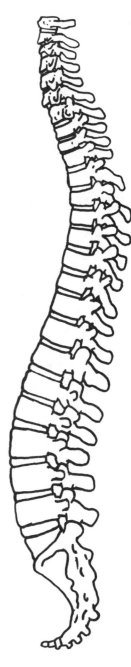

Properly aligned spine
(side view)

posture is a recipe for chronic pain and serious long-term damage.

For your body's sake, then, it is essential to practice proper posture as much as possible in all activities of daily life. This means not only when standing, sitting, or lying around but also when lifting objects, working at a computer, or washing dishes. (See **Chapter 12—Body Mechanics** for more information on the best way to perform many everyday activities.) It does not mean, however, avoiding sports and other vigorous activities that do, in the heat of the action, occasionally disrupt proper posture. Indeed, within limits, such movement is actually beneficial to the body, and as a rule, fitness and sports activities are highly recommended. Still, sports and other activities that disrupt proper posture repeatedly or for long periods should be avoided. (See **Chapter 16—Sports.**)

Proper posture comes naturally to few people. In fact, for some, including those with spinal deformities (like scoliosis), it may be difficult or even impossible to attain proper posture at all. Others may need corrective equipment—including specialized shoes, supports, chairs, or mattresses—to do so. For most people, however, it is simply a matter of careful cultivation.

Cultivating proper posture does take some doing and may even require the assistance of a physical therapist. The minimal requirements of proper posture are a reasonable degree of strength and endurance in the body's muscles and flexibility in the body's muscles, tendons, and ligaments—especially those of the back. This ensures that a properly aligned spine can be held in place over the course of a day; it also allows the neck to support the weight of the head without slumping or slouching. (See **Chapter 15—Strength, Endurance, and Flexbility** for a good program for enhancing these qualities.) Proper posture also requires that you keep your body weight within an appropriate range for your height and build to diminish any forces that would pull the spine out of place. (See **Chapter 13—Body Weight.**) But above all, it requires a clear awareness of what proper posture is and a conscious attention to practicing it. Below is a more thorough presentation of how to recognize and attain proper posture in the three most common positions: standing, sitting, and lying down.

Standing Posture

When you are standing, proper posture is the straight vertical alignment of your body from the top of your head through your body's center to the bottom of your feet. Viewed from the front and back of your body, this alignment represents a straight line that divides the body in half from the face down the middle of the breast bone to between the knees and feet.

Posture Practice 1

The exercise below is a demonstration of correct standing posture. To improve your posture, try practicing it two or three times a day.

1. Stand with your back against a wall. Place your heels about 6 inches from the wall and about 6 inches apart from each other. Keep your weight evenly distributed. Arms are relaxed at your sides. Keep your ankles straight, your feet pointed straight ahead, and your kneecaps facing front.

2. Bring your head back to touch the wall. Tuck your chin as if a string were attached to the middle of the back of your head; pretend the string is being pulled up. Pull up and in with the muscles in the lower abdomen, trying to flatten the stomach and bringing your lower back closer to the wall. Gently straighten your upper back by lifting your chest and bringing your shoulders back and down against the wall.

3. Hold this position for 10 seconds, breathing normally. Relax and repeat three or four times.

Viewed from the side, this alignment displays a straight line from the ear lobe to the shoulder to points just behind the hip joint and in front of the knee and ankle joints.

To maintain the spine's neutral position, the head should be held erect with the chin gently pulled back—as if you were pushing the very top of your head up to the ceiling. Some people find it helpful to imagine that there's a string attached to the top of their head, pulling them straight up. Proper alignment of the spine, however, is not even possible without proper alignment of the hips, knees, ankles, and feet, which needs to be achieved as well. (This is covered more fully in **Chapter 11—Gait.**)

A slouched or slumped-forward position increases the stress on vertebral disks. But the ramrod-straight "military" posture—with the lower back forward, shoulder blades winged backward, head pushed back—is no better; it demands excessive muscle activity along the spine. Both of these postures may lead to low back and neck pain and sometimes further problems as well.

Because your standing posture can also be influenced by the shoes you wear, choosing the right shoes is essential. High-heeled shoes, to take the most dramatic example, force the body into a forward position and thrust your lower back forward and your upper back backward just to maintain balance. The result is increased stress on the low back and, more likely than not, pain. (See **Chapter 14—Footwear.**)

Sitting Posture

Much of the standing posture principles apply to sitting as well: sit in a manner that allows you to maintain the gentle curves of your back, and hold your head erect with the chin gently pulled back. Slumping—characterized by an exaggerated thoracic curve and a drooping head—is particularly discouraged. Surprising though it may seem, sitting is actually more stressful on the lower back than standing; slumping magnifies this stress many times over.

Your choice of seat can make a big difference in promoting proper posture. A firm-backed chair is always the best option, especially when you are sitting for long periods. Sit back far enough so that your lower spine makes contact with the back of the chair. (If this is difficult or uncomfortable, you're probably sitting in the wrong chair.) A lumbar cushion or pillow can often transform an insufficiently supportive chair into an acceptable one; just make sure the cushion doesn't force your lower back into an exaggerated arching position. An inflatable lumbar support—a great idea for

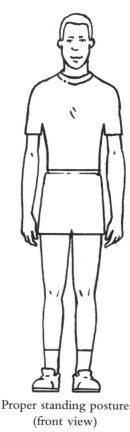

Proper standing posture
(front view)

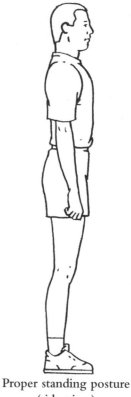

Proper standing posture
(side view)

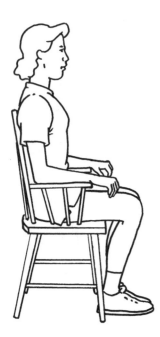

Proper sitting posture

Posture Practice 2

This is a demonstration of correct sitting posture. To improve your posture, try practicing it two or three times a day.

1. Sit in a supportive straight-back chair, with both feet flat on the floor and your back resting against the chair. Arms are relaxed with hands on your lap or on armrests. Hold your head erect. Tuck your chin in as if a string were attached to the middle of the back of the head; pretend the string is being pulled up.

2. Pull up and in with the muscles in the lower abdomen, trying to flatten the stomach. Gently straighten the upper back, lifting the chest. Bring shoulders back and down against the chair.

3. Hold this position for 10 seconds, breathing normally and keeping the rest of the body relaxed. Relax and repeat three or four times.

people with chronic low back pain—can be taken just about anywhere.

Armrests promote proper posture by providing some support for the neck and shoulders. The height of the seat should allow for the feet to be flat on the floor and the knees to be just about hip level. Backless seats are not recommended.

A wide range of chairs, especially office chairs, is now on the market designed with the features necessary to promote proper posture. The better among them are also adjustable in seat height and angle of seat back. But the market has a variety of more gimmicky, "ergonomic" offerings as well, such as chairs that you kneel into and perch on. While these products do seem to help some people, in many cases they may not provide the support the back needs for prolonged sitting.

When sitting on a seat, place your feet flat on the floor directly in front of you—or, if it's more comfortable, on a footrest.

Sitting on a flat surface, like a floor or lawn or bed, is discouraged because it tends to cause the spine to slump. If you do sit on a flat surface, however, try to have your back well supported (against a wall, for example) and keep the knees bent with a pillow or other soft support set beneath them. Sitting cross-legged with the back supported is also fine.

Lying-Down Posture

Maintaining the neutral position of the spine while lying down, whether for sleeping or simply for resting, requires not just the adoption of an appropriate position but the proper choice of surface and proper use of head support as well. As with standing and sitting, the goal is to keep your spine in the neutral position—but horizontally.

This is nearly impossible to achieve without a reasonably firm surface to lie on. A surface that's too soft—whether it's a mattress, couch, or water bed—allows your body to sink down in the middle, no matter what position you lie down in. This is a major cause of muscle soreness and joint stiffness, among other problems. A firm mattress, futon, or bedroll provides more support for the spine; water beds are also fine, as long as they are filled up enough to provide a firm surface. If you're stuck with a too-soft mattress, try placing a ½- to ¾-inch sheet of plywood between the mattress and the box spring, or place the plywood on top of the mattress with a sheet of "egg crate" foam on top of the board. The floor also provides plenty of support—although it may be a bit difficult to sleep on; a camping pad or 2-inch foam mattress may make it more comfortable.

The right pillow is important, no matter what your sleeping surface. It shouldn't put your head at an angle—that is, hold it too high or too low—which puts enormous strain on your neck. Don't "overpillow" your head. And remember that pillows don't last forever; replace them when they no longer support your head properly. Your best bet is a specially designed contoured pillow that supports the natural curve of your neck. It should be neither too firm nor too rigid.

Of the three common lying-down positions—on your side, on your back, and face down—lying on your side is most recommended. This should be done with the knees bent toward the chest and a large, firm pillow placed between the legs. This position is especially preferable if the sleeping surface is soft.

If you find it more comfortable to lie on your back, you should set one or two pillows under your knees (although this is not recommended if you have arthritis of the knees). Your hands can be placed on your lower stomach to help relax the upper back and shoulders. On a soft mattress, however, lying on your back means effectively being in a slouch—for a full one-third of the day if you sleep this way.

Lying on your stomach is not a good idea, regardless of the surface. It tends to arch the lumbar spine and usually pushes the neck to the limit of its range of motion on one side. It's almost certain to cause back and neck strain, even for brief periods (like lying on the beach), but especially if you sleep this way all night. If you're a habitual stomach sleeper, try lying on your back or side and placing long pillows to either side to prevent you from rolling over during the night. If that fails, place a firm pillow under your stomach and hips to decrease the arch of your back.

Posture Practice 3

One of the best ways to improve your posture, whether standing or sitting, is also one of the most old-fashioned. Simply balance a small pillow on the top of your head and go about your routine activities—walking, working at a desk, doing the dishes—for several minutes. (It helps if the pillow has tweedy or nubby texture to keep it from falling off too easily.) The results are instantaneous: from the moment you begin, you do have proper posture. And if you repeat the exercise at least once a day over a period of weeks, proper posture will likely become an automatic part of your daily life.

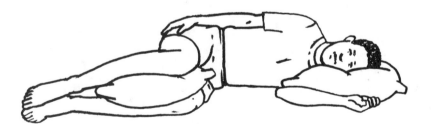

Proper lying-down posture—on side

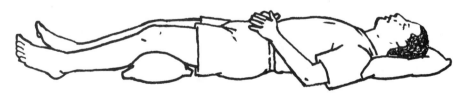

Proper lying-down posture—on back

Checking Your Posture

The best way to check your posture is to get a postural examination from a physical therapist. You can, however, make a preliminary check of your typical standing posture, which may allow you to determine if a professional examination and evaluation are necessary. To do this thoroughly, you'll need a full-length mirror, a wall, a Polaroid camera, and a little help from a friend.

1. Standing directly in front of a full-length mirror, use the following checklists to evaluate your posture:

PROPER POSTURE

- Head is held straight, eyes level.
- Shoulders are level.
- Spaces between your arms and body are equal.
- Hips are level.
- Kneecaps face straight ahead.
- Ankles and feet are straight.

POOR POSTURE

- Head tilts to one side or forward.
- One shoulder is lower than the other.
- Spaces between your arms and body are unequal.
- One hip is higher than the other.
- Either or both of your knees turn in or out.
- Ankles and feet roll in (pronate), so that your weight is on the inner borders of your feet.

If your posture displays any of the warning signs, your spine may not be properly aligned down the middle of the body.

2. Stand with your back to a wall, your heels about 6 inches from the wall. Place one hand behind your neck, with the back of that hand against the wall. Place the other hand behind your lower back, with the palm against the wall. If there's enough space between your body and the wall to move your hands forward and back more than 1 inch, the curves of your spine are probably not in proper alignment.

3. Have a friend take a full-length Polaroid photograph of you from a side view. Use the following checklists to evaluate your posture:

PROPER POSTURE

- Head is held erect.
- Chin is parallel to the floor.
- Shoulder is directly below your ear.
- Chest is held moderately elevated and the upper back erect.
- Abdomen is flat.
- Lower back has a slight forward curve.
- Knees are straight.

POOR POSTURE

- Head slumps forward.
- Chin tilts up with the head held back.
- Shoulders are drooped forward, pulled back, or raised too high.
- Chest is sunken in and shoulders are rounded.
- Abdomen sags.
- Lower back is too flat (no gentle curve), or it curves forward excessively into a hollow back.
- Knees bend forward or are thrown backward into a locked position.

If your posture displays any of the warning signs, your spine is probably not properly maintaining its three natural curves.

CHAPTER ELEVEN

Gait

One of the most common sources of everyday stress—especially of stress to the lower body—is the simple act of walking. Walking, after all, involves placing your entire body weight on one and then the other leg and foot each time you take a step. Furthermore, walking is a repetitive activity, calling on the same muscles, joints, and other structures to engage in the same motions over and over again. And given all the walking we are inclined to do during the course of a normal day, these stresses can start to accumulate.

Although walking does cause stress, there is no reason that, when done within normal limits, this stress should add up to any real problems. Whether it does depends in large measure on the nature of your "gait."

Your gait is your own particular style of walking. Whether you shuffle your feet, have a bouncy step, stride forward with purpose, or move gingerly, that is an aspect of your gait. As with fingerprints, everyone has his or her own unique gait. Although your gait may evolve somewhat over the course of your lifetime, from day to day it tends to remain constant.

Your gait is of great significance to your well-being because, like posture, it largely determines the distribution of the stress of walking to the various parts of your legs and feet. A "proper gait" channels this stress in a way that the muscles, joints, and other structures are well equipped to handle.

As it turns out, there is no single proper gait; proper gaits come in an infinite variety of styles. Nevertheless, all these gaits do display a number of common basic qualities. Without going into elaborate detail about the highly complex mechanics of gait, these basic qualities may be summed up as follows:

- With each step the heel is first to make contact with the ground, followed by the bottom of the foot in a rolling motion, followed by the ball of the foot and the toes, which propel the body on to the next step.
- When on the ground, the bottom of the foot is tilted neither inward (overpronating) nor outward (oversupinating).
- The legs move in a rhythmic fashion, displaying no "hitch."
- The legs move symmetrically, displaying an even stride length.
- Both knees point forward, turned neither inward nor outward.

Standing

Although improper alignment of the legs does the most damage when you walk or run, it can also cause trouble when you are simply standing. The sheer weight of your upper body, even when not moving, places stress on the hips, knees, ankles, and feet. And if there is improper alignment in one or more of these areas, that stress is sure to be distributed in a troublesome fashion.

Just as significantly, improperly aligned legs can have the effect of disrupting your posture, with ill effects on your back, neck, shoulders—even down to your toes. Pronated feet, for example, can lead to inward movement of the knees and altered hip alignment, leading ultimately to an altered alignment of the spine. A shortened leg may have a similar effect. (See Chapter 10—Posture for more information.)

- The pelvis remains level and rotates smoothly with each step, not moving excessively either up and down or side to side.
- The arms swing rhythmically and evenly backward and forward to counterbalance the movements of the legs.
- The body maintains good posture.

Needless to say, even if you have a proper gait, you will not display these qualities with each and every step you take. If you walk on a beach or other uneven surface or clamber through a rocky field, your gait is sure to be a bit more awkward; indeed, it has to be awkward in order to handle such challenges. The question is whether your typical gait possesses the above qualities.

A gait that typically fails to possess these qualities is, simply put, an improper gait. And the more of these qualities it lacks or the more conspicuously it lacks them, the more likely it is to do your body some damage.

Not surprisingly, the health of your feet is especially dependent on your gait. An improper gait makes them vulnerable to corns and calluses, bunions and bunionettes, mallet toes and hammer toes, plantar fasciitis (damage to the tissue on the bottom of the foot), and a range of other problems both major and minor. But the rest of the leg may pay a significant price for an improper gait as well. The hips are susceptible to bursitis; the upper legs and knees to iliotibial band syndrome; the knees to

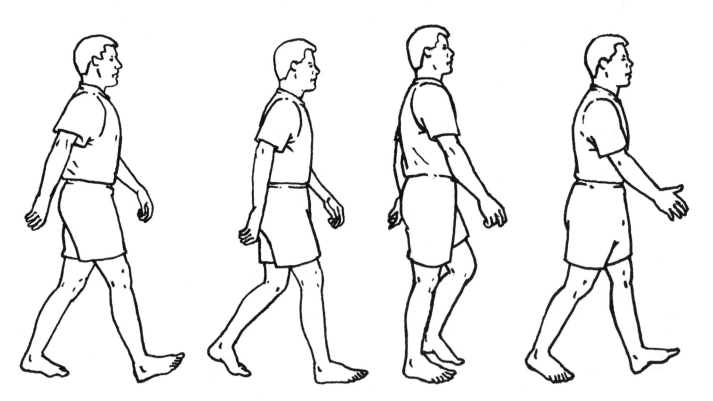

Proper gait

chondromalacia patellae (damage to the cartilage under the kneecap); and the front of the ankle to shin splints. All are at risk of various degrees of strain and sprain. An improper gait may even disrupt the alignment of your spine, with implications for your back, neck, shoulders, and down to your toes. (See **Chapter 10—Posture**.)

Depending on the nature of your gait deficiency, the problems caused by an improper gait during walking generally do not present themselves in the short term. Often it takes many years of walking in a particular manner before injuries start to appear.

And whatever risks can be ascribed to an improper walking gait apply doubly to an improper running gait—largely because the forces that travel down the legs and through the feet with each step are far greater. Many of the injuries mentioned above are, in fact, considerably more common results of running deficiencies than of walking deficiencies. And unlike walking injuries, running-related injuries tend to present themselves quite readily.

For these reasons, it is essential to practice a proper gait both while walking and while running. Fortunately, for most people this is not a difficult matter; a proper gait is relatively common, and an improper one is relatively rare.

Still, an improper gait is not always easy to overcome, often because there is some sort of minor deformity in the lower extremities, inherited or otherwise. If, for example, one leg is slightly shorter than the other, there will be uneven stresses on the joints. Varus deformity (bow leg), valgus deformity (knock knee), hallux valgus (bunion), or low arch are other examples of misalignments that may prevent a proper gait. If you suffer from such a condition, you may need specialized shoes or an orthotic insert to normalize your gait. In such instances, however, it may not be possible to attain a proper gait at all.

Another cause of improper gait is poor posture. A spine that is not well aligned may distribute too much of your body weight to one side or too far forward. During walking and running, this poor alignment may disrupt your whole gait. Good posture, then, is really a prerequisite of a proper gait—though it, too, is not always possible to attain. (For more information on developing good posture, see **Chapter 10—Posture**.)

A familiar cause of an improper gait, especially a temporary one, is the wrong shoes. Some shoes cause your feet to overpronate (roll excessively to the inside of the foot) or oversupinate (roll excessively to the outside of the foot), leading to disruptions of proper alignment all the way up the leg. If you use running shoes that have this effect, the consequences may be particularly severe. Ill-fitting shoes may also affect your gait indirectly: if they

Calling All Runners

Because the stress of serious regular running (or even of high-intensity walking) can take a considerable toll on the legs and feet, the chances of injury—and of serious injury—due to an improper gait are much greater than they are for the less active individual. If you are a runner and feel you may be developing problems, it is highly recommended that you consult your physical therapist about getting a gait analysis. A gait analysis will allow the physical therapist to identify any trouble spots in your running style and provide you with appropriate advice for minimizing the risk of injury. Your physical therapist may also help you select suitable running shoes (or orthotic device if necessary).

Checking Your Gait

The best way to check your gait is to get a gait analysis from a physical therapist. You can, however, make a preliminary check of your typical gait, which may allow you to determine if a professional examination and evaluation are necessary. To do so, all you'll need is a full-length mirror.

1. Walk directly toward the mirror, checking that:
   - Your knees remain straight.
   - Your body displays an overall symmetry.
   - Your arms swing rhythmically to counterbalance legs.
   - Your hips are level.
   - You feel like you are "walking tall."

2. Walk past the mirror, checking that:
   - Your heel is the first part of your foot to make contact with the ground.
   - You "roll off" the toes, ending with the big toe.
   - Your steps are of equal length.

cause your feet pain, you might alter your gait to minimize the discomfort. (For more information, see **Chapter 14 — Footwear**.)

Still another cause of an improper gait is an injury to the leg or foot. Whether it is a major injury, like a knee sprain that causes you to limp, or a minor one, like a corn that leads you to favor one side of the foot, the outcome may be a temporary disruption of your gait. Ironically, the very injuries that lead you to alter your gait are often themselves the product of an improper gait. The result is a vicious cycle in which an improper gait leads to injury, which leads to a further disruption of the gait, which leads to further injury, and so on.

Finally, an improper gait may simply be a function of bad habits. In such instances simply learning how to practice a proper gait, under the guidance of a physical therapist, may be all that is needed.

CHAPTER TWELVE

Body Mechanics

"Body mechanics" is a somewhat ungainly term for a relatively straightforward concept. The term refers broadly to the way in which we use our bodies and the different parts of our bodies as we go about the day-to-day business of living. Whether or not we hold our backs straight when brushing our teeth or lean on our elbows when reading or use a wrist rest when typing at a keyboard or run with our feet turned inward or carry heavy loads in a backpack—all these issues are issues of body mechanics. And how they are resolved has significant consequences.

This is because, for all its remarkable versatility, the body is still a somewhat delicate piece of machinery. While its various components—the bones, ligaments, muscles, tendons, disks, bursae, and other structures—make the body capable of impressive physical feats, they do have their limits. And if we use our bodies in ways that place too much stress on one or more of these structures, they can easily be damaged. It is essential, then, to your body's general health and well-being that you practice "proper body mechanics"—body mechanics that keep the stresses within a manageable range.

This is, of course, easier said than done. After all, proper body mechanics are not always immediately identifiable. Just because a particular practice is painless doesn't mean that it represents proper body mechanics. Indeed, many practices that feel just fine are actually quite harmful, and the ill effects may make themselves felt hours, days, or—if the practice becomes a habit—even months or years later. It may, for example, take a long evening of watching television with your chin resting comfortably in your palm before your jaw feels the unpleasant consequences. (On the other hand, a practice that doesn't feel right is almost certainly not proper body mechanics.) At any rate, some practices may do their damage even before you've had a chance to find out if they're painless; by the time you've reached into the back seat to retrieve a bag of groceries, for example, you may have already given your back a severe strain.

Furthermore, the familiar itinerary of everyday life—with its workplace duties, household chores, sports, and similar activities—offers almost unlimited opportunities to use the body improperly. Everything from sitting at a desk to painting a ceiling to swinging a golf club has the capacity to cause injury. And in the absence of clear knowledge of how best to tackle these common challenges, poor body mechanics are almost inevitable, at least occasionally.

Although it would be impossible to create a comprehensive rule book containing appropriate body mechanics for each and every human activity, the following catalogue of do's and don'ts covers some of the most common. (Actually, there are many more don'ts than do's, a reflection in part of the many creative ways in which people have found to do themselves harm.) The guidelines do overlap a bit—and a few are also reiterated in **Chapter 16—Sports** and **Chapter 17—Work**. Some affect just a single body part, like the jaw or the elbow; others affect quite a few. But all are very much worth heeding in the interest of keeping your body healthy.

Do maintain proper posture while standing, sitting, or lying down. Failure to do so can cause trouble for your back, neck, jaw, shoulders, and—when standing—even your feet. See **Chapter 10—Posture** for detailed information.

Don't lean forward from the hips during standing activities, like washing dishes, shaving, brushing your teeth, or dressing. This disrupts the posture and stresses the back, especially the lower back. It may also affect the neck and shoulders. If working for short periods of time over a low sink or counter, it's much better to bend the knees and lower the body, keeping the back straight. If this tires your legs, take a few breaks. Or try sitting on a stool if working for long periods. Whenever possible, bring your body close enough to a mirror to avoid leaning over. If the bathroom sink prevents that, consider installing a mirror with an extending arm so that you can bring the mirror to your face and not vice versa. You may need to start wearing your glasses or contact lenses during these activities.

Don't stand in a fixed position for prolonged periods, as when waiting in line or preparing a meal. Even with good posture, holding the back and head upright is very stressful on the back and neck muscles; it can also be quite hard on the muscles and ligaments of the feet and may place excessive pressure on the feet. If possible, put one foot up on a footstool while standing. Shift your weight frequently from side to side. And take occasional breaks to sit or lie down and to stretch the back.

Don't lean forward during seated activities such as writing, eating, or driving. This disrupts good posture and stresses the back, neck, and shoulders, just as leaning forward while standing does. When working at a table or desk, be sure your chair is pulled in close to the table; when driving, adjust the seat so

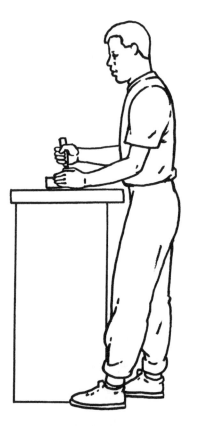

Proper body mechanics during standing activity

that you can assume a neutral position at the steering wheel, not reach for it.

Don't sit for prolonged periods, as when working at a computer, travelling in a train or airplane, or watching a movie. Even with good posture, this is more stressful on the back than standing for long periods. If you must sit for long periods, take a break every hour or so to stand up, walk around, and stretch the back if possible.

Don't pull heavy objects to move them, as when moving furniture. This may put the back and neck at risk, just as lifting improperly does. Always push objects whenever possible, keeping the knees slightly bent and the neck and back in alignment.

Do lift even moderately heavy objects using proper techniques: Assume a neutral position with good posture and the head erect. Put one foot slightly behind the other and bend the knees to lower your body to the object. With the arms slightly bent at the elbow, the wrists straight, and the stomach and chin in, use your legs and hips, rather than your back, to lift. Keep a heavy object close to you and centered. Bending over with the knees straight to lift may cause serious trauma, such as a herniated disk in the back. Keeping the arms straight may hyperextend the elbow. Bending the wrists puts too much stress on the area and leaves it vulnerable to ligament, muscle, and tendon strain, as well as nerve compression.

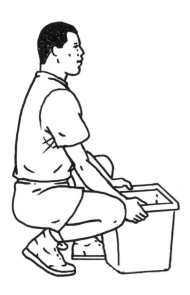
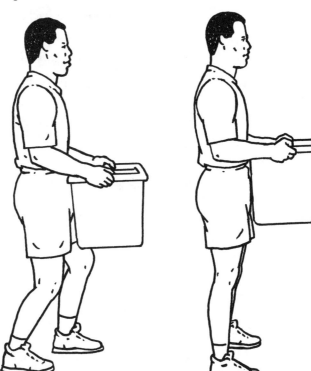

Proper lifting technique

Don't carry heavy loads in your arms, as when transporting boxes of books or bags of groceries. No matter how efficient your carrying technique, heavy loads have the potential to be extremely stressful on the back and many other parts of the body as well. Whenever possible, split a heavy load into several lighter loads and make multiple trips. Or if the load cannot be split, get someone to give you a hand. If you must carry a heavy load in your arms, be sure to hold it close to your body.

Don't carry weight unevenly to one side of the body, as when wearing a heavy purse over the shoulder, lugging a full suitcase in one hand, or even holding a big bag of groceries under one arm. This may result in so-called "carrier's tilt," or malalignment of the back and neck to one side, which causes stress and fatigue in the low back, neck, and shoulder. If possible, redistribute the weight into two smaller bags, one for each arm or shoulder. Or opt for a backpack.

Don't twist your trunk while reaching for or picking up something, as when retrieving an item from the back seat of the car or unloading the washing machine into the dryer. This is a common cause of back muscle strain, spasm, and disk problems. Instead, bend your knees, move your feet, and turn your whole body.

Do use a backpack to carry weight. Worn on both shoulders, with the straps relatively loose, a backpack channels the stress down to your hips. Compared with other methods of carrying weight, this considerably minimizes the chances of injury to your more vulnerable back, neck, and shoulders. Still, even a backpack should not be made too heavy.

Don't sit up or otherwise prop your body up in bed or on the floor, as when reading or watching television. This can be punishing on the back and neck and often other areas as well. If you insist on sitting up, at least be sure to sit with your back set against the headboard or wall and a few pillows below your knees. If reading, lay the book on a pillow or mini desk on your lap to avoid bending or hunching forward. And if you tend to prop yourself up in a contorted position, change the position often.

Don't crane your neck forward during standing or seated activities, as when putting on makeup or working at a computer. This disrupts your neck posture and may be very stressful on the neck. To prevent this, apply the same recommendations that apply to leaning forward during standing or seated activities (which often accompanies neck craning): when standing, bend your knees and lower your body to the work surface; if looking in the mirror, bring your body close or buy an extending mirror; if seated, pull your seat forward; and always wear your glasses or contact lenses.

Don't hold the neck in a fixed position for a prolonged period, as when working at a computer or watching a movie. This requires a constant contraction of the muscles and stresses the neck. Take occasional breaks to stretch out the area.

Don't tilt the head up (even slightly) or down for a prolonged period. The former is common when watching a movie from the front row or working at a poorly positioned computer monitor; the latter is common when reading or working at a desk. Both of these disrupt your neck posture and may be very stressful on the neck and jaw.

Don't chew on hard or unforgiving items, like pencils, ice, hard candy, or large gobs of gum. It puts stress on the jaw muscles.

Don't clench your jaw (repeatedly or constantly) or grind your teeth. These widespread habits (also known as bruxism) place considerable stress on the temporomandibular joint and tend to put the jaw out of correct alignment. (If you grind your teeth at night, you should see your dentist.)

Don't rest your chin in the palm of your hand, as when watching television, reading, or sitting at a desk. This puts direct pressure on the jaw and TMJ and also may cause strain or damage to the soft tissue of the cervical region.

Don't cradle the telephone receiver between your ear and shoulder. This disrupts neck posture to the side and stresses your neck, jaw, and shoulder. Hold the phone in your hand or use a shoulder-rest attachment. If you talk on the phone for long periods of time, consider a headset receiver or a speaker phone.

Don't hook your arm over the back of a chair or car seat for an extended period of time; this pushes the shoulder beyond its normal range of motion.

Don't repeatedly raise your arm above shoulder level, as when pruning a tree or putting items on a high shelf. This may strain the rotator cuff and shoulder tendons. Use a ladder or other appropriate tools to make this unnecessary. If you must repeatedly raise the arm, make sure your shoulders are warmed up and stretched out beforehand; also take frequent breaks from the activity and, if possible, alternate hands.

Do learn and practice proper form in sports activities that involve throwing or swinging a racquet, bat, or other such equipment, including baseball, softball, tennis, racquetball, squash, and golf. Proper form—along with proper conditioning of the muscles—is the most reliable way to avoid a range of common shoulder, wrist, and especially elbow injuries (like "tennis elbow" and "golfer's elbow").

Don't lean on your elbow for a prolonged period, as when reading or watching television. This puts pressure on the elbow's sensitive olecranon bursa and may lead to bursitis. It can also cause cubital tunnel syndrome.

Don't repeatedly bend and straighten your arm, as when hammering or chopping wood. This may strain the area. If you must do so, make sure your elbows are warmed up and stretched beforehand; also take frequent breaks and try to alternate hands as much as possible.

Do use proper elbow and wrist support when typing at a keyboard. This includes armrests on your chair and a wrist rest on the desk. Failure to do so may lead to carpal tunnel syndrome. Also take frequent breaks to shake out and stretch the wrist and hand. (You may want to talk to your physician or physical therapist about getting a wrist brace.)

Don't hold a pen or pencil too tightly for prolonged periods. This is a sure recipe for "writer's cramp." If you must write for long periods, take frequent breaks to stretch and shake out the hand.

Don't hold the wrists in an excessively flexed position for a prolonged period, as when typing, knitting, or sewing. This "cocked" position, combined with repetitive motion, can lead to carpal tunnel syndrome or tendinitis.

Don't use tools or equipment that are poorly designed, are too large or too small for your hands, or vibrate too much. Such tools can lead to compensatory overuse of the wrist and hand muscles and joints, often resulting in muscle strain and joint dysfunction.

Do maintain a proper gait while walking or running, including during sports activities. Failure to do so can lead to trouble for your feet, ankles, knees, hips, and lower back; it may even disrupt your posture, with further negative consequences. See **Chapter 11—Gait** for detailed information.

Don't walk or run for prolonged periods unless the hip, knee, ankle, and foot have been fully warmed up and stretched beforehand. This is a primary cause of repetitive-motion injuries to all these areas. The risks increase when walking or running on uneven surfaces, like a rocky path.

Don't squat for prolonged periods. This increases the compressive forces on the hip and knee joints.

Don't sit on the floor with the knees turned in and feet splayed out to the sides; this compresses the knee joints and stresses the ligaments.

Do wear knee pads during activities performed on the knees, such as gardening or cleaning. Continuously leaning on unpadded knees puts pressure on the sensitive prepatellar bursae and may lead to bursitis.

Do wear appropriate shoes. They can save your feet a great deal of trouble, from corns to bunions, especially when you are running. They may also have considerable impact on your posture and gait. See **Chapter 14—Footwear** for detailed information.

CHAPTER THIRTEEN
Body Weight

Body weight and body composition are vital components of overall fitness. Obesity is a major risk factor for heart disease. In addition, excess body weight can put considerable stress on many of the body's joints, including the back, hips, knees, ankles, and feet. It can also make proper posture difficult to maintain, with unfavorable implications for other parts of the body as well. (See **Chapter 10—Posture**.)

For these reasons (as well as for your general health and wellness), it's important to remain within your appropriate weight range. There are a number of different approaches to determining your appropriate weight range. One simple way, used by co-author Marilyn Moffat, is with a mathematical formula.

For men the formula works as follows: Start with 106 pounds for the first 5 feet of height and add 6 additional pounds for each additional inch of height; your proper weight should be no more than 10 percent above this figure and no more than 10 percent below. For example, if you are 5 feet 9 inches, you start with 106 pounds for the first 5 feet and add 6 more pounds for each of the additional 9 inches, or 54 more pounds. The total is 160 pounds. Ten percent of 160 pounds is 16 pounds. So your weight should be no more than 176 pounds (and no less than 144 pounds).

For women, start with 100 pounds for the first 5 feet of height and add 5 pounds for each additional inch; again, your proper weight should be no more than 10 percent above or below this figure. If you are 5 feet 4 inches, then you start with 100 pounds for the first 5 feet and add 5 more pounds for each of the additional 4 inches, or 20 pounds. The total is 120 pounds. Ten percent of 120 pounds is 12 pounds. So your weight should be no more than 132 pounds (and no less than 108 pounds).

For quick reference, you can use the **Healthy Weight Range Chart**, which is based on this formula, on page 140.

If you find that you are above a healthy weight range for your height, you may be putting your body at risk of injury. You should seek professional assistance in devising a tailored weight-reduction program.

Healthy Weight Range Chart

HEIGHT	WEIGHT (IN POUNDS) MEN	WEIGHT (IN POUNDS) WOMEN
5'0"	95 to 117	90 to 110
5'1"	101 to 123	95 to 116
5'2"	106 to 130	99 to 121
5'3"	112 to 136	104 to 126
5'4"	117 to 143	108 to 132
5'5"	122 to 150	112 to 138
5'6"	128 to 156	117 to 143
5'7"	133 to 163	122 to 148
5'8"	139 to 169	126 to 154
5'9"	144 to 176	130 to 160
5'10"	149 to 183	135 to 165
5'11"	155 to 189	140 to 170
6'0"	160 to 196	144 to 176
6'1"	166 to 202	148 to 182
6'2"	171 to 209	153 to 187
6'3"	176 to 216	158 to 192

CHAPTER FOURTEEN

Footwear

It should hardly be surprising that one of the most important steps you can take toward having healthy feet is wearing the right shoes. Many of the most common foot problems—from bunions to corns and calluses—can be traced directly to poorly fitting or inappropriate everyday footwear. Foot (and ankle) problems are also common consequences of engaging in vigorous activities with insufficiently supportive and shock-absorbing athletic shoes.

Less obvious is that your choice of footwear may have implications for other parts of the body. In part this is because shoes play a major role in determining your gait, that is, your particular manner of walking and running. And your gait, in turn, has an impact not only on your feet and ankles, but on your knees, hips, and lower back as well. An improper gait may lead to a wide range of strains, sprains, and other disorders—especially during sports or similar activities. (See **Chapter 11—Gait** for more information.)

There are several ways in which shoes can negatively affect your gait. If your shoes fit poorly and cause pain, you might alter your gait in a subtle way to minimize the discomfort—walking on the outside of the foot, for example, to avoid putting pressure on a callous. But the wrong shoes also can affect your gait directly by throwing off the foot's normal alignment.

The wrong shoes may even disrupt your posture, forcing you to arch your spine too far forward, backward, or to the side just to stay upright. And this can have repercussions for the back, neck, shoulders, and feet (and your knees and hips as well). (See **Chapter 10—Posture** for more information.)

For this reason it is important to know how to recognize good-quality footwear that is well suited to your particular feet, both for everyday and athletic usage. When you are buying shoes, after all, knowledgeable salespeople are not always available.

There is no guarantee you will be able to find shoes that fit correctly. In that case you may require custom-made shoes or custom-made orthotics, inserts and molds designed to more properly accommodate a shoe to your foot. Consult your physical therapist for guidance.

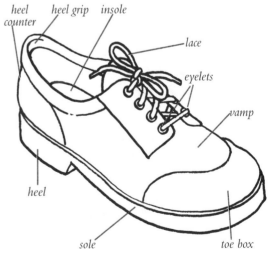

Parts of a shoe

Everyday Shoes

The two main qualities you should look for in everyday shoes are fit and support. If the shoes aren't comfortable when you try them on, don't buy them. No amount of "breaking them in" is going to make the wrong shoes fit correctly: if they don't fit right now, they won't fit right a year from now—and your feet will be a lot worse for the wear.

As a rule, it's a good idea to favor lace-up shoes, especially if you already have foot problems. Lace-ups give you more control over fit than slip-ons.

A few other considerations when buying everyday shoes:

Insole: The insole should match the arch of your foot, whether high, flat, or normal. A high arch will require extra cushioning; a flat arch may require an orthotic insert (a buildup inside the shoe) to provide support and limit motion.

Sole: The sole should be flexible enough to bend easily at the forefoot. Crepe soles add cushion and shock absorption, increasing comfort during standing and walking.

Heel: The heel should be low. High heels, whether on women's shoes or men's boots, put pressure on the arch and the ball of the foot. They also throw your posture out of alignment.

Vamp: Like the sole, the vamp should bend easily at the forefoot.

Material: Breathable, natural materials such as leather, suede, or cotton canvas are preferable to synthetics or plastic. The latter seal in heat and moisture, creating an ideal environment for fungal or bacterial infections. Also, softer materials (such as suede) are recommended for feet with bunions or other minor deformities. (On the other hand, if you tend to overpronate or oversupinate, you should avoid very soft leather or canvas and other materials that are nonsupportive.)

Toe box: The toe box should provide plenty of wiggle room for the toes in both depth and width. Pointed toe boxes, common in women's shoes and cowboy boots, should be avoided; they're likely to cause corns, calluses, bunions, hammer toes, claw toes, and other problems.

Heel grip: The heel grip should hold the heel snugly in place. But it should cause no friction with the skin, which can lead to blisters and other problems.

Athletic Shoes

Good athletic shoes have many of the same qualities as good everyday shoes. But because athletic shoes must protect the feet—and the body generally—from the shocks and stresses of vigorous activity, they require extra cushioning and support.

Because the care of the foot is so important to overall health, serious athletes should consult a physical therapist before buying athletic shoes. In addition to providing guidance, the physical therapist may perform a gait analysis (often on videotape) to help maximize the athlete's performance and to identify any problems.

Do be aware that there is little correlation between cost and quality when it comes to athletic shoes. So don't assume that the more expensive shoes are better. Check the quality of the workmanship and stitching yourself.

A few other considerations when buying athletic shoes:

Insole: As with everyday shoes, the insole should match the arch of your foot, whether high, flat, or normal. A high arch will require extra cushioning; a flat arch may require an orthotic device (usually a buildup inside the shoe) to provide extra support and limit motion.

Sole: The sole should be made from a foam material to provide cushioning during activity, but also firm enough to provide support. When pressed, the sole should bend at the forefoot rather than at the midfoot. The shank, directly under the arch, should be stiff and make complete contact with the ground. If it doesn't, the shoe may not offer enough support.

Heel: The heel should be made from a foam material to provide shock absorption. If the arch is low, a firm heel counter will add some support.

Material: Breathable materials such as leather and cotton canvas are preferable to synthetics or plastic; the latter materials hold in heat and moisture and create an ideal environment for fungal or bacterial infections.

Eyelets: The shoe should feature alternating eyelets for support. These allow the laces to create a crisscross pattern, which provides extra support and strength.

Laces: Laces should be round (like spaghetti) rather than flat. They should be laced through eyelets in the shape of webs or loops (similar to those of hiking boots) to better distribute the pressure on the top of the foot.

Toe box: The toe box should provide plenty of wiggle room for the toes in both depth and width.

Heel grip: The heel grip should hold the heel snugly in place. A padded cuff at the top opening may provide a firmer grip and cause less friction on the skin.

For most casual athletes a standard, all-purpose athletic shoe—a "cross-trainer"—should suffice. Other, more serious athletes, however, should take advantage of the specialized shoe options available.

Runners should select a shoe with enhanced shock absorption; the shoe should be flexible and lightweight enough, however, to minimize the

Getting the Right Fit

Whatever kind of shoes you're buying, here's a bit of advice for making sure the shoe fits.

- Don't rely on shoe sizes alone—they can vary widely among manufacturers and styles.
- Always try on both shoes before you buy. Most people have feet that vary slightly in size; use the larger of the two sizes as your guide.
- Your feet tend to swell slightly as the day progresses. Shop late in the day to get an accurate feel of the shoes you're trying on.
- Before visiting the store, trace the outline of your feet on a sheet of paper while standing. At the store, place any shoes you are considering over the outline; you'll see instantly if the shoes are too small and if they match the shape of your foot.
- Always have your feet measured while you're standing.
- Wear athletic socks when trying on athletic shoes to get an accurate fit.

stress on the Achilles tendon and calf muscles. Walkers should look for similar shock absorption in the heel. Athletes whose sports are played on a court surface (tennis and other racquet sports, basketball, volleyball) should choose shoes with a midsole that provides increased forefoot stability to reduce stress on the ankles. High-top shoes are worth considering for anyone who has problems with ankle stability. (Also, athletes whose sports require cleated shoes, like football and soccer, are less prone to injury with shorter cleats.)

In general, women should buy a true woman's athletic shoe, not simply a downsized man's shoe labeled as a woman's athletic shoe. A correctly made woman's shoe has a narrower foot and a narrower heel; this prevents the heel from slipping during athletic competition. (Exceptions to this rule are sometimes made if you have foot problems—such as bunions—that require shoes with more toe room or if you use an orthosis.)

CHAPTER FIFTEEN

Strength, Endurance, & Flexibility

The challenges of everyday life make considerable demands on the body. Carrying briefcases, putting away groceries, pulling weeds, opening jars, closing windows, chewing meat, climbing stairs, even sitting or standing for long periods: all of these seemingly innocent activities (and many, many more) actually put the joints, muscles, tendons, and other structures under genuine, if relatively low-level, stress.

As long as the various body parts are equipped to handle this stress—in other words, as long as they possess adequate strength, endurance, and flexibility—there is no reason why it should lead to injury. If, however, they are unequipped to handle the stress, it is altogether possible that, in the short or long run, one or more of them will indeed suffer strain, sprain, tendinitis, or worse.

Although different people naturally possess strength, endurance, and flexibility in varying degrees, for most of us, especially as we age, it takes work to attain and then maintain these qualities at a level compatible with everyday life. And while simply including moderate amounts of physical activity in your daily life can itself be highly beneficial, proper conditioning generally requires some sort of regular exercise program.

Chapter 18—Strength and Endurance Exercises and **Chapter 19—Flexibility Exercises** together constitute a broad pool of many dozens of exercises from which such a program may be drawn. There are practically unlimited ways of combining these exercises to create an effective regimen. It would be impossible to provide a regimen perfectly tailored for everyone. Your program must really be a function of several unique factors, including your existing fitness status and your comfort level with particular exercises. That said, below are some basic guidelines on getting started.

No exercise regimen can be expected to provide the necessary overall protection if it neglects any of the major body parts: namely, the back, neck, shoulder, elbow, wrist/hand, hip, knee, and ankle/foot. (Unless your

Cardiovascular Conditioning

A regular program of aerobic activities that get the heart pumping and the lungs working is an important complement to your strength, endurance, and flexibility exercise regimen. Such activities have important benefits for the heart, the lungs, and other parts of the body. For more information on this vital matter, see Appendix B— Cardiovascular Conditioning.

jaw gives you trouble, it probably need not be included in your exercise regimen.) Each body part, after all, faces distinct challenges and needs strength, endurance, and flexibility of its own. The text for all the exercises in Chapters 18 and 19 delineates clearly the body part(s) to which it is targeted; each chapter also features a cross-listing of the exercises by body part.

It is also essential that, for each of these body parts, all of the principal muscles, tendons, and ligaments receive appropriate attention. With the knee, for example, this means working with the muscles, tendons, and ligaments of both the front and the back of the thigh and those of the back of the lower leg as well. As it turns out, many exercises service more than one body part. Those that provide strength in the abdomen, for example, may benefit both the neck and the back. The text for all the exercises in Chapters 18 and 19 indicates in general terms the muscles, tendons, and ligaments affected; it is important to pay attention to this information in developing your exercise program.

A full, effective body maintenance program should add up to 50 or so exercises. This might seem like a considerable number, but, in fact, the exercises themselves are quite brief. Working through your program should not take more than 45 minutes to one hour. (You may also save time by doing flexibility exercises for two different parts of the body simultaneously, such as the jaw and the wrist/hand.)

Although it is possible to train with an emphasis on strength rather than endurance, and (to some degree) vice versa, the exercises in Chapter 18 are designed to accomplish both of these ends simultaneously—if they are done right. As a rule, these exercises require a certain minimum number of repetitions to optimize their strengthening impact. Although this number may vary from one exercise to another and from one person to another, for most people this number is 10 to 15 repetitions. Beyond this number, the additional *strengthening* benefit is likely to be minimal.

This number, however, is rarely enough to provide sufficient *endurance*, which requires that the muscles be worked over time. For optimum strength and endurance-building impact, then, the "set" of 10 to 15 repetitions generally ought to be repeated three times. Needless to say, these target numbers might be difficult at first; you may have to work up to these levels by exercising regularly over a period of weeks, beginning with fewer repetitions.

Several of the strength and endurance exercises in Chapter 18 require the use of dumbbells or ankle weights to provide the necessary resistance. Needless to say, in any given exercise, there is no single weight level proper for everyone; people are simply not all capable of lifting the same amounts. Still, in order for these exercises to help prepare the body for its everyday demands, a certain minimum amount is necessary. This amount may range considerably, depending on the individual and the muscle group being trained. (For example, while 10 to 12 pounds might suit a bicep exercise, 6 to 8 pounds might be more appropriate for a deltoid exercise.) Still, for most people, 5 to 15 pounds makes for a sensible minimum range. With any given exercise you should lift as much weight as you comfortably can while still being able to perform the target number of repetitions. Again, some people may need to work up to this level, starting with either lighter weights or fewer repetitions. (For the purposes of basic maintenance, there is no need to use heavier weights; the aim here is not bodybuilding.) In cases where the use of weights is marked as optional, weights are recommended most highly for those who find that the exercise, without weights, is simply too easy to do.

Flexibility exercises, like endurance exercises, require that the muscles, tendons, and ligaments in question be stretched over time. Generally, however, a single set of 10 repetitions with a 10-second hold each is plenty. Alternatively, however, you may opt for a set of 3 repetitions with a 30-second hold each.

With flexibility exercises, the number of repetitions and the duration of the hold may also be determined somewhat on a case-by-case basis. If the muscles, tendons, and ligaments in a particular part of your body do not feel tight when you work with them, you may not need to spend much time on those stretches; on the other hand, if the body part feels excessively tight, you may want to concentrate on the area more. Each time you exercise, you may adjust your program accordingly.

For effective body maintenance, you should work through a full program of exercises three to five times per week. (The alternate days could be used for cardiovascular conditioning.) However, exercises using weights should be done on no more than three non-successive days per week. So if you choose to exercise four or five days per week, leave out the weight training exercises on those extra days.

To help prevent muscle strains or tears, exercise sessions should be preceded by 5 to 10 minutes of light aerobic activity, like walking or cycling. During this aerobic activity, take care to move your arms so that the upper body warms up too. To cool down, follow your exercise regimen with a few more minutes of light aerobic activity. (You can also combine your exercise sessions with cardiovascular conditioning, doing 5 to 10 minutes of warmup, 20 minutes or so of cardiovascular conditioning, and 5 to 10 minutes of cooldown—followed by some quick stretches—before beginning your exercise regimen.) If you have

Ordering Your Exercises

There are a few rules of thumb regarding the order in which you perform the various exercises in your routine:

• Work the major regions of the body—the upper body, the lower body, and the torso—one at a time.

• Within any region of the body, start with the larger muscles or muscle groups, then move on to the smaller ones. The muscles of the upper leg, for example, should be worked before those of the lower leg.

• As much as possible, try also to work muscle groups that are "opposite" one another in succession. For example, after working the biceps muscles (in the front of the upper arm), move on to the triceps muscles (in the back of the upper arm).

• For each of these muscle groups, do the appropriate strength and endurance exercise(s) and then the appropriate flexibility exercise(s). Alternatively, you may do all your strength and endurance exercises first, and then all your flexibility exercises.

pain of any sort (other than mild temporary stiffness and soreness), you should consult your physical therapist or physician before attempting any of the exercises. And, of course, if you experience sharp or severe pain while engaging in any of these exercises, stop what you're doing at once.

The box, **"Body Maintenance Program,"** below, offers one example of a basic exercise regimen. You may wish to use this as a starting-off point or to develop your own regimen based on the principles outlined above. Either way, as you become familiar with the exercises, feel free to experiment and vary your routine. Indeed, experimentation is much encouraged, since it is a good way to head off getting bored with your conditioning program.

Again, these programs and the exercises in Chapters 18 and 19, as a whole, are designed to produce strength, endurance, and flexibility for everyday life, including normal vigorous activities. Serious athletes, heavy physical laborers, and other very active individuals, however, may wish to develop these qualities to a higher degree—either throughout the body or in regions particular to their activity. They may be able to do so with these exercises; but it would be better if they worked in consultation with a physical therapist or physician. Some useful information along these lines can be found in **Chapter 16—Sports**.

It should be noted that exercises that develop strength, endurance, and flexibility—either throughout the body or in one particular area—are commonly prescribed by physical therapists as part of the rehabilitative process for a wide range of problems. If you do have a problem, you should never try to address it yourself with exercises except in consultation with a physical therapist; otherwise, you are likely to do further damage.

Body Maintenance Program

The exercises presented below together make up a conditioning program specifically tailored to provide the levels of strength, endurance, and flexibility your body needs to meet the challenges of everyday life. Detailed instructions and appropriate illustrations for each exercise can be found in Chapter 18—Strength and Endurance Exercises and Chapter 19—Flexibility Exercises. Exercises marked with an asterisk (*) require weights.

This program is directed principally toward fitness novices, although it will certainly benefit even more experienced individuals. It is, however, but one of an infinite number of equally effective combinations of exercises. So particularly as you become familiar with these exercises, feel free to substitute your own alternatives.

Be sure to read this chapter in its entirety before engaging in these exercises. It contains many tips, explanations, and cautions with which you must be familiar in order to make safe and effective use of this conditioning regimen.

STRENGTH AND ENDURANCE EXERCISES

Abdominal Crunch with Hands to Knees (page 175)
Back • Neck

Rotation Crunch with Hands at Ears (page 179)
Back • Neck

Easy Push-Up (page 182)
Back • Neck • Shoulder

Leg and Arm Extension (page 183)
Back • Hip • Knee

Shoulder Shrug* (page 184)
Back • Neck

Seated Butterfly Lift* (page 187)
Back • Shoulder

Neck Strengthener (page 188)
Neck

Neck Flexor (page 189)
Neck

Lateral Neck Flexor (page 190)
Neck

Bench Press* (page 194)
Shoulder

Butterfly* (page 194)
Shoulder

Shoulder Pullover* (page 195)
Shoulder

External Shoulder Rotation* (page 196)
Shoulder

Internal Shoulder Rotation* (page 197)
Shoulder

Overhead Press* (page 197)
Shoulder

Front Arm Lift* (page 198)
Shoulder • Back

Side Arm Lift* (page 199)
Shoulder

Upright Row* (page 199)
Shoulder

Biceps Curl* (page 200)
Elbow

Vertical Triceps Extension* (page 201)
Elbow

Palm-Down Wrist Extension* (page 203)
Wrist/Hand

Palm-Up Wrist Flexion* (page 203)
Wrist/Hand

Finger Extension (page 205)
Wrist/Hand

Lateral Leg Lift (page 206)
Hip • Knee

Inner Leg Lift (page 207)
Hip • Knee

Kickback (page 209)
Hip • Knee • Back

Step Squat (page 216)
Knee • Hip • Back

Bent-Knee Calf Raise (page 217)
Knee • Hip • Ankle/Foot

Standing Knee Curl (page 219)
Knee • Hip

Standing Toe Raise (page 220)
Ankle/Foot

FLEXIBILITY EXERCISES

Basic Low Back Stretch (page 226)
Back • Neck

Cross-Legged Spine Stretch (page 229)
Back • Hip • Knee

Advanced Spinal Twist (page 232)
Back

Cobra Stretch (page 235)
Back • Hip

Neck Rotation (page 239)
Neck

Assisted Lateral Neck Stretch (page 240)
Neck

Fan Stretch (page 247)
Shoulder

Shoulder Release (page 252)
Shoulder

Triceps Stretch (page 253)
Elbow • Shoulder

Palm-Up Wrist/Finger Extension (page 255)
Wrist/Hand

Palm-Down Wrist/Finger Flexion (page 255)
Wrist/Hand

Lying Hip Flexor Stretch (page 261)
Hip

V-Sit Stretch (page 263)
Hip • Back

Buttocks Stretch (page 265)
Hip

Hamstring/Hip Stretch (page 268)
Hip • Knee

Standing Quad Stretch (page 272)
Hip • Knee

Runner's Stretch (page 274)
Ankle/Foot • Knee

Calf Stretch with Flexed Knee (page 275)
Ankle/Foot

Lower Leg Lengthener (page 277)
Ankle/Foot

Foot Circles (page 278)
Ankle/Foot

Sports

Regular, moderate exercise in any form is a great way to improve and sustain overall health. Whether jogging, walking, cross-country skiing, or gardening, exercise gets your heart pumping and body moving and contributes to a longer, healthier life. It also provides an opportunity to maximize the function of the muscles, tendons, and ligaments and to enable the joints to be brought to the ends of their normal range of motion; this has the short-term benefit of making the body less susceptible to soreness and stiffness and the long-term benefit of diminishing the chances of osteoarthritis and other degenerative ailments.

But while being active is highly beneficial, it does also increase the risk of injury, especially if you're out of shape and don't adequately prepare your body before you take the field. Before you play, then, it is recommended that you take the time to warm up and run through a regimen of flexibility exercises for your entire body, focusing in particular on the areas you use the most during your chosen sport or activity (see the box, **"Pre-Game Prep,"** on page 161).

For the recreational athlete, this pre-game approach does need to be coupled with a regular long-term exercise program to build and maintain strength and endurance in the muscles, as well as flexibility in the muscles, tendons, and ligaments. Notwithstanding the widespread belief that you should play a sport to get in shape, you do, in fact, have to get in shape to play a sport. (For more information, see **Chapter 15—Strength, Endurance, and Flexibility**.) Serious athletes will need to take this a step further, building additional strength, endurance, and/or flexibility in those body parts central to their chosen activity. For this it is a good idea to consult with a physical therapist.

Common sense is the best line of defense against injury. If you don't engage in sports or similar physical activities regularly, it is important not to push yourself too much when you do. And if you do experience any pain whatsoever, stop what you're doing at once.

Below is an alphabetical catalog of some popular individual and team sports featuring advice to help you prevent injuries and play it safe.

Stay Active

Although sports alone cannot provide all the necessary strength, endurance, flexibility, and cardiovascular conditioning you need, they are nonetheless highly beneficial to your overall health. Indeed, the U.S. Surgeon General has determined that regular physical activity helps prevent both cardiovascular disease and musculoskeletal problems and can generally improve an individual's quality of life. APTA stands firmly behind these findings.

Individual Sports

Aerobics: At one time aerobic exercise was a punishing "no pain, no gain" activity. Since then aerobics has evolved into a gentler, low-impact activity that provides an excellent workout with minimal risk of injury.

The two "musts" of aerobics are good shoes and a cushioned surface to move on. Shoes designed for aerobics and cross-training are both acceptable footwear choices (see **Chapter 14—Footwear**). If you take an aerobics class at a health club or gym, the class will almost certainly be held on an appropriate surface; if you work out at home, you'll need to make sure you're exercising on a properly cushioned floor surface.

It's a good idea to do your warm-up to some relaxed or moderately paced music before moving on to a full-body stretch (see the box, **"Pre-Game Prep,"** on page 161). Pay particular attention to your back, hips, knees, and ankles. Let the tempo of your music direct the pace of your workout: start at a slower pace, gradually working up to a faster beat over the course of a 20- to 30-minute workout, then cool down for 5 minutes with something more relaxed.

The only hard-and-fast rule of aerobics is to keep one foot on the floor at all times. This will soften the impact of the other foot when it hits the floor (because you won't be making any flying leaps) and reduce the chance of injury.

Bicycling: Bicycling—stationary or moving—delivers a first-class aerobic workout; it's also a great way to strengthen your lower body and control your weight. If you are properly conditioned, cycling puts little strain on your knees (especially in comparison to running or jogging), and if you use proper riding form, injuries are fairly rare. For individuals with arthritis in the knees, a recumbent bike provides an ideal way to get fit with minimal stress.

Correct fit is of paramount concern when selecting a bicycle, whether you choose a racing, touring, off-road (mountain biking), or stationary model. It's essential that you get expert advice before you buy. Riding a bicycle that doesn't fit your body can make you vulnerable to an array of repetitive-motion injuries, especially in the knee and hip regions. When riding, it's important to remember not to rest too much of your weight on your wrists; this can lead to wrist and hand trouble. Standing up and biking on your toes may be very stressful to the feet. Be certain your bike seat is adjusted to the proper height to protect your knees from injury, and always wear a helmet certified by the American National Standards Institute (ANSI), the American Society for Testing and Materials (ASTM), and/or the Snell Memorial Foundation.

To prepare for a bike ride, first warm up with a few minutes of gentle riding. Then do an overall body stretch, paying extra attention to stretching your back, neck, knees, and hips (see the box, **"Pre-Game Prep,"** on page 161). Serious bikers may find it necessary to condition their bodies off the bike as well. Good cross-training options include running, walking, and swimming.

Golf: Although golf is a difficult sport to master, it accommodates people of many different levels of skill and strength. In addition, the continued evolution of the golf club has made the sport more accessible to beginners and easier on your body parts.

It's smart to take some lessons from a professional before heading for the course. A professional will teach you how to develop the correct swing so you can avoid "golfer's elbow," an inflammation of the muscles and tendons along the inside of the forearm, and other strains that may result from improper form.

Before you play, do a short walking or running warm-up, followed by a regimen of stretches for your entire body, paying particular attention to your back, neck, shoulders, elbows, wrists, and hands (see the box, **"Pre-Game Prep,"** on page 161). Serious golfers should be mindful of conditioning the back and upper body while off the golf course in order to protect themselves from repetitive-motion injuries.

If you decide to buy golf clubs, buy from a golf pro if possible. He or she will be able to determine the best club to fit your physical characteristics, and this will help you prevent unnecessary injuries.

Martial Arts: Martial arts, such as tai-chi and karate, have now entered the American mainstream. These ancient disciplines, with their exquisitely calibrated and balanced movements, are relatively safe activities—if practiced properly. The martial arts require virtually no equipment other than a flat surface to work out on, but they do require lessons to learn the sport. (Some do use protective pads and headgear.)

Tai-chi especially can be performed by people of all ages, even the very elderly, with almost no risk of injury. Other popular martial arts, such as karate, jujitsu, and tae kwon do, may involve direct physical contact (more so than tai-chi), and injuries (especially to the hands, knees, and toes) are a possibility. Be sure to warm up and then stretch your entire body before starting a workout to prevent any unnecessary injuries (see the box, **"Pre-Game Prep,"** on page 161).

Rowing: Rowing—either on the water or on a rowing machine—is an effective way to build upper-body strength while getting a cardiovascular workout at the same time. It can, however, bring about repetitive-motion injuries, especially to the back, shoulders, elbows, and wrists. To avoid such injuries, serious rowers should do strength and endurance conditioning to those body parts that work the hardest during rowing.

Rowing doesn't require any special training, but if you row on the water, you do need gloves to protect your hands from blisters and shoes with a good nonskid sole. Because rowing works mainly your upper body, you should—after a brief warm-up—stretch those body parts, such as your back, neck, shoulders, elbows, wrists, and hands, during an overall body stretch (see the box, **"Pre-Game Prep,"** on page 161).

Running: Running is an efficient way to burn calories and achieve cardiovascular fitness. Unfortunately, running injuries are common, especially to the lower back, hips, knees, shins, ankles, and feet. And while the recovery rate is high—at least in the short term—it's also true that running may accelerate the natural wear-and-tear process in these body parts. Many runners suffer chronic problems in one or more of these regions.

Well-made, supportive running shoes are crucial to preventing running injuries. (For information on buying shoes, see **Chapter 14—Footwear**.) Just as important as the right shoes is the right warm-up routine. A brief period of light jogging or running in place, followed by overall stretches and focused back and lower-extremity stretching to your hips, knees, ankles, and feet, is essential (see the box, **"Pre-Game Prep,"** on page 161).

If you're a serious runner (or intend to become one), you should precondition your body with weight training and see a physical therapist, who can help you achieve your potential and avoid injury by performing a gait analysis, a detailed study of your particular running style. A gait analysis is also a must for any runner who is experiencing pain or reduced function to pinpoint the problem.

Skating (in-line, roller, and ice): Skating provides a strong cardiovascular workout while honing your coordination and agility; it's also a favored method of cross-training for skiers and cyclists.

The main danger with skating is falling or crashing. In order to reduce your chances of injury, always wear a helmet certified by the American National Standards Institute (ANSI), the American Society for Testing and Materials (ASTM), and/or the Snell Memorial Foundation (SNEL). You should also be sure to wear wrist, elbow, and knee protectors. The elbow and knee protectors should be covered with hard plastic shields, not fabric. If you fall, fabric pads may shred and leave your skin exposed. Wear padded, fingerless leather gloves and padded bicycle shorts, which can help protect your pelvis and tailbone in case you fall.

Before you put on your skates, warm up with an aerobic routine (like running or walking) and an all-over body stretch; skating is particularly hard on your hips, knees, ankles, and feet, so give these body parts a good stretch before you start to skate (see the box, **"Pre-Game Prep,"** on page 161).

Skiing (cross-country and alpine): Cross-country skiing provides an unsurpassed aerobic workout while working every major muscle group—all with minimal stress on the joints. Cross-country skiing is virtually risk-free, unlike its more glamorous cousin, alpine (downhill) skiing, which produces a fairly steady procession of knee sprains, torn ligaments, leg fractures, and other injuries.

Equipment that fits you correctly is important to preventing injuries in both cross-country and downhill skiing. Rent before you buy equipment, and then buy only from a dealer with expert salespeople. Lessons are a must, especially with downhill skiing, so that you learn proper form and can avoid both traumatic and repetitive-motion injuries.

Finally, remember to do a brief aerobic warm-up and a full-body stretch before hitting the slopes or trails. Your stretches should focus on all of your major body parts, since skiing gives you a full body workout (see the box, **"Pre-Game Prep,"** on page 161). If you're a serious skier and you plan to spend a good deal of time on skis this winter, be sure to prepare your body off-season with weight and endurance training.

Swimming: Swimming provides a superior aerobic workout that's extremely gentle on the joints. It's an activity that's appropriate for top athletes, as well as those who are elderly, injured, disabled, or out of shape.

Swimming injuries usually involve the shoulders. As an "overhead" sport, swimming may subject your shoulders to the same level of wear and tear as pitching a baseball or playing tennis. If you develop shoulder pain or instability, your physical therapist may suggest substituting a more gentle stroke (such as the breaststroke) for a more explosive one (such as the butterfly). Swimmers with low back problems may also wish to avoid face-down strokes like the crawl, breaststroke, and butterfly in favor of the back-stroke or sidestroke.

Before swimming, you can warm up by walking or jogging in the shallow end of the swimming pool, then do an all-over body stretch (in or out of the pool) plus focused stretching of your back, neck, shoulders, and hips (see the box, **"Pre-Game Prep,"** on page 161). Serious swimmers need to condition their bodies with weight training and flexibility exercises to build strength and increase their range of motion.

Tennis and Other Racquet Sports: Racquet sports, such as tennis, racquetball, squash, and badminton, cause injuries that are almost always related to overuse, with the elbows, shoulders, and knees most at risk. "Tennis elbow," an inflammation of the muscles and tendons along the outside of the forearm, is the classic ailment and can result from playing any racquet sport. Soreness, inflammation, and lack of stability in the shoulder may also occur. And the bouncing, lunging, twisting movements of racquet games can precipitate a number of back and knee ailments.

The risk of injury can be minimized by a brief warm-up (such as a few minutes of gentle volleying with your partner), followed by stretching your entire body, with focused stretching of your shoulders, elbow, wrists, hands, knees, ankles, and feet (see the box, **"Pre-Game Prep,"** on page 161). Being limber is particularly important for racquet-sport players because of the erratic movements required; to play tennis "cold" after being sedentary is to risk tendinitis, microscopic tears to the muscles, and worse.

Taking tennis lessons from a professional is a must, not only to learn the techniques of the game but also to acquire the proper form. Good form in tennis means trying to avoid twisting the trunk of the body when reaching for the ball. The twisting motion can put extra stress on your back and neck, so conditioning of those body parts when off the court is important. Your racquet should be of a size and weight well suited to you; a properly fitted grip is also recommended. Consult an expert when selecting a racquet. Comfortable, supportive footwear is also a must in tennis. Tennis shoes or properly cushioned cross-trainers are both good choices. (See **Chapter 14—Footwear.**)

Walking: Walking is hands down one of the easiest ways to maintain cardiovascular fitness. When you walk, start off at a moderate pace and walk for a few minutes to warm up; then stop to do some stretches for your entire body, focusing on your back, hips, knees, ankles, and feet (see the box,

"Pre-Game Prep," on page 161).

If you've been sedentary, you'll need to adjust your pace and the distance you walk, gradually working up to a faster pace and/or longer distance. Walkers should make sure to wear shoes with enhanced shock absorption in the heel (see **Chapter 14—Footwear**).

Carrying hand weights to work your upper body is generally not recommended because it can interfere with your stride, which involves swinging your arms fairly vigorously. It can also cause shoulder injury, especially if the weights are too heavy. And never use ankle weights; they make a proper gait impossible and may cause repetitive-motion or stress injuries.

For people who are already active, "power walking" can be a good way to increase cardiovascular fitness. Proper postural alignment, form, stride, pumping of the arms, and footwear are essential.

Weight Training: Weight training is an activity that can be practiced by people of all levels of fitness. It improves muscle tone, increases strength and flexibility, and improves overall general health, which makes it an important part of any fitness regimen.

Weight training can be done with free weights, such as barbells or dumbbells, or on any of the various specialized machines commonly found in gyms and health clubs. Heavy weights lifted a low number of repetitions build big bulky muscles (and enhance strength); lighter weights lifted a high number of repetitions tone and shape the muscles (and enhance endurance). When you begin a weight-training program, it's important to start out by lifting lighter weights and gradually work your way up to heavier weights as you become stronger and more confident.

Bodybuilding with heavy weights should always be done with a spotter. When you first begin training with weights, it's important to work with an expert to learn the proper form to use when lifting. It's easy to injure yourself if you're lifting improperly, and traumatic injuries, such as biceps ruptures, tendinitis, or rotator cuff tears, are common. These injuries can be avoided by properly preparing your body with a short warm-up and a series of all-over body stretches before you start to train (see the box, **"Pre-Game Prep,"** on page 161).

Yoga: Yoga has grown in popularity enormously in recent years. This ancient Indian practice for achieving a balance of mind and body has now spread to the Western world, bringing enhanced flexibility, stress relief, and peace of mind. There are several different schools of yoga thought, but the one most commonly practiced in the United States is called hatha yoga.

The practice of yoga involves a series of postures combined with controlled breathing techniques. Every posture in yoga has an opposite position to balance it. While yoga is not an aerobic exercise, it does help the practitioner develop strength, flexibility, and endurance in the muscles, as well as improve circulation and alignment of the spine.

Beginners should learn yoga from an experienced yoga teacher. The teacher will lead you through a series of postures and help you achieve the proper positions and breathing patterns. Once you learn the positions, you can practice yoga on your own, as it's a great way to stretch your body and relieve stress at any time.

Because yoga itself is a stretching activity, there is no particular warm-up routine to prescribe. You may, by all means, do some light all-over body stretching before beginning yoga, but in a class the teacher will slowly guide you into the postures. Breathing exercises and meditation usually begin and end a yoga workout.

There is no special equipment required in yoga, except for a comfortable mat to work on and some loose-fitting clothes. Special shoes are not required, either; in fact, most people prefer to do yoga while barefoot.

Team Sports

Baseball and Softball: Baseball and softball are considered "overhead" sports because the arm is raised above shoulder level during throwing and pitching (although underhand pitching is more common in softball). The muscles in the wrists, hands, elbows, and shoulder regions, particularly in the rotator cuff, are subject to repetitive-motion injuries. This can lead to soreness, tendinitis, and microscopic tearing of the muscles used in throwing, which makes conditioning of the shoulder and elbow with flexibility exercises and strength training a must for serious baseball and softball players.

Sliding into base is the most frequent cause of traumatic injuries in baseball or softball; strains are also common.

Before playing baseball or softball, make sure to give your entire body a good warm-up and stretching (see the box, **"Pre-Game Prep,"** on page 161). Pay particular attention to your back, since the twisting and bending movements common in baseball put extra demands on the it. Also focus your stretching on your neck, wrists, hands, ankles, and feet, which will improve your flexibility and reduce your risk of injury.

Basketball: Basketball combines coordination, agility, endurance, and bursts of speed. It's a great form of exercise for the millions of people who think of a pickup game with friends as more fun than a traditional workout.

Because basketball is considered an "overhead" sport, repetitive-motion and overuse injuries to the shoulders are not uncommon. Other injuries range from dislocated shoulders to ankle sprains; even stress fractures can occur in the feet because of the lack of "give" in basketball court flooring, which makes appropriately cushioned and (preferably) high-top sneakers imperative for basketball (see **Chapter 14 — Footwear**).

Warming up with a brief run and stretching the entire body is a must in any basketball player's regimen and crucial before a game or practice. Stretches should focus on the shoulders, back, wrists, hands, hips, knees, ankles, and feet (see the box, **"Pre-Game Prep,"** on page 161).

For serious basketball players, the game can be very physical. Although basketball is not classified as a contact sport, today's players are bigger, taller, stronger, and faster than ever before, while the size of the basketball court remains the same. The result is a game that ranks right up there with football in terms of its physical demands on the body, so serious players should condition the complete body, in addition to giving focused attention to the upper body and shoulders.

Football and Rugby: A complete list of football and rugby injuries would be almost encyclopedic; they range from muscle strain to rotator cuff problems to anterior cruciate ligament (ACL) injuries to torn Achilles tendons. You can lower your risk of injury by playing touch football or flag football, but if you play tackle football, sooner or later you're going to get hurt. As with any type of contact sport, you need to wear protective gear in the form of pads and a helmet to protect your body from harsh blows. If wearing cleated shoes, the cleats should be short to avoid getting caught in the turf—a certain recipe for traumatic injury to the knees or ankles.

A solid warm-up is essential before playing or practicing for football or rugby. Be sure to warm up by running or using another similar exercise, and stretch every major body part; all of them will surely be used in the course of a game (see the box, **"Pre-Game Prep,"** on page 161).

Cross-training is essential for the fitness of serious football and rugby players; running, bicycling, cross-country skiing, swimming, and rowing are all good choices. Weight lifting and agility drills are also highly recommended to build muscle strength, power, endurance, and the ability to change direction quickly while moving.

Hockey (ice and roller): Hockey lives up to its reputation as a fast and sometimes brutal sport. Even in casual games players may skate at high speeds and collisions are common, so it's necessary for hockey players to wear protective gear such as wrist protectors, elbow protectors, and kneepads. Skull fractures and concussions are among the most serious traumatic hockey injuries, making it absolutely essential to wear a helmet. Dental and facial injuries are also common, but many of them can be prevented by wearing mouth guards and face masks.

Fear of falling and getting hurt keeps some people from pursuing this rough sport, but it's easy to learn techniques that minimize danger. Before putting on your skates, warm up with a brief, brisk walk or run, then stretch your entire body, paying particular attention to your wrists, hips, knees, ankles, and feet (see the box, **"Pre-Game Prep,"** on page 161). Make sure that the skates you wear fit snugly but not uncomfortably. You should be able to wiggle your toes, but your heels shouldn't move inside the boot as you move your legs.

Because hockey is such a rough sport, serious players should be sure to condition their entire bodies with weight training off the ice, focusing on the muscles in the back and lower extremities.

Soccer: Soccer can accommodate players of all shapes, sizes, and skill levels. As a fast-paced, nonstop running sport played on a huge field, it provides an excellent aerobic workout.

Soccer is a rough sport. Injuries run the gamut from common sprains and tendinitis to fractures and even concussion. Shin guards are worn to protect the lower part of the leg. If you wear cleated shoes, stick with short cleats to protect against traumatic ankle and knee injuries.

As with all sports, proper warm-up and overall stretching prior to play are a must. Because soccer uses mainly the lower part of the body, give extra attention during stretching to your low back, hips, knees, ankles, and feet (see the box, **"Pre-Game Prep,"** on page 161).

For serious soccer players, training should include running for endurance, sprinting, agility drills, and strengthening exercises for the legs and neck.

Volleyball: Common volleyball injuries are ankle sprains, finger jams, and overuse injuries, such as tendinitis. And because volleyball is an "overhead" sport, strains to the rotator cuff and other shoulder injuries may occur. In order to avoid such repetitive-motion injuries and strains, strengthening of the upper body is imperative for the serious volleyball player. Another must is good footwear with a thin, well-cushioned mid-sole to reduce the amount of stress placed on the ankles and feet (see **Chapter 14—Footwear**).

It's also important to learn proper hitting form in order to minimize the chances of forearm bruises, jammed fingers, and similar injuries.

Before joining a game of volleyball, start with a brief aerobic warm-up of walking or light jogging, then stretch your entire body, paying particular attention to your neck, shoulders, elbows, wrists, and hands (see the box, **"Pre-Game Prep,"** below).

Pre-Game Prep

The program of flexibility outlined below is specifically tailored to provide overall flexibility for the body before engaging in sports and other vigorous activities. Detailed instructions and appropriate illustrations for each exercise can be found in Chapter 19—Flexibility Exercises. As you become familiar with the exercises, feel free to experiment and vary your routine.

No matter what sport or activity you choose, it's a good idea to address every body part by performing 3 repetitions of each of the exercises with a 10-second hold. Those body parts most heavily called upon in your particular sport, however, should be treated to 1 or 2 more repetitions. Further useful information along these lines can

be found throughout this chapter.

Your pre-game stretching regimen should take approximately 10 to 15 minutes to complete. To help prevent muscle strains or tears, be sure to precede your exercises with at least 5 minutes of light aerobic activity. This can take the form of running, walking, or cycling, although it may vary according to your chosen sport.

If you have pain of any kind (other than mild temporary stiffness and muscle tightness), you should consult your physical therapist or physician before attempting any of these exercises. And, of course, if you experience sharp or severe pain during any of these exercises, stop what you're doing at once.

Basic Low Back Stretch (page 226)
Back • Neck

Cross-Legged Spine Stretch (page 229)
Back • Hip • Knee

Advanced Spinal Twist (page 232)
Back

Cobra Stretch (page 235)
Back • Hip

Neck Rotation (page 239)
Neck

Assisted Lateral Neck Stretch (page 240)
Neck

Fan Stretch (page 247)
Shoulder

Shoulder Release (page 252)
Shoulder

Triceps Stretch (page 253)
Elbow • Shoulder

Palm-Up Wrist/Finger Extension (page 255)
Wrist/Hand

Palm-Down Wrist/Finger Flexion (page 255)
Wrist/Hand

Lying Hip Flexor Stretch (page 261)
Hip

V-Sit Stretch (page 263)
Hip • Back

Buttocks Stretch (page 265)
Hip

Hamstring/Hip Stretch (page 268)
Hip • Knee

Standing Quad Stretch (page 272)
Hip • Knee

Runner's Stretch (page 274)
Ankle/Foot • Knee

Calf Stretch with Flexed Knee (page 275)
Ankle/Foot

Lower Leg Lengthener (page 277)
Ankle/Foot

Foot Circles (page 278)
Ankle/Foot

CHAPTER SEVENTEEN
Work

Most of us have little choice but to work for a living. Unfortunately, our jobs can be extremely stressful on the muscles and joints. Day after day we make demands on our bodies, often for eight or more hours at a stretch. Repeated motions or continual stress can lead to overuse or even traumatic injuries. Active occupations, from assembly-line to construction work, are riskiest, but office jobs cause more than their fair share of trouble. Nor is maintaining a household free of risk.

There are many things you can do to minimize the possibility of job-related injuries, regardless of your line of work. One of these is to take regular five-minute breaks throughout the day to relieve the stress on those parts of your body that the job taxes most heavily. Another is to warm up and stretch those same body parts before you start your workday and then to periodically stretch them again throughout the day—at the same time, perhaps, that you take your regular breaks (see the box, **"Workday Prep,"** on page 166). These approaches do need to be coupled with a regular long-term exercise program to build and maintain strength and endurance in the muscles, as well as flexibility in the muscles, tendons, and ligaments. (For more information, see **Chapter 15—Strength, Endurance, and Flexibility.**)

Each particular job, of course, makes its own unique set of demands on the body. And while it would be impossible comprehensively to lay out the challenges of and precautions for the vast variety of occupations, it is possible to offer advice based on some of the kinds of tasks we are commonly called on to perform at work. Your job may require just one of these tasks, or it may require several, in which case it is important to follow the advice offered for each task. Either way, this information may be critical to your workplace well-being. (You should also read **Chapter 12—Body Mechanics,** which touches on some of the points made below and offers other useful hints.)

Active Jobs

Many jobs involve repeated or continual **bending** forward at the waist. This includes everything from dishwashing to drafting to baggage handling.

Bending, however, disrupts good posture and may be very stressful on the back, especially the lower back, as well as the neck and even shoulders—all of which should be the focus of your stretching routine. But the best way to avert trouble is to find ways to avoid bending altogether; it is important to maintain good standing posture as much as possible (see **Chapter 10— Posture**). If you are working at a low surface or counter, see if you can raise the surface; drafting tables, for example, are generally adjustable. If not, bend your knees to lower your body and keep your back straight or, if possible, sit on a lower stool.

Lines of work that involve **lifting and carrying** heavy objects, such as construction, furniture moving, warehouse work, and homemaking (for example, carrying groceries), make major demands on the body, even putting it at risk of serious traumatic injury. The back is especially at risk, but so, too, are the neck, shoulders, elbows, wrists, and hands. All these body parts need to be stretched thoroughly and repeatedly throughout the workday. But lifting is most threatening if done improperly. Never bend over to lift with the knees and arms straight; this is a recipe for herniated disks and for ligament, muscle, and tendon strains. Instead, put one foot slightly behind the other and bend the knees to lower your body to the object (it's not necessary to do a full squat). With the arms slightly bent at the elbow, the wrists straight, and the stomach and chin in, use your legs and hips, rather than your back, to lift. Keep a heavy object close to you and centered. Also, when moving a heavy object, it's better to push it than to pull it.

Assembly-line work, shelf stacking, meat cutting, and many other jobs involve **repetitive arm or hand motions**—like bending and straightening the arm or clasping and unclasping the hand. Especially if the motion called for is awkward, the result can be strain and other injury to the elbows, wrists, and hands. Make sure these body parts are carefully and regularly stretched, and shake out your arms and hands during your breaks. Because a too-high work surface can increase the stress, adjust it if necessary. Also, keep your elbows low and close to the body; vary your movements to avoid excessive repetition; and alternate hands whenever possible. And if your job leads you to bump or lean on your elbow frequently, as in plumbing, you should consider wearing elbow pads to avoid cubital tunnel syndrome and other such injuries.

The shoulders are at risk of rotator cuff strains and other injuries in jobs that involve **raising the arms overhead**, especially raising them repeatedly, as in house painting and carpentry. Focus your stretching on the shoulders, and, as much as possible, minimize your need to perform overhead tasks by adjusting your workplace. Use stepladders and lower work shelves. If you must raise your arms, try alternating the arm you use.

Occupations that involve **standing** for long periods—like sales, teaching, police work, and nursing, among others—may be stressful on the back and neck, as well as, of course, the ankles and feet. All these body parts should be the focus of your workday stretches. Be sure as well to practice good standing posture (see **Chapter 10—Posture**). Avoid standing in a fixed position; shift your weight frequently back and forth between your feet. Even placing one foot up on a box or footstool may relieve stress on your back and neck. For your feet's sake, it's a good idea to wear appropriately supportive and well-cushioned shoes (see **Chapter 14—Footwear**); a padded mat under your feet may also reduce the stress on your soles. During your breaks, be sure to shake out your feet and ankles.

Office Jobs

Desk jobs—and other long-term sitting occupations, like driving (or even air-traffic control)—may not be terribly active, but they do have their own set of risks. Sitting in the same position for hours on end is itself a common cause of back and neck stress. Slouching or leaning forward in your seat only adds to the pressure on your lower back. The familiar habits of craning your neck forward or tilting your head up to look at a computer screen, dropping your head down to read or write, or holding a telephone receiver to your ear with your shoulder can all be very hard on your neck. In some instances the stress may extend all the way to the jaw or shoulders. Working for extended periods at a keyboard can also lead to injuries like carpal tunnel syndrome in the wrists and hands, especially if they are held in a flexed position.

To avoid problems in such jobs, it is important first of all to develop and maintain good sitting posture (see **Chapter 10—Posture**). Good posture requires a firm-backed chair, ideally one with armrests for added shoulder and neck support. Sit back in the chair, with your knees just about level with your hips and your feet resting comfortably on the floor. If necessary, you may put a small box or footstool beneath your feet. An adjustable seat makes it easy to find the right level. And be sure to pull the chair into your desk to avoid leaning forward.

If you work at a computer, the monitor should be placed directly in front of you, slightly below eye level. If your monitor rests on top of your CPU, it's probably too high; try placing the CPU in another configuration—on

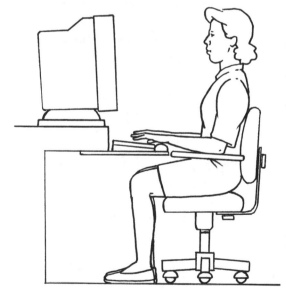

Proper workstation setup

the floor, perhaps, or next to the monitor. Adjusting the height of your chair or desk is another option.

The keyboard should be placed on the desk directly in front of you at about waist level. When typing, your upper arm and forearm should form a right angle, and your wrists should maintain a neutral position, flexed neither up nor down. Specialized wrist braces are available to help you hold this position. It's also useful to set a padded wrist rest in front of your keyboard. Armrests on your chair are especially important if you work at a keyboard.

Finally, be sure to focus your stretching on the back, neck, and shoulders and, if you work at a keyboard, your wrists and hands as well. During your breaks, walk around and shake out your wrists and hands.

Workday Prep

The flexibility exercises listed below are designed to prevent the buildup of on-the-job stress in the various parts of your body—especially in the upper back, neck, and shoulders (for office workers) and the back and legs for those who do heavy lifting. Detailed instructions and appropriate illustrations for each exercise can be found in Chapter 19—Flexibility Exercises. (As you become familiar with the exercises below, you may wish to experiment with other flexibility exercises.)

The particular exercises you adopt should be tailored to the nature of your own job; choose just those exercises that benefit the body parts most heavily taxed over the course of your workday. Useful information along these lines can be found throughout this chapter.

Run through a set of the appropriate exercises before beginning work—3 to 5 repetitions of each, with a 10-second hold—and every few hours or so thereafter. To help prevent muscle strains or tears, be sure to precede your first round of exercises with at least 5 minutes of light aerobic activity; a brisk walk around the workplace is fine.

If you have pain of any kind (other than mild temporary stiffness and tightness), you should consult your physical therapist or physician before attempting any of these exercises. And, of course, if you experience sharp or severe pain during any of these exercises, stop what you're doing at once.

Seated Low Back Stretch (page 228)
Back

Seated Spinal Twist (page 231)
Back

Side Stretch (page 232)
Back • Shoulder

Stretch and Reach (page 234)
Back

Corner Stretch (page 236)
Back • Shoulder

Raised-Arm Neck Flex (page 238)
Neck

Neck Rotation (page 239)
Neck

Seated Neck Twist (page 238)
Neck

Assisted Lateral Neck Stretch (page 240)
Neck

Neck Circles (page 241)
Neck

Shoulder Roll (page 243)
Shoulder

Shoulder Release (page 252)
Shoulder

Elbow Stretch (page 253)
Elbow

Triceps Stretch (page 253)
Elbow • Shoulder

Palm-Up Wrist/Finger Extension (page 255)
Wrist/Hand

Palm-Down Wrist/Finger Flexion (page 255)
Wrist/Hand

Lunge Stretch (page 262)
Hip

Butterfly Stretch (page 263)
Hip

Buttocks Stretch (page 265)
Hip

Hip Abductor Stretch (page 265)
Hip

Standing Hamstring Stretch (page 271)
Hip

Standing Quad Stretch (page 272)
Hip • Knee

Calf Stretch with Flexed Knee (page 275)
Ankle/Foot

Lower Leg Lengthener (page 277)
Ankle/Foot

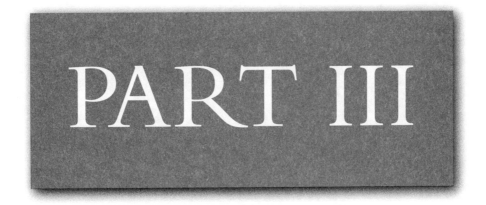

PART III

Strength & Endurance Exercises

The dozens of exercises in this chapter represent some of the many strengthening and endurance-building exercises for body maintenance and repair. They can be drawn upon in various combinations to create part of a regular regimen for taking care of your body. For more advice along these lines and a suggested basic exercise regimen, see **Chapter 15—Strength, Endurance, and Flexibility.**

These exercises may also serve as part of a rehabilitation program for a wide range of problems. They should be used for this purpose, however, only under the supervision of a physical therapist.

Although each exercise should be repeated several times to be effective, there is no blanket rule for the number of repetitions appropriate for any particular individual in any particular case. If you are using these exercises as part of a regular maintenance regimen, three sets of 10 repetitions each is a good target number. However, when starting an exercise program, you may have to begin gently with a single set with as few as two or three repetitions and gradually build up. This is the most effective way to prevent undue soreness or injury.

If you are using these exercises as part of a rehabilitative program, the number of repetitions should be determined in consultation with your physical therapist.

A number of the exercises in this chapter use or offer the option of using hand or ankle weights to increase resistance. The typical hand weight is a small dumbbell. (A soup can may also be used for the purpose.) The typical ankle weight is a weighted cuff that loops around the ankle. Some of these cuffs are adjustable, allowing for weight to be added or removed.

Cautions

If you have pain (other than simple stiffness or soreness) in any part of your body, a history of health trouble, or an existing medical condition (including pregnancy), it is essential to check with your physical therapist before attempting any of these exercises. And if you experience pain, instability, tingling, or numbness in any part of your body—or if you feel dizzy—during any exercise, you should stop doing it at once to avoid the possibility of injury.

When using weights, be sure to choose a weight light enough that it permits you to perform the exercise smoothly and slowly, without jerky motions. Pay careful attention to the breathing instructions noted within each exercise. It is essential not to hold your breath when exercising; this may restrict blood flow to your heart and increase your blood pressure.

Before engaging in any weight-based exercises, it is a good idea to consult an expert to ensure that you do not injure yourself by lifting too much weight or by lifting improperly.

`BACK • NECK`

BASIC ABDOMINAL STRENGTHENER

Targets the muscles in the abdomen.

1. Lie on your back with your knees bent and your feet flat on the floor. Keep your stomach tight and your neck straight to maintain proper alignment. Keep your arms at your sides, palms down. Inhale.

2. Tightening your stomach, press your low back toward the floor. Exhale as you press your low back down. Hold the position for 5 to 10 seconds, breathing evenly. Repeat.

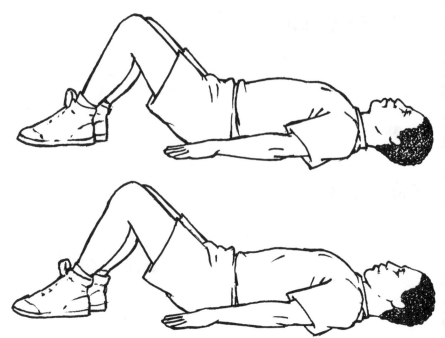

`BACK • NECK`

ABDOMINAL CRUNCH WITH ARMS AT SIDES

Targets the muscles in the abdomen.

1. Lie on your back with your knees bent and your feet flat on the floor. Keep your stomach tight, your neck straight, and the small of your back pressed toward the floor to maintain proper alignment. Keep your arms at your sides, palms down. Inhale.

2. With your stomach tight and chin tucked, slowly lift just your head and shoulders up, keeping your arms next to your sides (not down on the floor), until the upper part of your shoulder blades lifts off the floor. (Do not use your arms to push yourself up.) Exhale as you lift. Hold the position for 5 to 10 seconds, breathing evenly. Return slowly to the starting position.

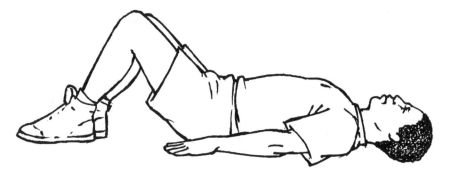

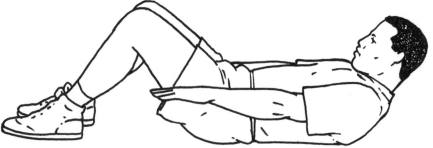

BACK • NECK

ABDOMINAL CRUNCH WITH HANDS TO KNEES

Targets the muscles in the abdomen and the front of the neck.

1. Lie on your back with your knees bent and your feet flat on the floor. Keep your stomach tight, your neck straight, and the small of your back pressed toward the floor to maintain proper alignment. Keep your arms at your sides, palms down. Inhale.

2. With your stomach tight and chin tucked, lift just your head and shoulders up, lifting and reaching your hands toward your knees until the upper part of your shoulder blades lifts off the floor. Exhale as you lift. Hold the position for 5 to 10 seconds, breathing evenly. Return slowly to the starting position.

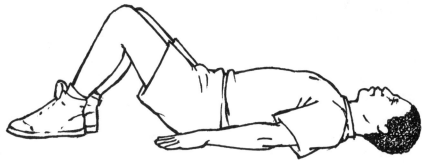

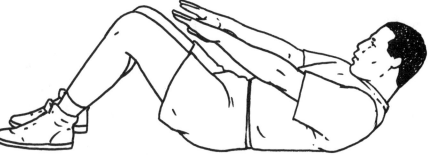

BACK • NECK

ABDOMINAL CRUNCH WITH CROSSED ARMS

Targets the muscles in the abdomen and the front of the neck.

1. Lie on your back with your knees bent and your feet flat on the floor. Keep your stomach tight, your neck straight, and the small of your back pressed toward the floor to maintain proper alignment. Cross your arms over your chest. Inhale.

2. With your stomach tight and chin tucked, slowly lift just your head and shoulders up until the upper part of your shoulder blades lifts off the floor. Exhale as you lift. Hold the position for 5 to 10 seconds, breathing evenly. Return slowly to the starting position.

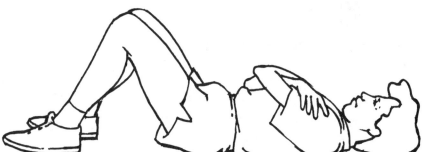

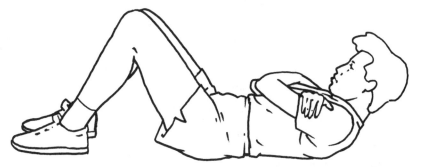

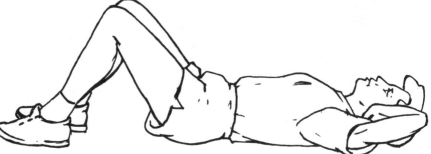

`BACK • NECK`

ABDOMINAL CRUNCH WITH HANDS AT EARS

Targets the muscles in the abdomen and the front of the neck.

1. Lie on your back with your knees bent and your feet flat on the floor. Keep your stomach tight, your neck straight, and the small of your back pressed toward the floor to maintain proper alignment. Place your hands beside your ears with your elbows angled out. Inhale.

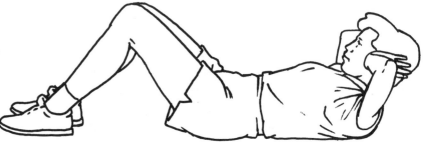

2. With your stomach tight and chin tucked, slowly lift just your head and shoulders up until the upper part of your shoulder blades lifts off the floor. Exhale as you lift. Hold the position for 5 to 10 seconds, breathing evenly. Return slowly to the starting position.

`BACK • NECK`

ABDOMINAL CRUNCH WITH RAISED ARMS

Targets the muscles in the abdomen and the front of the neck.

1. Lie on your back with your knees bent and your feet flat on the floor. Keep your stomach tight, your neck straight, and the small of your back pressed toward the floor to maintain proper alignment. Raise your arms straight overhead. Keep your upper arms next to your ears and your palms up. Inhale.

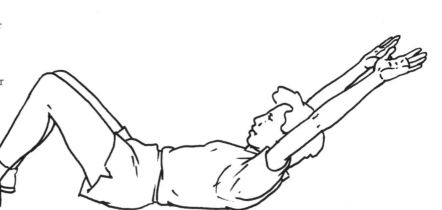

2. With your stomach tight and chin tucked, slowly lift just your head and shoulders up until the upper part of your shoulder blades lifts off the floor. Your arms should remain by your ears. Exhale as you lift. Hold the position for 5 to 10 seconds, breathing evenly. Return slowly to the starting position.

BACK • NECK

KNEE-TO-CHEST ABDOMINAL CRUNCH WITH HANDS TO KNEES

Targets the muscles in the abdomen and the front of the neck.

1. Lie on your back with your knees bent and your feet flat on the floor. Keep your stomach tight, your neck straight, and the small of your back pressed toward the floor to maintain proper alignment. Keep your arms at your sides, palms down. Inhale.

2. With your stomach tight and chin tucked, slowly raise your head and shoulders up, lifting and reaching your arms toward your knees, until the upper part of your shoulder blades lifts off the floor; then lift one knee toward your chest. Exhale as you lift. Hold the position for 5 to 10 seconds, breathing evenly. Return slowly to the starting position.

3. Repeat, lifting the other knee toward your chest.

You may also perform this exercise using other arm positions (arms at sides, crossed arms, hands at ears, raised hands) as illustrated on pages 174–176.

BACK • NECK • HIP

EXTENDED-LEG ABDOMINAL CRUNCH WITH HANDS TO KNEES

Targets the muscles in the abdomen and the front of the neck.

1. Lie on your back with your knees bent and your feet flat on the floor. Keep your stomach tight, your neck straight, and the small of your back pressed toward the floor to maintain proper alignment. Keep your arms at your sides, palms down. Inhale.

2. With your stomach tight and chin tucked, slowly raise your head and shoulders up, lifting and reaching your arms toward your knees, until the upper part of your shoulder blades lifts off the floor; then extend one leg into the air so that it's at a 45-degree angle. Exhale as you lift. Hold the position for 5 to 10 seconds, breathing evenly. Return slowly to the starting position.

3. Repeat, extending the other leg.

You may also perform this exercise using other arm positions (arms at sides, crossed arms, hands at ears, raised hands) as illustrated on pages 174–176.

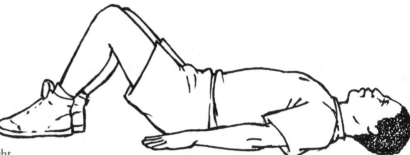

BACK • NECK

ROTATION CRUNCH WITH ARMS AT SIDES

Targets the muscles in the front and sides of the abdomen and neck.

1. Lie on your back with your knees bent and your feet flat on the floor. Keep your stomach tight, your neck straight, and the small of your back pressed toward the floor to maintain proper alignment. Keep your arms at your sides, palms down. Inhale.

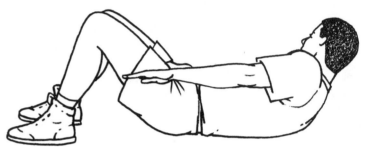

2. With your stomach tight, chin tucked, and arms next to your sides (not down on the floor), slowly lift just your head and shoulders up at an angle so that your left shoulder blade lifts off the floor. (Do not use your arms to push yourself up.) Exhale as you lift. Hold the position for 5 to 10 seconds, breathing evenly. Return slowly to the starting position.

3. Repeat on the opposite side (lifting your right shoulder blade off the floor).

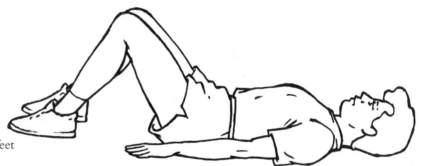

BACK • NECK

ROTATION CRUNCH WITH HANDS TO KNEES

Targets the muscles in the front and sides of the abdomen and neck.

1. Lie on your back with your knees bent and your feet flat on the floor. Keep your stomach tight, your neck straight, and the small of your back pressed toward the floor to maintain proper alignment. Keep your arms at your sides, palms down. Inhale.

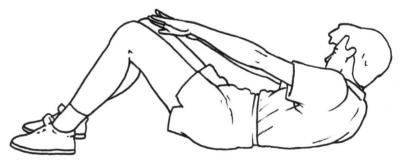

2. With your stomach tight and chin tucked, reach both of your hands to the outside of your right knee, slowly lifting just your head and shoulders up on an angle so that your left shoulder blade lifts off the floor. Exhale as you lift. Hold the position for 5 to 10 seconds, breathing evenly. Return slowly to the starting position.

3. Repeat on the opposite side (reach for your left knee so that your right shoulder blade lifts off the floor).

BACK • NECK

ROTATION CRUNCH WITH CROSSED ARMS

Targets the muscles in the front and sides of the abdomen and neck.

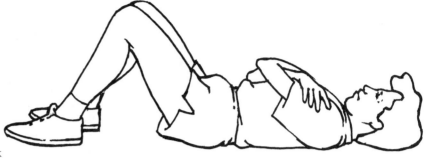

1. Lie on your back with your knees bent and your feet flat on the floor. Keep your stomach tight, your neck straight, and the small of your back pressed toward the floor to maintain proper alignment. Cross your arms over your chest. Inhale.

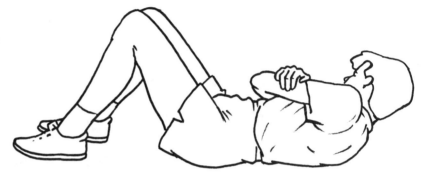

2. With your stomach tight and chin tucked, slowly lift just your head and shoulders up on an angle toward your right knee until your left shoulder blade lifts off the floor. Exhale as you lift. Hold the position for 5 to 10 seconds, breathing evenly. Return slowly to the starting position.

3. Repeat on the opposite side (lift your right shoulder toward your left knee).

BACK • NECK

ROTATION CRUNCH WITH HANDS AT EARS

Targets the muscles in the front and sides of the abdomen and neck.

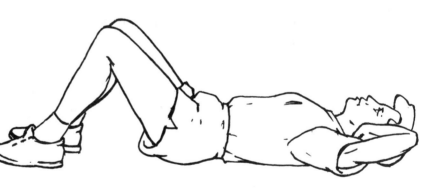

1. Lie on your back with your knees bent and your feet flat on the floor. Keep your stomach tight, your neck straight, and the small of your back pressed toward the floor to maintain proper alignment. Place your hands beside your ears with your elbows angled out. Inhale.

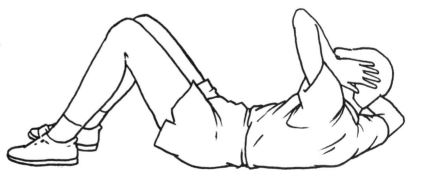

2. With your stomach tight and chin tucked, slowly lift just your head and shoulders up on an angle toward your right knee until your left shoulder blade lifts off the floor. Exhale as you lift. Hold the position for 5 to 10 seconds, breathing evenly. Return slowly to the starting position.

3. Repeat on the opposite side (lift your right shoulder toward your left knee).

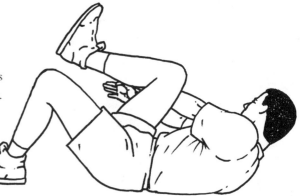

BACK • NECK

ROTATION CRUNCH WITH RAISED ARMS
Targets the muscles in the front and sides of the abdomen and neck.

1. Lie on your back with your knees bent and your feet flat on the floor. Keep your stomach tight, your neck straight, and the small of your back pressed toward the floor to maintain proper alignment. Raise your arms overhead. Keep your upper arms next to your ears and your palms up. Inhale.

2. With your stomach tight, chin tucked, and upper arms next to your ears, slowly lift just your head and shoulders up on an angle toward your right knee until your left shoulder blade lifts off the floor. (Do not use your arms to thrust yourself up.) Exhale as you lift. Hold the position for 5 to 10 seconds, breathing evenly. Return slowly to the starting position.

3. Repeat on the opposite side (lift your right shoulder toward your left knee).

BACK • NECK

KNEE-TO-CHEST ROTATION CRUNCH WITH HANDS TO KNEES
Targets the muscles in the front and sides of the abdomen and neck.

1. Lie on your back with your knees bent and your feet flat on the floor. Keep your stomach tight, your neck straight, and the small of your back pressed toward the floor to maintain proper alignment. Keep your arms at your sides, palms down. Inhale.

2. With your stomach tight and chin tucked, slowly raise your head and shoulders up at an angle, lifting and reaching your hands toward the outside of your right knee, until the upper part of your left shoulder blade lifts off the floor; then lift your right knee toward your chest. Exhale as you lift. Hold the position for 5 to 10 seconds, breathing evenly. Return slowly to the starting position.

3. Repeat on the opposite side (lifting your right shoulder blade off the floor and bringing your left knee toward your chest).

You may also perform this exercise using other arm positions (arms at sides, crossed arms, hands at ears, raised hands) as illustrated on pages 178–180.

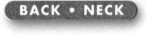

BACK • NECK

EXTENDED-LEG ROTATION CRUNCH WITH HANDS TO KNEES

Targets the muscles in the front and sides of the abdomen and neck.

1. Lie on your back with your knees bent and your feet flat on the floor. Keep your stomach tight, your neck straight, and the small of your back pressed toward the floor to maintain proper alignment. Keep your arms at your sides, palms down. Inhale.

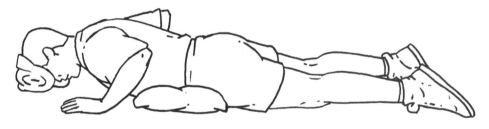

2. With your stomach tight and chin tucked, reach both of your hands to the outside of your right knee, slowly lifting just your head and shoulders up on an angle until your left shoulder blade lifts off the floor. Straighten your right leg out in the air so it's at a 45-degree angle. Exhale as you lift. Hold the position for 5 to 10 seconds, breathing evenly. Lower your leg and return slowly to the starting position.

3. Repeat on the opposite side (reach both hands toward your left knee while straightening the left leg).

You may also perform this exercise using other arm positions (arms at sides, crossed arms, hands at ears, raised hands) as illustrated on pages 178–180.

BACK • NECK

THE COBRA

Targets the muscles in the abdomen, back, and neck.

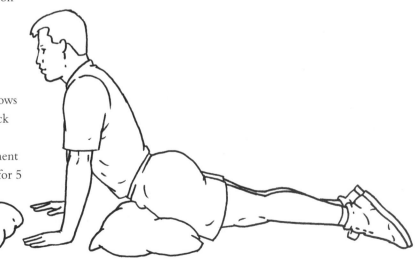

1. Lie on your stomach with your forehead resting on the floor. (You may use a towel roll under your forehead.) Place a large pillow under your stomach. Keep your hands flat on the floor at shoulder level. Inhale.

2. Push up onto your hands, straightening your elbows and arching your spine backward. Be sure not to lock your elbows into extension, and try to keep your stomach tight and neck straight so that good alignment is maintained. Exhale as you lift. Hold the position for 5 to 10 seconds, breathing evenly. Return slowly to the starting position.

`BACK • NECK • SHOULDER`

EASY PUSH-UP
Targets the muscles in the back, abdomen, neck, and arms.

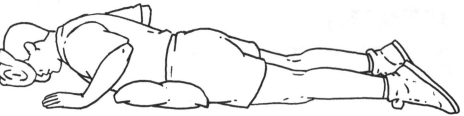

1. Lie on your stomach with your forehead resting on the floor. (You may use a towel roll under your forehead.) Place a large pillow under your stomach. Keep your hands flat on the floor at shoulder level. Inhale.

2. Perform a push-up from the on-knees position, straightening your elbows as you push up. Be sure not to lock your elbows into extension, and try to keep your stomach tight and neck straight so that good alignment is maintained. Exhale as you lift. Hold the position for 5 to 10 seconds, breathing evenly. Return slowly to the starting position.

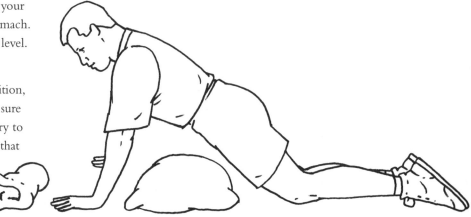

`BACK • NECK • SHOULDER`

ADVANCED PUSH-UP
Targets the muscles in the chest, back, abdomen, neck, and arms.

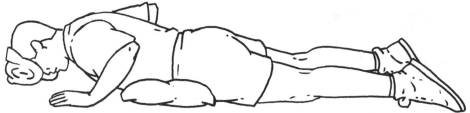

1. Lie on your stomach with your forehead resting on the floor. (You may use a towel roll under your forehead.) Place a large pillow under your stomach. Keep your hands flat on the floor at shoulder level. Inhale.

2. Perform a push-up with your legs extended, straightening your elbows as you push up. Be sure not to lock your elbows into extension, and try to keep your stomach tight and neck straight so that good alignment is maintained. Exhale as you lift. Hold the position for 5 to 10 seconds, breathing evenly. Return slowly to the starting position.

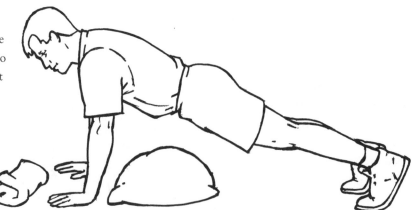

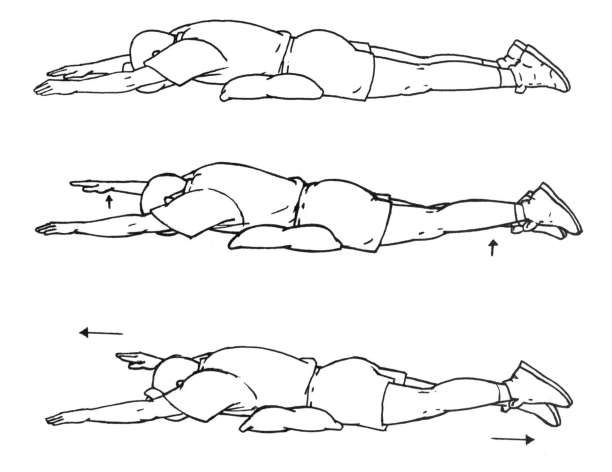

BACK • HIP • KNEE

LEG AND ARM EXTENSION

Targets the muscles in the back, arms, hips, and back of the knees.

Note: *This exercise may be done with ankle weights and/or hand weights (see page 171).*

1. Lie on your stomach with your forehead resting on the floor. (You may use a towel roll under your forehead.) Place a large pillow under your stomach. Raise your arms overhead and place them on the floor in front of you. Inhale.

2. Slowly lift one arm and the opposite leg up at the same time about 1 inch off the floor. Then pull your arm and leg away from each other. Try to keep your stomach tight and neck straight so that proper alignment is maintained. Exhale as you lift your arm and leg. Hold the position for 5 to 10 seconds, breathing evenly. *Do not hold the position if using weights.*

3. Bring your arm and leg toward each other again and return slowly to the starting position.

4. Repeat, using the opposite arm and leg.

BACK • NECK

SHOULDER SHRUG

Targets the muscles in the upper back and neck.

Note: *This exercise uses hand weights (see page 171).*

1. Sit all the way back on a sturdy, armless chair, feet up on a small footstool, with your shoulders down and relaxed and your arms at your sides (the back of the chair should be straight and positioned near a wall, if possible). Keep your stomach in, chin tucked, gaze forward, and head upright. Inhale.

2. Shrug your shoulders. Exhale as you bring up your shoulders. Inhale as you return slowly to the starting position.

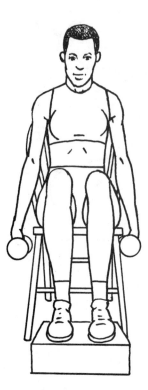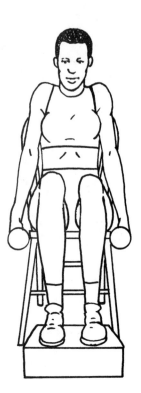

BACK • SHOULDER

BACK EXTENSOR

Targets the muscles in the upper back and shoulders.

1. Sit all the way back on a sturdy, armless chair, feet up on a small footstool, with your shoulders down and relaxed (the back of the chair should be straight and positioned near a wall, if possible). Keep your stomach in, chin tucked, gaze forward, and head upright. Place your hands behind your head, fingers clasped and elbows angled out. Inhale.

2. Pulling your stomach in, simultaneously push your elbows back as you pinch your shoulder blades together. Exhale as you pinch your shoulder blades. Hold the position for 5 to 10 seconds, breathing evenly. Return slowly to the starting position.

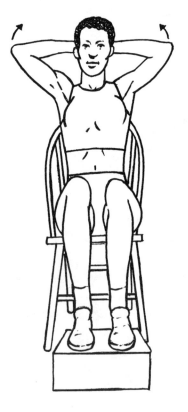

BACK

PRAYING-HANDS BACK TIGHTENER
Targets the muscles in the middle and upper back.

1. Sit all the way back on a sturdy, armless chair, feet up on a small footstool, with your shoulders down and relaxed (the back of the chair should be straight and positioned near a wall, if possible). Keep your stomach in, chin tucked, gaze forward, and head upright. Place your arms in an "A" position, fingers interlaced as if praying. Inhale.

2. Keeping your shoulders relaxed (not hunched) and your stomach in, slowly bring your elbows back as you pinch your shoulder blades together. (Your hands should open up a little.) Exhale as you pinch your shoulder blades. Hold the position for 5 to 10 seconds, breathing evenly. Return slowly to the starting position.

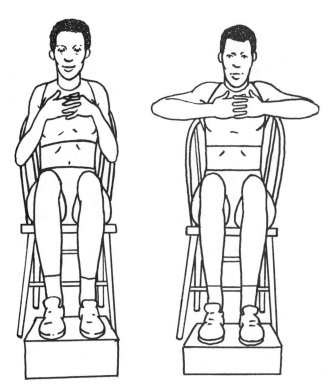

BACK • SHOULDER

BACK AND ARM EXTENSOR
Targets the muscles in the upper back and shoulders.

1. Stand with your knees slightly bent and your arms up to shoulder level, with your palms facing the ceiling. Keep your stomach in, chin tucked, gaze forward, head upright, and knees slightly bent. Inhale.

2. Pulling both arms back, with your thumbs leading, slowly pinch your shoulder blades together. Exhale as you pinch your shoulder blades. Hold the position for 5 to 10 seconds, breathing evenly. Return slowly to the starting position.

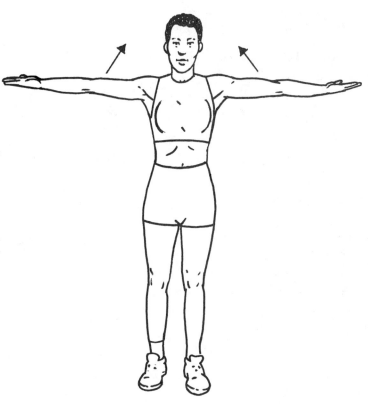

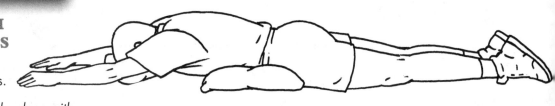

BACK • SHOULDER

BACK LIFT WITH SQUARED ARMS

Targets the muscles in the upper back and shoulders.

Note: *This exercise may be done with hand weights (see page 171).*

1. Lie on your stomach with your forehead resting on the floor. (You may use a towel roll under your forehead.) Place a large pillow under your stomach. Place your arms on the floor in a square "U" position, palms down. Inhale.

2. Slowly lift only your arms up, keeping your elbows soft. Try to keep your stomach tight and neck straight so that proper alignment is maintained. Exhale as you lift your arms. Hold the position for 5 to 10 seconds, breathing evenly. *Do not hold the position if using weights.* Return slowly to the starting position.

You may also lift and lower one arm at a time.

BACK • NECK • SHOULDER

BACK LIFT WITH EXTENDED ARMS

Targets the muscles in the neck, back, and shoulders.

Note: *This exercise may be done with hand weights (see page 171).*

1. Lie on your stomach with your forehead resting on the floor. (You may use a towel roll under your forehead.) Place a large pillow under your stomach. Raise your arms overhead. Keep your upper arms next to your ears and your palms down. Inhale.

2. Slowly lift only your arms up, keeping your elbows soft. Try to keep your stomach tight and neck straight so that proper alignment is maintained. Exhale as you lift your arms. Hold the position for 5 to 10 seconds, breathing evenly. *Do not hold the position if using weights.* Return slowly to the starting position.

You may also lift and lower one arm at a time.

BACK LIFT WITH OPEN ARMS

Targets the muscles in the upper and lower back.

Note: *This exercise may be done with hand weights (see page 171).*

1. Lie on your stomach with your forehead resting on the floor. (You may use a towel roll under your forehead.) Place a large pillow under your stomach. Raise your arms overhead. Keep your arms slightly out to the sides in a "Y" position, palms down. Inhale.

2. Slowly lift only your arms up, keeping your elbows soft. Try to keep your stomach tight and neck straight so that proper alignment is maintained. Exhale as you lift your arms. Hold the position for 5 to 10 seconds, breathing evenly. Do not hold the position if using weights. Return slowly to the starting position.

You may also lift and lower one arm at a time.

BACK • SHOULDER

SEATED BUTTERFLY LIFT

Targets the muscles in the middle and upper back and arms.

Note: *This exercise uses hand weights (see page 171).*

1. Sit all the way back on a sturdy, armless chair, feet up on a small footstool, with your shoulders down and relaxed (the back of the chair should be straight and positioned near a wall, if possible). Keep your stomach in, chin tucked, gaze forward, and head upright. Lean forward over your knees and let your arms hang down. Inhale.

2. Slowly lift your arms out to the sides, bringing the weights up to shoulder height. Exhale as you lift your arms. Inhale as you return slowly to the starting position.

You may also lift and lower one arm at a time.

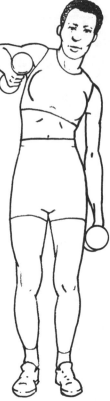
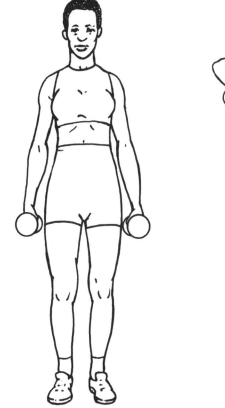

BACK • SHOULDER

SIDE BEND

Targets the muscles in the upper and mid back, shoulders, and arms.

Note: *This exercise uses hand weights (see page 171).*

1. Stand with your legs 6 to 8 inches apart, knees slightly bent, and the weights in your hands. Keep your stomach in, chin tucked, gaze forward, and head upright. Place your arms at your sides with your palms facing inward. Inhale.

2. Slowly bend your body at the waist to one side as you bring the weight on other side up under your armpit. Exhale as you bend to the side. Inhale as you return slowly to the starting position.

3. Repeat on the opposite side.

NECK

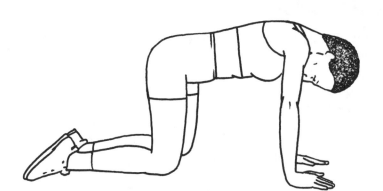

NECK STRENGTHENER

Targets the muscles in the back of the neck and upper back.

1. Kneel down on your hands and knees, with your head dropped down toward your chest and your stomach in. Inhale.

2. Lift your head up until it's even with your shoulders, keeping your chin in. Exhale as you lift your head. Hold the position for 5 to 10 seconds, breathing evenly. Return slowly to the starting position.

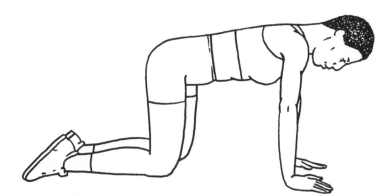

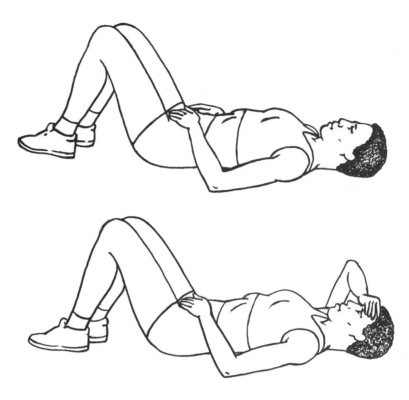

NECK

NECK FLEXOR
Targets the muscles in the front of the neck.

1. Lie on your back with your knees bent and your feet flat on the floor. Keep your stomach tight, your neck straight, and the small of your back pressed toward the floor to maintain proper alignment. Keep your hands on your lower abdomen and your shoulders down and relaxed. Inhale.

2. With the palm of your hand against your forehead, attempt to slowly bring your chin to your chest while you resist the motion (head does not move) with the pressure of your hand. Exhale as you resist the pressure. Hold the position for 5 to 10 seconds, breathing evenly, then gently release the pressure.

NECK

NECK ROTATOR
Targets the muscles on the sides of the neck.

1. Lie on your back with your knees bent and your feet flat on the floor. Keep your stomach tight, your neck straight, and the small of your back pressed toward the floor to maintain proper alignment. Keep your hands on your lower abdomen and your shoulders down and relaxed. Inhale.

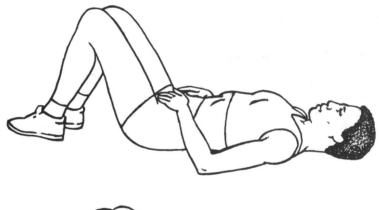

2. With the palm of one hand against your cheek, attempt to slowly turn your head (ear lobe to shoulder) toward the same shoulder while you resist the motion (head does not move) with the pressure of your hand. Exhale as you turn your head. Hold the position for 5 to 10 seconds, breathing evenly, then gently release the pressure.

3. Repeat on the opposite side.

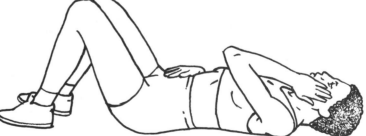

NECK

LATERAL NECK FLEXOR
Targets the muscles in the sides of the neck.

1. Lie on your back with your knees bent and your feet flat on the floor. Keep your stomach tight, your neck straight, and the small of your back pressed toward the floor to maintain proper alignment. Keep your hands on your lower abdomen and your shoulders down and relaxed. Inhale.

2. With the palm of one hand against your head, attempt to slowly tilt your head (ear lobe to shoulder) toward the same shoulder while you resist the motion (head does not move) with the pressure of your hand. Exhale as you tilt your head. Hold the position for 5 to 10 seconds, breathing evenly, then gently release the pressure.

3. Repeat on the opposite side.

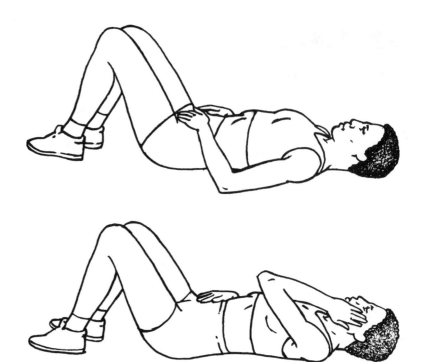

NECK

SIDEWAYS NECK FLEXOR
Targets the muscles in the sides of the neck.

1. Lie on one side with your head on your forearm and your knees bent toward your chest. Inhale.

2. Pulling your stomach in, lift your head slowly toward the ceiling. Exhale as you lift your head. Hold the position for 5 to 10 seconds, breathing evenly. Return slowly to the starting position.

3. Repeat on the opposite side.

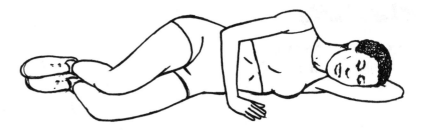

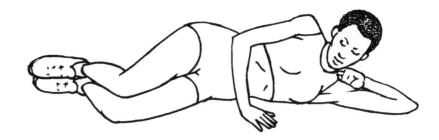

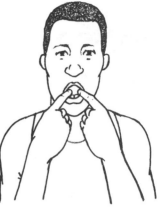

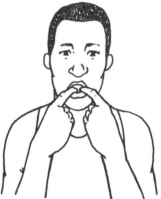

JAW

JAW CLOSER

Targets the muscles that close the mouth.

Note: *This exercise should be done in front of a mirror.*

1. Sit all the way back on a sturdy, armless chair, feet up on a small footstool, with your shoulders down and relaxed (the back of the chair should be straight and positioned near a wall, if possible). Keep your stomach in, small of back pressed toward the back of the chair, chin tucked, gaze forward, and head upright. Place both of your index fingers in your mouth on your bottom teeth.

2. Open your mouth and then slowly resist closing your mouth with the pressure from your index fingers. Inhale and exhale through your nose throughout the entire exercise. Hold the position for 5 to 10 seconds, breathing evenly. (Stop this exercise if you hear an increasing number of clicks.)

JAW

JAW OPENER

Targets the muscles that open the mouth and move it from side to side.

Note: *This exercise should be done in front of a mirror.*

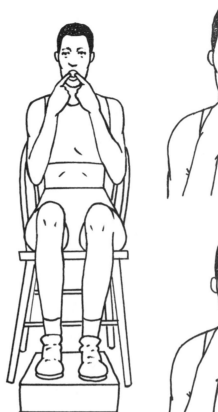

1. Sit all the way back on a sturdy, armless chair, feet up on a small footstool, with your shoulders down and relaxed (the back of the chair should be straight and positioned near a wall, if possible). Keep your stomach in, small of back pressed toward the back of the chair, chin tucked, gaze forward, and head upright. Place both of your hands on your lower jaw, fingers facing back.

2. Hold your lower jaw on both sides with your thumbs under your jaw and your index fingers alongside your cheeks. Slowly resist opening your mouth and moving it to the left and right. Inhale and exhale through your nose throughout the entire exercise. Hold the position for 5 to 10 seconds, breathing evenly.

3. Repeat in each direction.

JAW

JAW STRENGTHENER
Targets the muscles in the jaw.

Note: *This exercise should be done in front of a mirror.*

1. Sit all the way back in a sturdy, armless chair, feet up on a small footstool, with your shoulders down and relaxed (the back of the chair should be straight and positioned near a wall, if possible). Keep your stomach in, small of back pressed toward the back of the chair, chin tucked, gaze forward, and head upright.

2. With your tongue on the roof of your mouth and your jaw relaxed (not clenched), make a "clucking" sound with your tongue. Breathe in and out through your nose during the entire stretch.

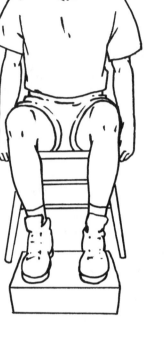

SHOULDER • BACK • NECK

KNEELER WITH EXTENDED ARM
Targets the muscles in the shoulders, upper back, and neck.

Note: *This exercise can be done with light hand weights (see page 171).*

1. Kneel down on your hands and knees. Keep your stomach in, chin tucked, gaze downward, and head and neck in alignment. Inhale.

2. Slowly lift one arm up in the air alongside your ear. Exhale as you lift your arm. Hold the position for 5 to 10 seconds, breathing evenly. *Do not hold the position if using weights.* Return slowly to the starting position.

3. Repeat on the opposite side.

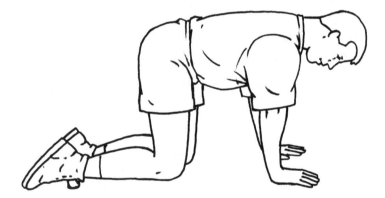

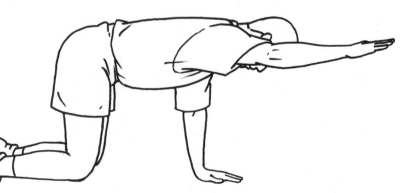

SHOULDER • BACK • NECK

KNEELER WITH SIDE ARM

Targets the muscles in the shoulders, upper back, and neck.

Note: *This exercise can be done with light hand weights (see page 171).*

1. Kneel down on your hands and knees. Keep your stomach in, chin tucked, gaze downward, and head and neck in alignment. Inhale.

2. Slowly lift one arm up and straight out to the side of your body. Exhale as you lift your arm. Hold the position for 5 to 10 seconds, breathing evenly. *Do not hold the position if using weights.* Return slowly to the starting position.

3. Repeat on the opposite side.

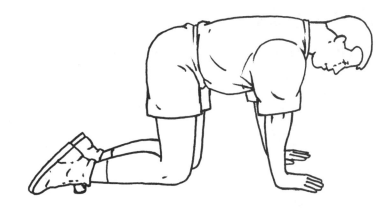

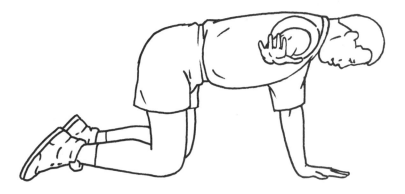

SHOULDER • BACK • NECK

KNEELER WITH REVERSE ARM

Targets the muscles in the shoulders, upper back, and neck.

Note: *This exercise can be done with light hand weights (see page 171).*

1. Kneel down on your hands and knees. Keep your stomach in, chin tucked, gaze downward, and head and neck in alignment. Inhale.

2. Slowly lift one arm up and straight back, pointing it toward your foot. Exhale as you lift your arm. Hold the position for 5 to 10 seconds, breathing evenly. *Do not hold the position if using weights.* Return slowly to the starting position.

3. Repeat on the opposite side.

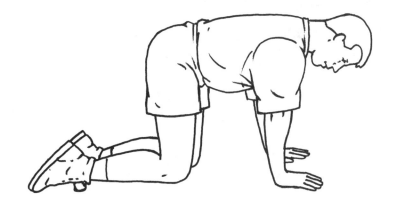

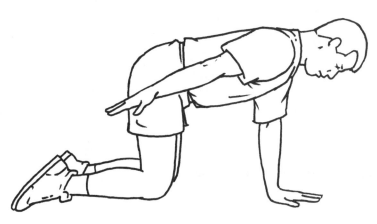

SHOULDER

BENCH PRESS

Targets the muscles in the shoulders, arms, and chest.

Note: *This exercise uses hand weights (see page 171).*

1. Lie on your back on a bench (or the floor) with your knees bent and your feet flat on the bench, shoulders down and relaxed. Grasp the weights in your hands and bend your elbows at a 90-degree angle, palms facing toward your feet, stomach tight, and neck straight. Keep your low back pressed toward the bench. Do not arch your back. Inhale.

2. Slowly lift both arms straight up in the air, keeping your elbows soft. Exhale as you lift your arms. Inhale as you return slowly to the starting position.

You may also lift and lower one arm at a time.

SHOULDER

BUTTERFLY

Targets the muscles in the chest and the back of the upper arms.

Note: *This exercise uses hand weights (see page 171).*

1. Lie on your back on a bench (or the floor) with your knees bent and your feel flat on the bench, shoulders down and relaxed. Grasp the weights in your hands and extend your arms straight up in the air with your elbows soft, stomach tight, neck straight, and palms facing each other. Keep your low back pressed toward the bench. Do not arch your back. Inhale.

2. Slowly lower your arms out to the sides, keeping your elbows slightly bent as you do so. (If you are lying on the floor instead of a bench, do not touch your arms to the floor.) Exhale as you lower your arms. Inhale as you return slowly to the starting position.

You may also lift and lower one arm at a time.

SHOULDER

SHOULDER PULLOVER

Targets the muscles in the shoulders, upper arms, upper chest, and upper back.

Note: *This exercise uses a single hand weight (see page 171).*

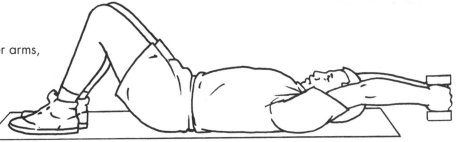

1. Lie on your back on a bench with your knees bent and your feet flat on the bench, shoulders down and relaxed. Keeping your stomach tight and neck straight, extend your arms alongside your ears (do not lock your elbows) and use both hands to hold a single weight. Keep your low back pressed toward the bench. Do not arch your back. Inhale.

2. Slowly lift the weight, keeping your arms straight, thumbs pointing toward your head, until the weight is directly overhead. Exhale as you lift your arms. Inhale as you return slowly to the starting position.

BACK · SHOULDER

HORIZONTAL SHOULDER ABDUCTION

Targets the muscles in the shoulders, upper and mid back, and arms.

Note: *This exercise uses hand weights (see page 171).*

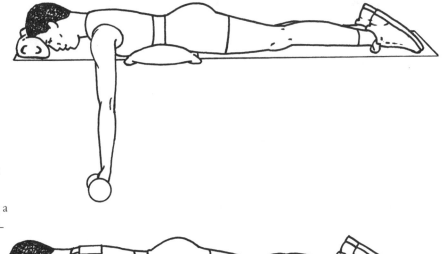

1. Lie on your stomach on a bench with your legs extended and one shoulder and arm positioned near the edge of the bench. Place a pillow under your stomach and rest your forehead on the bench or on a towel roll. Keeping your stomach tight, let your arm hang down off of the bench with your hand holding a single weight. The palm of your hand should face forward. Inhale.

2. Slowly lift the weight out to shoulder height, keeping your arm straight throughout the exercise. Exhale as you lift your arm. Inhale as you return slowly to the starting position.

3. Repeat on the opposite side.

SHOULDER • BACK

THE ROWER

Targets the muscles in the back, upper back, and shoulders.

Note: *This exercise uses hand weights (see page 171).*

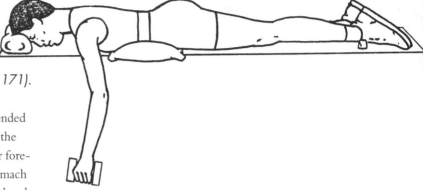

1. Lie on your stomach on a bench with your legs extended and one shoulder and arm positioned near the edge of the bench. Place a pillow under your stomach and rest your forehead on the bench or on a towel roll. Keeping your stomach tight, let your arm hang down off the bench with your hand holding a single weight. Inhale.

2. Slowly lift the weight, bending your arm back and up in a rowing motion and squeezing your shoulder blade (your arm should remain close to your body). Exhale as you lift your arm. Inhale as you return slowly to the starting position.

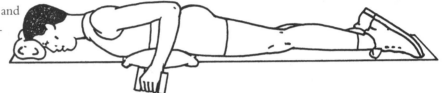

3. Repeat on the opposite side.

SHOULDER

EXTERNAL SHOULDER ROTATION

Targets the muscles in the shoulders and the middle and upper back.

Note: *This exercise uses hand weights (see page 171).*

1. Lie on your side with your knees bent and a pillow under your head. Holding a weight, bend your top arm at the elbow and place it at your side. The weight should be in front of your stomach at waist level. Inhale.

2. Keeping your top arm glued to your side (you may place a towel or pillow between your side and elbow), slowly rotate your arm up so the weight is almost facing the ceiling. Exhale as you rotate your arm. Inhale as you return slowly to the starting position.

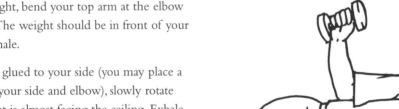

3. Repeat on the opposite side.

INTERNAL SHOULDER ROTATION

Targets the muscles in the shoulders and the middle and upper back.

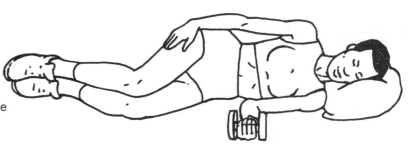

Note: *This exercise uses hand weights (see page 171).*

1. Lie on your side with your knees bent and a pillow under your head. Rest your top arm on your body and place a weight in your lower hand, bending the elbow at a 90-degree angle. The weight should be almost on the floor. Inhale.

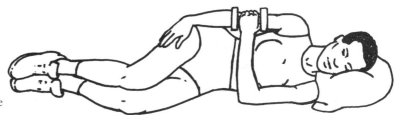

2. Slowly rotate your bottom arm up so the weight comes across your stomach at waist level. Exhale as you rotate your arm. Inhale as you return slowly to the starting position.

3. Repeat on the opposite side.

SHOULDER • BACK

OVERHEAD PRESS

Targets the muscles in the shoulders, arms, and upper back.

Note: *This exercise uses hand weights (see page 171).*

1. Sit all the way back on a sturdy, armless chair, feet up on a small footstool, with your shoulders down and relaxed (the back of the chair should be straight and positioned near a wall, if possible). Keep your stomach in, chin tucked, gaze forward, and head upright. Raise the weights to the top of your shoulders, palms facing forward, elbows pointing outward. Inhale.

2. Lift the weights straight up and have them meet directly overhead. (Do not lock your elbows.) Exhale as your lift your arms. Inhale as you slowly lower the weights back to your shoulders by bending your elbows.

You may also lift and lower one arm at a time.

SHOULDER

FRONT ARM LIFT

Targets the muscles in the shoulders, arms, chest, and upper back.

Note: *This exercise uses hand weights (see page 171).*

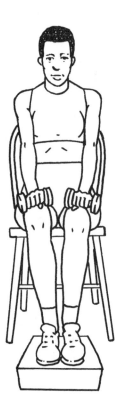
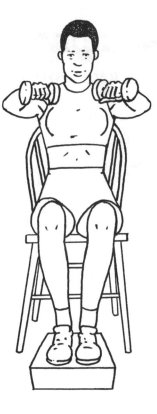

1. Sit all the way back on a sturdy, armless chair, feet up on a small footstool, with your shoulders down and relaxed (the back of the chair should be straight and positioned near a wall, if possible). Keep your stomach in, chin tucked, gaze forward, and head upright. The weights should rest on top of your thighs, with your palms facing down, and your arms straight. Inhale.

2. Slowly lift both your arms up in front, keeping your elbows slightly bent and shoulders down, until the weights are as close to shoulder height as comfortable, making sure to keep your shoulders down. Exhale as you lift your arms. Inhale as you return slowly to the starting position.

You may also lift and lower one arm at a time.

SHOULDER

ANTERIOR ARM LIFT

Targets the muscles in the shoulders, arms, chest, and upper back.

Note: *This exercise uses hand weights (see page 171).*

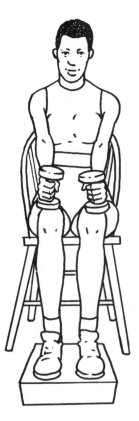
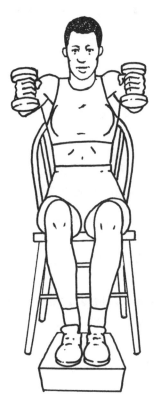

1. Sit all the way back on a sturdy, armless chair, feet up on a small footstool, with your shoulders down and relaxed (the back of the chair should be straight and positioned near a wall, if possible). Keep your stomach in, chin tucked, gaze forward, and head upright. The weights should rest on top of your thighs, with your palms facing inward, and your arms straight. Inhale.

2. Slowly lift both your arms up in front, keeping your elbows slightly bent, until the weights are as close to shoulder height as comfortable, making sure to keep your shoulders down. Exhale as you lift your arms. Inhale as you return slowly to the starting position.

You may also lift and lower one arm at a time, or have your palms facing upward instead of inward.

SHOULDER

SIDE ARM LIFT

Targets the muscles in the shoulders and upper back.

Note: *This exercise uses hand weights (see page 171).*

1. Sit all the way back on a sturdy, armless chair, feet up on a small footstool, with your shoulders down and relaxed (the back of the chair should be straight and positioned near a wall, if possible). Keep your stomach in, chin tucked, gaze forward, and head upright. The weights should be down at your sides, with your palms facing inward, and your elbows slightly bent. Inhale.

2. Keeping your shoulders down, slowly lift both your arms out to the sides until the weights are as close to shoulder height as comfortable. Exhale as you lift your arms. Inhale as you return slowly to the starting position.

You may also lift and lower one arm at a time, or have your palms facing forward, with the thumbs pointed toward the ceiling, as you lift.

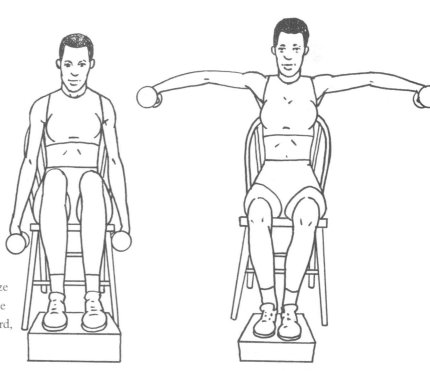

SHOULDER

UPRIGHT ROW

Targets the muscles in the upper back, shoulders, and elbows.

Note: This exercise uses hand weights (see page 171).

1. Stand with one knee on a sturdy, armless chair and the other leg at the side of the chair with your knee bent slightly. Keeping your stomach tight and neck straight, bend your body slightly forward and support yourself by resting your forearm on the back of the chair. Grasp the weight in the other hand and let your arm hang straight down to the side of the chair. Inhale.

2. Slowly lift the weight, bending your elbow back above shoulder height toward the ceiling. Exhale as you lift your arm. Inhale as you return slowly to the starting position.

3. Repeat on the opposite side.

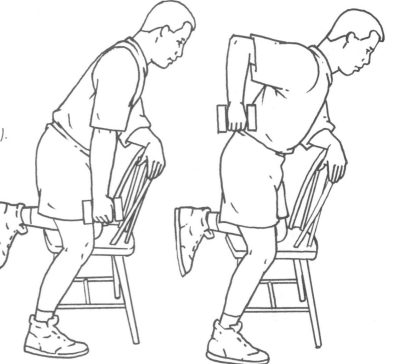

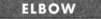

BICEPS CURL

Targets the muscles in the front of the upper arms and wrists.

Note: *This exercise uses hand weights (see page 171).*

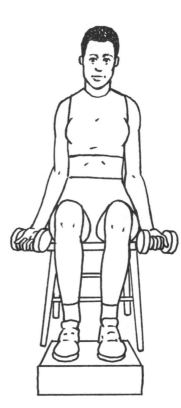
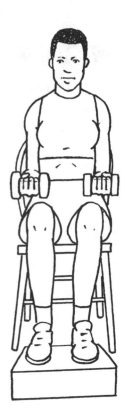

1. Sit all the way back on a sturdy, armless chair, feet up on a small footstool, with your shoulders down and relaxed (the back of the chair should be straight and positioned near a wall, if possible). Keep your stomach in, chin tucked, gaze forward, and head upright. The weights should be down at your sides, with your palms facing forward, and your elbows straight but soft. Inhale.

2. Slowly bend your elbows and bring the weights up to a 90-degree angle. Exhale as you lift your arms. Inhale as you return slowly to the starting position.

You may also lift and lower one arm at a time.

ELBOW

HAMMER CURL

Targets the muscles in the front of the upper arms.

Note: *This exercise uses hand weights (see page 171).*

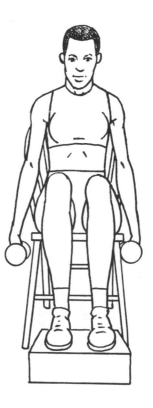
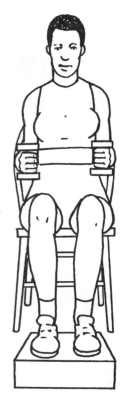

1. Sit all the way back on a sturdy, armless chair, feet up on a small footstool, with your shoulders down and relaxed (the back of the chair should be straight and positioned near a wall, if possible). Keep your stomach in, chin tucked, gaze forward, and head upright. The weights should be down at your sides, with your palms facing inward, and your elbows straight but soft. Inhale.

2. Slowly bend your elbows while keeping your palms facing inward, and bring the weights up to a 90-degree angle. Exhale as you lift your arms. Inhale as you return slowly to the starting position.

You may also lift and lower one arm at a time.

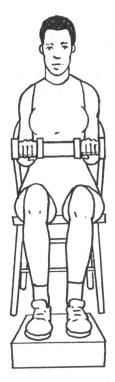

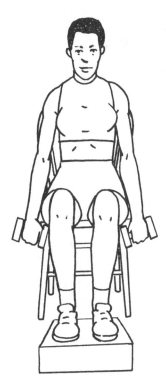

PALM-DOWN ARM CURL

Targets the muscles in the front of the upper arms
and wrists.

Note: *This exercise uses hand weights (see page 171).*

1. Sit all the way back on a sturdy, armless chair, feet up on a
small footstool, with your shoulders down and relaxed (the
back of the chair should be straight and positioned near a wall,
if possible). Keep your stomach in, chin tucked, gaze forward,
and head upright. The weights should be down at your sides,
with your palms facing backward, and your elbows straight but
soft. Inhale.

2. Slowly bend your elbows and bring the weights up to a
90-degree angle. Exhale as you lift your arms. Inhale as you
return slowly to the starting position.

You may also lift and lower one arm at a time.

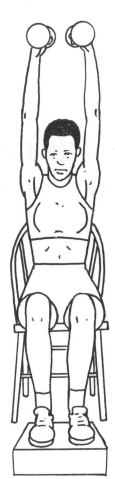

ELBOW

VERTICAL TRICEPS EXTENSION

Targets the muscles in the back of the upper arms.

Note: *This exercise uses hand weights (see page 171).*

1. Sit all the way back on a sturdy, armless chair, feet up on a
small footstool, with your shoulders down and relaxed (the
back of the chair should be straight and positioned near a wall,
if possible). Keep your stomach in, chin tucked, gaze forward,
and head upright. The weights should be behind your head,
with your palms facing each other, and your elbows close to
your head, pointing up. Inhale.

2. Slowly straighten your arms up (do not lock your elbows)
while keeping your palms facing inward. Exhale as you
straighten your arms. Inhale as you return slowly to the
starting position.

You may also lift and lower one arm at a time.

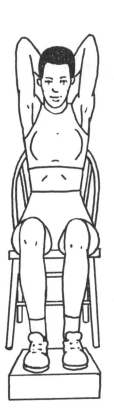

ELBOW • SHOULDER

STANDING TRICEPS EXTENSION

Targets the muscles in the elbows, arms, and back.

Note: *This exercise uses hand weights (see page 171).*

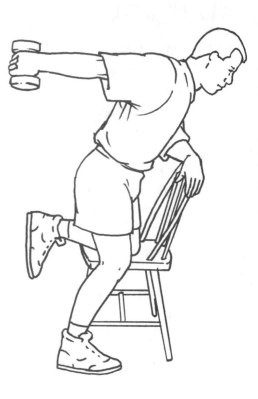

1. Stand with one knee on a sturdy, armless chair and the other leg at the side of the chair with your knee bent slightly. Keeping your stomach tight and neck straight, bend your body slightly forward and support yourself by resting your forearm on the back of the chair. Grasp the weight in the other hand and point your elbow back at or just above shoulder height toward the ceiling. Inhale.

2. Keeping your elbow soft, slowly straighten it. Exhale as you straighten your elbow. Inhale as you return slowly to the starting position.

3. Repeat on the opposite side.

ELBOW • SHOULDER

SEATED PRESS-UP

Targets the muscles in the elbows, arms, chest, and back.

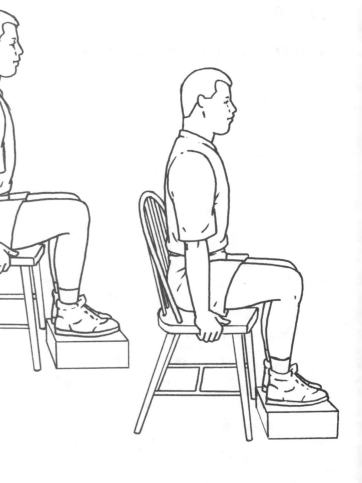

1. Sit on a sturdy, armless chair, feet up on a small footstool, with your shoulders down and relaxed (the back of the chair should be straight and positioned near a wall, if possible). Keep your stomach in, chin tucked, gaze forward, and head upright. With your hands, grasp the seat of the chair next to your hips. Inhale.

2. Keeping your spine straight, slowly lift your body up a few inches. Exhale as you lift your body. Hold the position for 5 to 10 second, breathing evenly. Return slowly to the starting position.

WRIST/HAND

PALM-DOWN WRIST EXTENSION
Targets the muscles in the wrists.

Note: *This exercise uses hand weights (see page 171).*

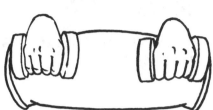

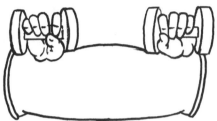

1. Sit all the way back on a sturdy, armless chair, feet up on a small footstool, with your shoulders down and relaxed (the back of the chair should be straight and positioned near a wall, if possible). Keep your stomach in, chin tucked, gaze forward, and head upright. Place a firm pillow on your lap. Keeping your elbows at your sides, bend them at a 90-degree angle. Place your forearms on the pillow with your wrists hanging over the edge of the pillow, holding the weights with your palms down. Inhale.

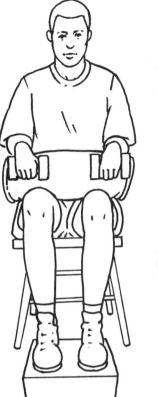

2. Extend both wrists up slowly, keeping your forearms on the pillow. Exhale as you bend your wrists. Inhale as you return slowly to the starting position.

You may also bend one wrist at a time.

WRIST/HAND

PALM-UP WRIST FLEXION
Targets the muscles in the wrists.

Note: *This exercise uses hand weights (see page 171).*

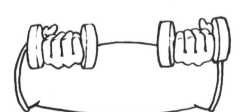

1. Sit all the way back on a sturdy, armless chair, feet up on a small footstool, with your shoulders down and relaxed (the back of the chair should be straight and positioned near a wall, if possible). Keep your stomach in, chin tucked, gaze forward, and head upright. Place a firm pillow on your lap. Keeping your elbows at your sides, bend them at a 90-degree angle. Place your forearms on the pillow with your wrists hanging over the edge of the pillow, holding the weights with your palms facing the ceiling. Inhale.

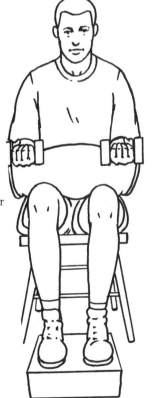

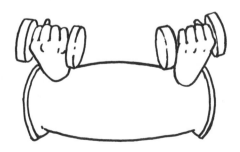

2. Bend both wrists up slowly, keeping your forearms on the pillow. Exhale as you bend your wrists. Inhale as you return slowly to the starting position.

You may also bend one wrist at a time.

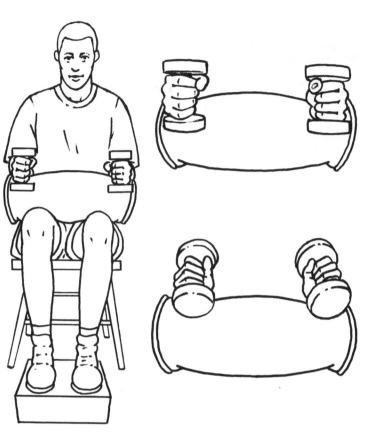

WRIST/HAND

RADIAL DEVIATION WITH THUMBS UP

Targets the muscles in the wrists.

Note: *This exercise uses hand weights (see page 171).*

1. Sit all the way back on a sturdy, armless chair, feet up on a small footstool, with your shoulders down and relaxed (the back of the chair should be straight and positioned near a wall, if possible). Keep your stomach in, chin tucked, gaze forward, and head upright. Place a firm pillow on your lap. Keeping your elbows at your sides, bend them at a 90-degree angle. Place your forearms on the pillow with your wrists hanging over the edge of the pillow, holding the weights with your thumbs pointing toward the ceiling. Inhale.

2. Bend both wrists up slowly, keeping your forearms on the pillow. Exhale as you bend your wrists. Inhale as you return slowly to the starting position.

You may also bend one wrist at a time.

WRIST/HAND

HAND GRIP

Targets the muscles in the fingers and hands.

Note: *This exercise uses a soft rubber ball.*

1. Sit all the way back on a sturdy, armless chair, feet up on a small footstool, with your shoulders down and relaxed (the back of the chair should be straight and positioned near a wall, if possible). Keep your stomach in, chin tucked, gaze forward, and head upright. Keeping your elbows at your sides, bend them at a 90-degree angle. Inhale.

2. Grasp a soft sponge, soft rubber ball, or foam ball in one hand and squeeze it as firmly as possible. Exhale as you squeeze your hand. Hold the position for 5 to 10 seconds, breathing evenly.

3. Repeat on the opposite side.

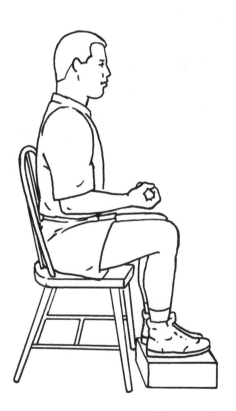

WRIST/HAND

FINGER EXTENSION

Targets the muscles in the fingers and hands.

Note: *This exercise uses a small, wide rubber band (about ¼" to ½" wide).*

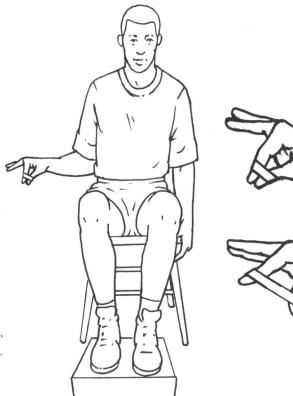

1. Sit all the way back on a sturdy, armless chair, feet up on a small footstool, with your shoulders down and relaxed (the back of the chair should be straight and positioned near a wall, if possible). Keep your stomach in, chin tucked, gaze forward, and head upright. Keeping your elbows at your sides, bend them at a 90-degree angle. With your palms facing in, wrap a rubber band around the thumb and index finger of one hand. Inhale.

2. Stretch your thumb and index fingers as far apart as possible, while keeping them straight. Exhale as you stretch your fingers. Hold the position for 5 to 10 seconds, breathing evenly.

3. Repeat the exercise with the band wrapped around your thumb and each of your other fingers.

4. Repeat on the opposite side.

WRIST/HAND

FINGER ABDUCTION

Targets the muscles in the fingers.

Note: *This exercise uses a small, wide rubber band (about ¼" to ½" wide).*

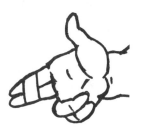

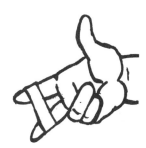

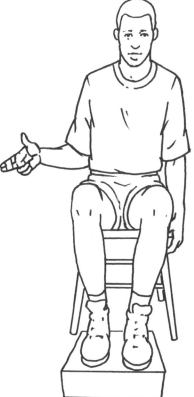

1. Sit all the way back on a sturdy, armless chair, feet up on a small footstool, with your shoulders down and relaxed (the back of the chair should be straight and positioned near a wall, if possible). Keep your stomach in, chin tucked, gaze forward, and head upright. Keeping your elbows at your sides, bend them at a 90-degree angle. With your palms facing in, wrap a rubber band around the index and third fingers of one hand. Inhale.

2. Spread your fingers into a "V" position. Exhale as you stretch your fingers. Hold the position for 5 to 10 seconds, breathing evenly.

3. Repeat the exercise with the band wrapped around your middle and fourth fingers and fourth and little fingers.

4. Repeat on the opposite side.

HIP

SEATED HIP FLEXION

Targets the muscles in the front of the hips.

Note: *This exercise can be done with ankle weights (see page 171).*

1. Sit up straight on a table and let your legs hang over the edge at your knees. Hold on to the edge of the table and keep your stomach in, chin tucked, gaze forward, and head upright. Inhale.

2. Bring one knee up toward your chest. Exhale as you lift your knee. Hold the position for 5 to 10 seconds, breathing evenly. *Do not hold the position if using weights.* Return slowly to the starting position.

3. Repeat on the opposite side.

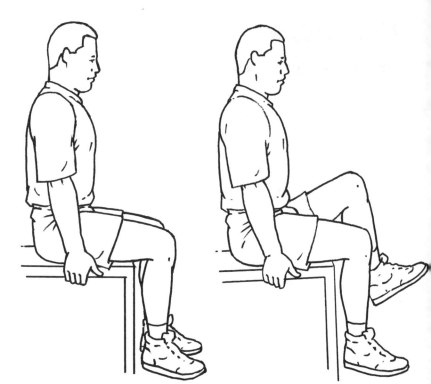

HIP · KNEE

LATERAL LEG LIFT

Targets the muscles in the hips and buttocks.

Note: *This exercise can be done with ankle weights (see page 171).*

1. Lie on your side with a pillow under your head. Keeping your stomach tight and neck straight, bend your bottom knee toward your chest and extend your top leg out straight. Inhale.

2. Slowly lift your top leg about 6 inches up off the floor. Exhale as you lift your leg. Hold the position for 5 to 10 seconds, breathing evenly. *Do not hold the position if using weights.* Return slowly to the starting position.

3. Repeat on the opposite side.

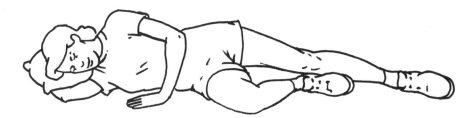

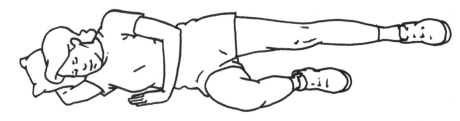

HIP • KNEE

INNER LEG LIFT

Targets the muscles in the inner thighs.

Note: *This exercise can be done with ankle weights (see page 171).*

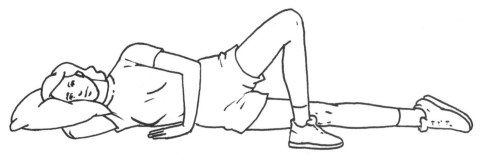

1. Lie on your side with a pillow under your head. Straighten your bottom leg out on the floor then bend your other leg and place your foot on the floor in front of the bottom knee. Inhale.

2. Slowly lift your bottom leg 4 to 5 inches off of the floor. Exhale as you lift your leg. Hold the position for 5 to 10 seconds, breathing evenly. *Do not hold the position if using weights.* Return slowly to the starting position.

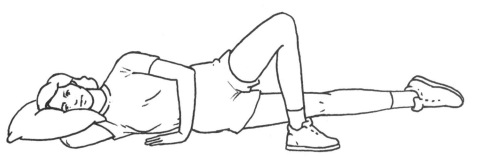

3. Repeat on the opposite side.

HIP

EXTERNAL HIP ROTATION

Targets the muscles in the hips and buttocks.

Note: *This exercise can be done with ankle weights (see page 171).*

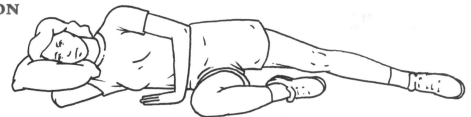

1. Lie on your right side with a pillow under your head. Keep your stomach tight and neck straight, bend your right knee toward your chest, and extend your left leg out straight. Inhale.

2. Slowly lift your left leg about 6 inches up off of the floor. Bend it at a 90-degree angle and then rotate the left thigh outward. Exhale as you lift your leg. Hold the position for 5 to 10 seconds, breathing evenly. *Do not hold the position if using weights.* Return slowly to the starting position.

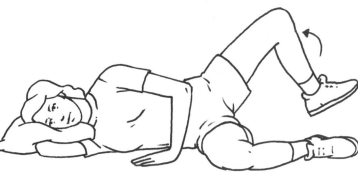

3. Repeat on the opposite side.

INTERNAL HIP ROTATION

Targets the muscles in the hips and buttocks.

Note: *This exercise can be done with ankle weights (see page 171).*

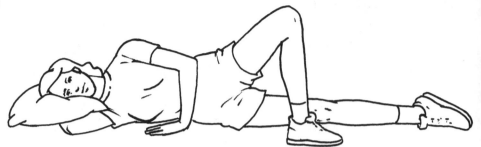

1. Lie on your left side with a pillow under your head. Keeping your stomach tight and neck straight, place your right foot on the floor in front of your left knee, and extend your left leg out straight. Inhale.

2. Slowly lift your left leg 2 to 3 inches up off the floor. Bend it at a 90-degree angle, and then rotate the left thigh inward. Exhale as you lift your leg. Hold the position for 5 to 10 seconds, breathing evenly. *Do not hold the position if using weights.* Return slowly to the starting position.

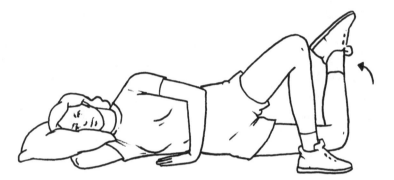

3. Repeat on the opposite side.

KNEE SQUEEZE

Targets the muscles in the inner thighs.

1. Lie on your back with your knees pointed up and your feet flat on the floor. Place a firm pillow or inflated ball between your knees. Keep your stomach tight, your neck straight, and the small of your back pressed toward the floor to maintain proper alignment. Keep your hands on your lower abdomen, shoulders down and relaxed. Inhale.

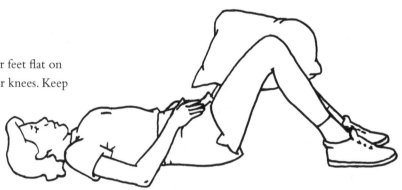

2. Squeeze your knees together as firmly as possible. Exhale as you squeeze your knees. Hold the position for 5 to 10 seconds, breathing evenly.

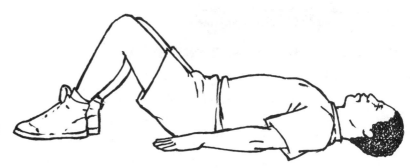

HIP • BACK

ABDOMINAL BRIDGE

Targets the muscles in the buttocks, thighs, abdomen, and back.

1. Lie on your back with your knees bent and your feet flat on the floor. Keep your stomach tight, your neck straight, and the small of your back pressed toward the floor to maintain proper alignment. Keep your arms at your sides, palms down. Inhale.

2. Keeping your stomach tight, perform a bridging movement by pinching your buttocks together as you lift them off the floor. Exhale as you lift your buttocks. Hold the position for 5 to 10 seconds, breathing evenly. Return slowly to the starting position.

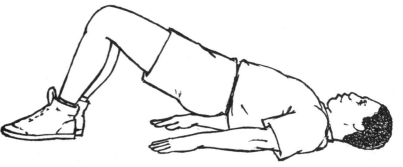

HIP • KNEE • BACK

KICKBACK

Targets the muscles in the buttocks, back, and upper thighs.

Note: *This exercise can be done with light ankle weights (see page 171).*

1. Kneel down on your hands and knees. Keep your stomach in, chin tucked, gaze downward, and head and neck in alignment. Inhale.

2. Slowly lift one leg out in the air, keeping your knee as straight as possible so your thigh is level with your body. Exhale as you lift your leg. Hold the position for 5 to 10 seconds, breathing evenly. *Do not hold the position if using weights.* Return slowly to the starting position.

3. Repeat on the opposite side.

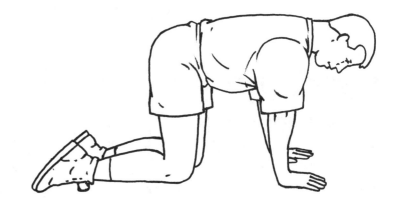

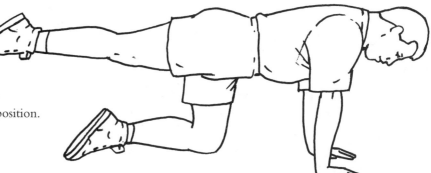

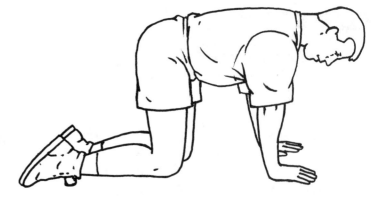

HIP • KNEE • BACK • NECK

KICKBACK WITH EXTENDED ARM
Targets the muscles in the hips, legs, arms, back, and neck.

Note: *This exercise can be done with ankle weights and/or hand weights (see page 171).*

1. Kneel down on your hands and knees. Keep your stomach in, chin tucked, gaze downward, and head and neck in alignment. Inhale.

2. Slowly lift one arm up in the air alongside your ear and, at the same time, lift the opposite leg out in the air, keeping your knee as straight as possible. Exhale as you lift your arm and leg. Hold the position for 5 to 10 seconds, breathing evenly. *Do not hold the position if using weights.* Return slowly to the starting position.

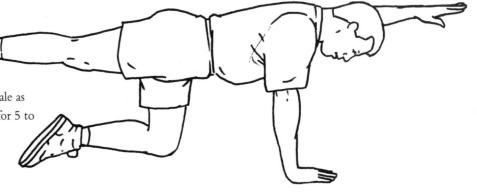

3. Repeat using the opposite arm and leg.

HIP • KNEE • BACK

KNEELER HIP HITCH
Targets the muscles in the buttocks, back, and back of the upper thighs.

Note: *This exercise can be done with light ankle weights (see page 171).*

1. Kneel down on your hands and knees. Keep your stomach in, chin tucked, gaze downward, and head and neck in alignment. Inhale.

2. Slowly lift one leg up with your knee bent at a 90-degree angle until your thigh is level with your body. Exhale as you lift your leg. Hold the position for 5 to 10 seconds, breathing evenly. *Do not hold the position if using weights.* Return slowly to the starting position.

3. Repeat on the opposite side.

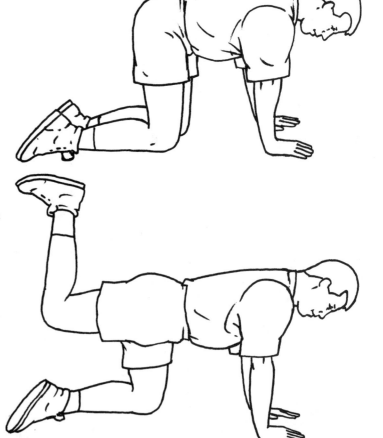

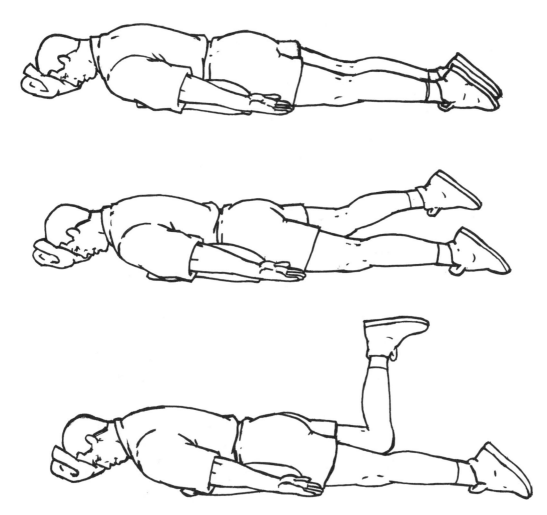

HIP • KNEE • BACK

HORIZONTAL HIP HITCH

Targets the muscles in the buttocks and the back of the upper thighs.

Note: *This exercise can be done with light ankle weights (see page 171).*

1. Lie on your stomach with your forehead resting on the floor. (You may use a towel roll under your forehead.) Place a large pillow under your stomach. Keep your arms at your sides, palms up. Inhale.

2. Lift one leg up 3 to 4 inches off the ground and then slowly bend the knee to a 90-degree angle. Try to keep your stomach tight and neck straight so that proper alignment is maintained. Exhale as you bend your knee. Hold the position for 5 to 10 seconds, breathing evenly. *Do not hold the position if using weights.* Slowly straighten your knee and return to the starting position.

3. Repeat on the opposite side.

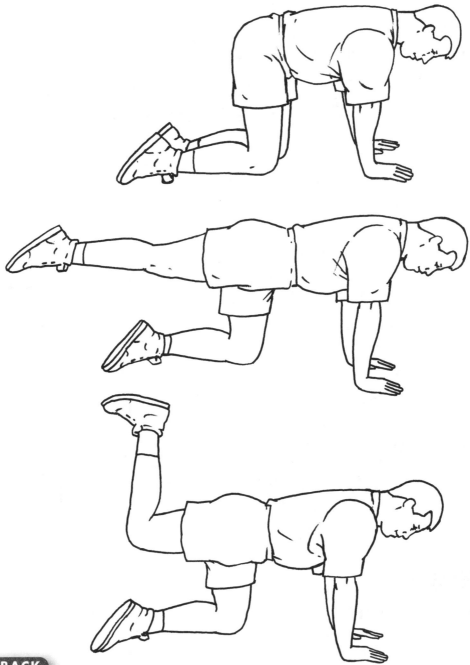

HIP • KNEE • BACK

HIP HITCH EXTENSION

Targets the muscles in the hips, back of the knees, back, and arms.

Note: *This exercise can be done with light ankle weights (see page 171).*

1. Kneel down on your hands and knees. Keep your stomach in, chin tucked, gaze downward, and head and neck in alignment. Inhale.

2. Slowly extend one leg back and up in the air until the knee is as straight as possible and your thigh is level with your body, then slowly bend your knee. Exhale as you bend your knee. Hold the position for 5 to 10 seconds, breathing evenly. *Do not hold the position if using weights.* Straighten your leg and return slowly to the starting position.

3. Repeat on the opposite side.

KNEE

QUAD KNEE PUSH

Targets the muscles in the front of the thighs.

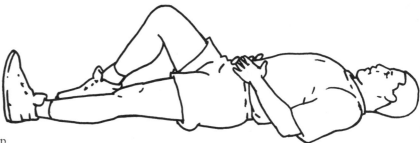

1. Lie on your back with one knee bent and the foot flat on the floor, the other leg extended out along the floor. Keep your stomach tight, your neck straight, and the small of your back pressed toward the floor to maintain proper alignment. Keep your hands on your lower abdomen, shoulders down and relaxed. Inhale.

2. Slowly push the knee of your extended leg into the floor as firmly as possible. Exhale as you push your knee down. Hold the position for 5 to 10 seconds, breathing evenly.

3. Repeat on the opposite side.

KNEE • HIP • BACK

STRAIGHT-LEG RAISE

Targets the muscles in the front of the thighs, hips, and abdomen.

Note: *This exercise can be done with ankle weights (see page 171).*

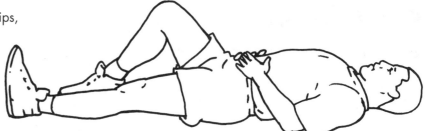

1. Lie on your back with one knee bent and the foot flat on the floor, the other leg extended out along the floor. Keep your stomach tight, your neck straight, and the small of your back pressed toward the floor to maintain proper alignment. Keep your hands on your lower abdomen, shoulders down and relaxed. Inhale.

2. Slowly lift the extended leg up in the air halfway between the floor and the top of your opposite knee. Exhale as you lift your leg. Hold the position for 5 to 10 seconds, breathing evenly. *Do not hold the position if using weights.* Return slowly to the starting position. Do not arch your back.

3. Repeat on the opposite side.

KNEE • HIP • BACK

SEATED KNEE EXTENSION

Targets the muscles in the front of the thighs, hips, and abdomen.

Note: *This exercise can be done with ankle weights (see page 171).*

1. Sit up straight on a table and let your legs hang over the edge at the knees. Hold on to the edge of the table and keep your stomach in, chin tucked, gaze forward, and head upright. Inhale. (If sitting straight is too uncomfortable for you, you can lean back slightly, arms behind you, keeping your head, neck, and back aligned and supporting your body on your hands.)

2. Slowly straighten one knee out. Exhale as you lift your knee. Hold the position for 5 to 10 seconds, breathing evenly. (Don't pull up on the edge of the table.) *Do not hold the position if using weights.* Return slowly to the starting position.

3. Repeat on the opposite side.

KNEE • HIP • BACK

SEATED STRAIGHT-LEG RAISE

Targets the muscles in the front of the thighs, hips, and abdomen.

Note: *This exercise can be done with ankle weights (see page 171).*

1. Sit on the floor with your hands on the floor behind your buttocks. Keep your stomach in, chin tucked, gaze forward, and head upright. Keep one leg straight and the other leg bent at the knee with your foot resting on the floor. Inhale.

2. Slowly lift the straight leg up in the air 6 to 8 inches. Exhale as you lift your leg. Hold the position for 5 to 10 seconds, breathing evenly. *Do not hold the position if using weights.* Return slowly to the starting position. (Alternatively, lift the leg up and back down as quickly as possible, or roll the leg outwardly and then lift up.) Do not lift your buttocks off the floor.

3. Repeat on the opposite side.

KNEE • HIP • BACK

BASIC VERTICAL SQUAT

Targets the muscles in the front of the thighs, buttocks, back, and abdomen.

Note: *This exercise can be done with hand weights (see page 171).*

1. Stand with your feet shoulder width apart and your hands at your sides, palms in. Keep your stomach in, chin tucked, gaze forward, head upright, and knees slightly bent. Inhale.

2. Slowly bend your knee one-quarter to one-half of the way down, being sure to keep your feet flat on floor and your buttocks moving backward so that you keep your knees behind or just directly over your ankle joints. Exhale as you lower your body. *Do not hold the position if using weights.* Hold the position for 5 to 10 seconds, breathing evenly. Return slowly to the starting position.

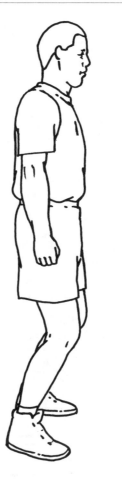
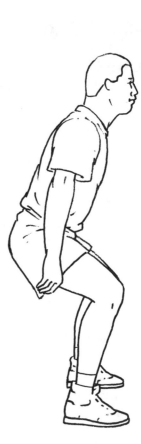

KNEE • HIP • BACK

WIDE-LEG VERTICAL SQUAT

Targets the muscles in the front of the thighs, buttocks, back, and abdomen.

Note: *This exercise can be done with hand weights (see page 171).*

1. Stand with your legs wider than shoulder width apart and your feet pointed slightly outward. Keep your stomach in, chin tucked, gaze forward, head upright, and knees slightly bent. Inhale.

2. Slowly bend your knees, being sure to keep your feet flat on the floor and your buttocks moving backward so that you keep your knees behind or just directly over your ankle joints. Exhale as you lower your body. Hold the position for 5 to 10 seconds, breathing evenly. *Do not hold the position if using weights.* Return slowly to the starting position.

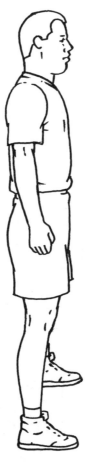
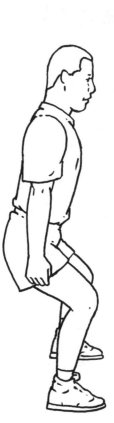

KNEE • HIP • BACK

STEP SQUAT

Targets the muscles in the front of the thighs, hips, back, and abdomen.

1. Stand on a step with one leg and place your other leg, slightly bent, partially on the step, but not touching the floor. Keep your stomach in, chin tucked, gaze forward, head upright, and knees slightly bent. Inhale.

2. Slowly bend the knee of your leg on the step, lowering your body down until your other foot is 2 to 4 inches below the step you are standing on. (Be sure that your buttocks move backward and your shoulders and body weight are at or behind your knee or ankle joints.) You can progressively lean forward (keeping your head, neck, and back aligned) and lower your foot farther toward the floor as you become more comfortable with this exercise, but your foot should not touch the floor. Exhale as you lower your body. Hold the position for 5 to 10 seconds, breathing evenly. Return slowly to the starting position.

3. Repeat on the opposite side.

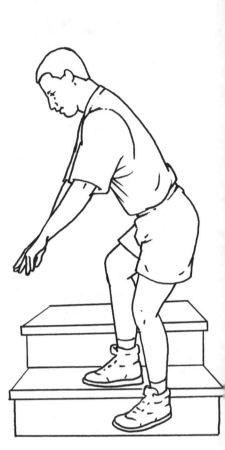

KNEE • HIP • BACK

WALL SQUATS

Targets the muscles in the front of the thighs, hips, back, and abdomen.

1. Stand on a nonskid surface with your back against a wall and your feet almost 2 feet away from the wall, 6 to 8 inches apart. Keep your stomach in, chin tucked, gaze forward, head upright, and knees slightly bent. Inhale.

2. Slowly slide your back down the wall to a near-sitting position, being sure that your knees are behind or just directly over your ankle joints (you should move your feet farther away from the wall if necessary to ensure this alignment). Exhale as you lower your body. Hold the position for 5 to 10 seconds, breathing evenly, working up to holding the position for 1 to 2 minutes. Return slowly to the starting position.

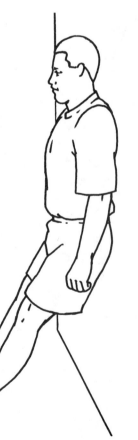

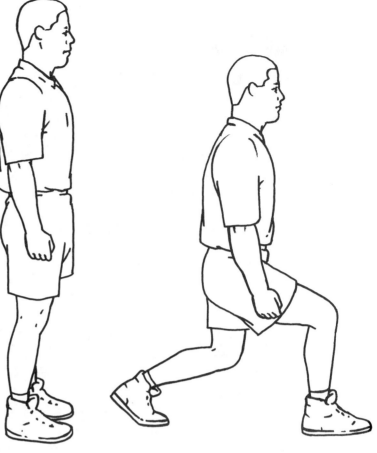

KNEE • HIP • BACK

BASIC FRONT LUNGE
Targets the muscles in the front of the thighs and hips.

Note: *This exercise can be done with hand weights (see page 171).*

1. Stand with your feet 6 to 8 inches apart. Keep your stomach in, chin tucked, gaze forward, head upright, and knees slightly bent. Inhale.

2. Step forward ("lunge") with one foot, being sure that your forward knee is behind or just directly over your ankle joint. Only lunge as far forward as you safely and comfortably can without pain, and be sure to let the heel of your back foot rise up off the floor as you perform the movement. Exhale as you lunge forward. Hold the position for 5 to 10 seconds, breathing evenly. *Do not hold the position if using weights.* Return slowly to the starting position.

3. Repeat on the opposite side.

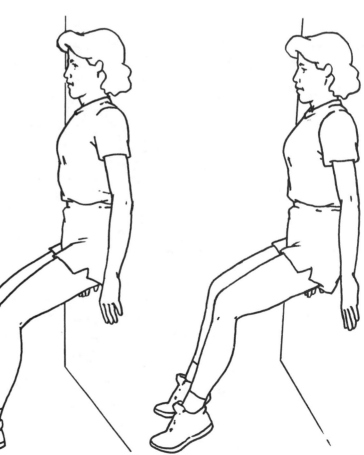

KNEE • HIP • ANKLE/FOOT

BENT-KNEE CALF RAISE
Targets the muscles in the front of the thighs, back of the calves, hips, back, and abdomen.

1. Stand with your back against a wall and your feet on a nonskid surface. Place your feet almost 2 feet away from the wall, 6 to 8 inches apart, with your back flat against the wall. Keep your stomach tight, gaze forward, head upright, and knees slightly bent. Bend your knees a third of the way down (be sure your knee joints are slightly behind or just over your ankle joints). Inhale.

2. Slowly rise up onto your toes, keeping your back flat against the wall. Exhale as you lift your body. Hold the position for 5 to 10 seconds, breathing evenly. Return slowly to the starting position.

KNEE • HIP • BACK

SIT-TO-STANDING SQUAT

Targets the muscles in the front of the thighs, hips, back, and abdomen.

1. Sit all the way back on a sturdy, armless chair with your shoulders down and relaxed (the back of the chair should be straight and positioned near a wall, if possible). Keep your stomach in, chin tucked, gaze forward, and head upright. Inhale.

2. Stand, lifting your body about ⅔ of the way up. Keep your back straight, stomach tight, neck straight, and knees slightly bent (be sure your knee joints are slightly behind or just over your ankle joints). Exhale as you lift your body. Hold the position for 5 to 10 seconds, breathing evenly. Return slowly to the starting position.

KNEE • HIP

KNEE CURL

Targets the muscles in the back of the thighs and calves.

Note: *This exercise can be done with ankle weights (see page 171).*

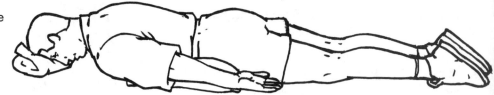

1. Lie on your stomach with your forehead resting on the floor. (You may use a towel roll under your forehead.) Place a large pillow under your stomach. Place your arms at your sides, palms up. Inhale.

2. Slowly bend one knee to a 90-degree angle. Keep your stomach tight and neck straight to maintain proper alignment. Exhale as you bend your knee. Hold the position for 5 to 10 seconds, breathing evenly. *Do not hold the position if using weights.* Return slowly to the starting position.

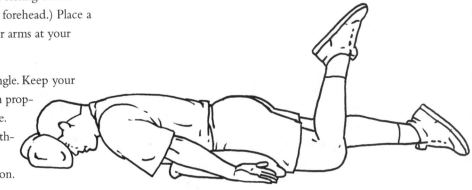

3. Repeat on the opposite side.

KNEE • HIP

STANDING KNEE CURL

Targets the muscles in the back of the thighs and calves.

Note: *This exercise can be done with ankle weights (see page 171).*

1. Stand with your feet shoulder width apart and hold on to the top of a dresser, countertop, or the back of a chair, keeping your stomach in, chin tucked, gaze forward, and head upright. Inhale.

2. Slowly bend one knee back to a 90-degree angle, being sure to keep your thighs even. Exhale as you bend your knee. Hold the position for 5 to 10 seconds, breathing evenly. *Do not hold the position if using weights.* Return slowly to the starting position.

3. Repeat on the opposite side.

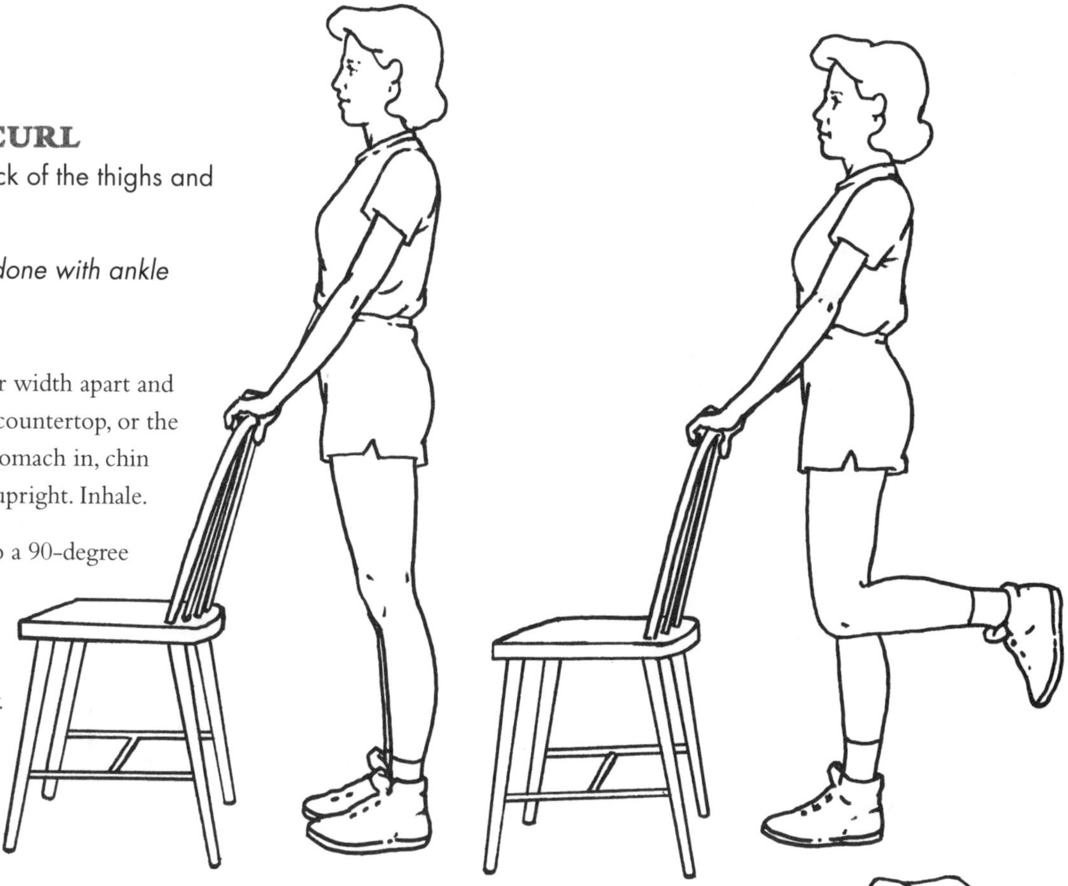

KNEE • ANKLE/FOOT

STANDING CALF LIFT

Targets the muscles in the calves.

1. Stand with your feet shoulder width apart and hold on to the top of a dresser, countertop, or the back of a chair, keeping your stomach tight and neck straight to maintain proper alignment. Inhale.

2. Slowly rise up onto your toes. Exhale. Hold the position for 5 to 10 seconds, breathing evenly. Return slowly to the starting position.

You may also lift and lower one foot at a time. (Simply keep the other heel slightly off the ground while doing the exercise.)

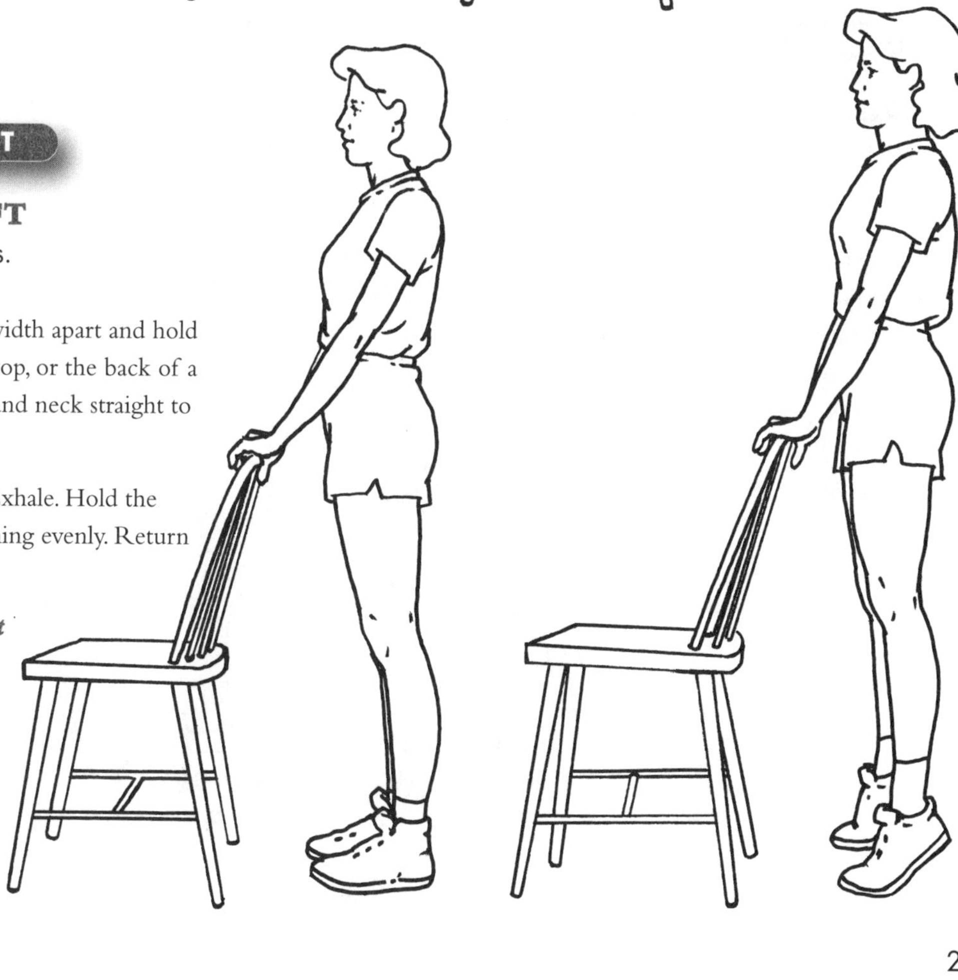

KNEE • ANKLE/FOOT

TOE WALK

Targets the muscles in the knees and calves.

1. Stand up straight, keeping your stomach tight and neck straight to maintain proper alignment. Inhale.

2. Walk on your tiptoes on a carpeted or nonskid surface for no more than 10 steps or 2 to 3 minutes.

ANKLE/FOOT

STANDING TOE RAISE

Targets the muscles in the shins.

1. Stand with your feet shoulder width apart and hold onto the top of a dresser, countertop, or back of a chair, keeping your stomach tight and neck straight to maintain proper alignment. Inhale.

2. Slowly lift your toes off the floor. Exhale. Hold the position for 5 to 10 seconds, breathing evenly. Return slowly to the starting position.

ANKLE/FOOT

TOE CURL
Targets the muscles in the toes.

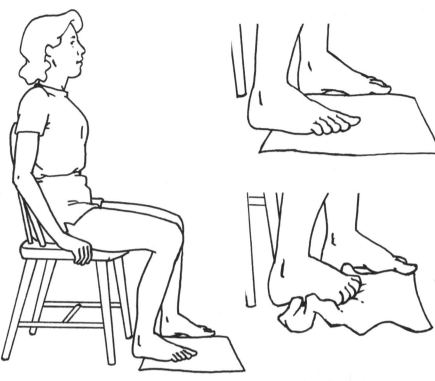

1. Sit all the way back on a sturdy, armless chair with your shoulders down and relaxed (the back of the chair should be straight and positioned near a wall, if possible). Keep your stomach in, chin tucked, gaze forward, and head upright. Placing a hand towel on the floor, rest your forefoot on the towel and your heel on the floor. Inhale.

2. Repeatedly curl your toes, bringing the towel into the arch of your foot. Exhale as you curl your toes.

3. Repeat on the opposite side.

ANKLE/FOOT

SEATED FOOT DORSIFLEXION
Targets the muscles in the calves and ankles.

Note: *This exercise can be done with weights fastened to the tops of your feet (see page 171).*

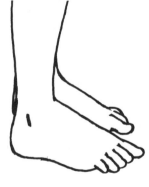

1. Sit on a table with your shoulders down and relaxed and your hands clasped to the edge of the desk. Keep your stomach in, chin tucked, gaze forward, and head upright. Inhale.

2. Without moving your legs, slowly flex your feet upward as high as they can go. Exhale as you lift your feet. Hold the position for 5 to 10 seconds, breathing evenly. *Do not hold the position if using weights.* Return slowly to the starting position.

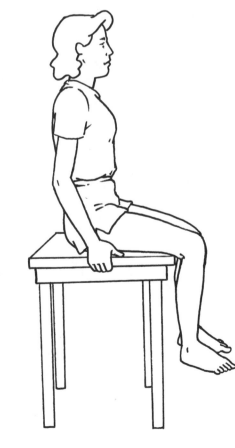

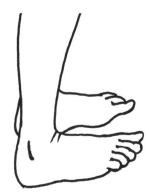

You can also flex and relax your feet one at a time.

ANKLE/FOOT

TOE/FOOT PRESS
Targets the muscles in the calves.

1. Sit on the floor with your legs stretched out in front of you. Keep your stomach in, chin tucked, gaze forward, and head upright. Inhale.

2. Placing the bottoms of your feet totally flat against a wall, push both feet into the wall, using your calf muscles. Exhale as you push. Hold the position for 5 to 10 seconds, breathing evenly.

You may also press one foot at a time.

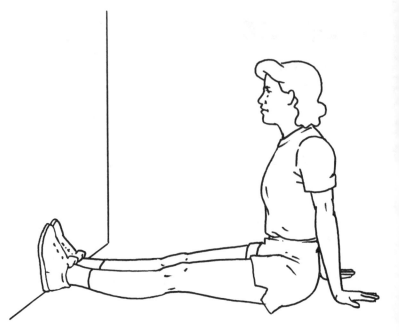

ANKLE/FOOT • HIP

ROPE JUMPING
Targets the muscles in the feet, ankles, the front of the thighs, and the hips.

Note: *This exercise should be done on a shock-absorbing floor (not concrete) and/or with cushioned footwear.*

1. Stand up straight, keeping your stomach tight and neck straight to maintain proper alignment. Inhale.

2. Holding the rope loosely in both hands, jump rope. Be sure to continue breathing throughout the exercise.

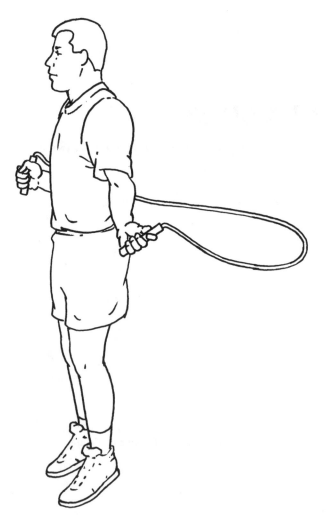

CHAPTER NINETEEN
Flexibility Exercises

The dozens of exercises in this chapter represent some of the many flexibility exercises for body maintenance and repair. They can be drawn upon in various combinations to create part of a regular regimen for taking care of your body. For more advice along these lines and a suggested basic exercise regimen, see **Chapter 15—Strength, Endurance, and Flexibility**.

Many of these flexibility exercises may also help prepare the body for sports, work, or other vigorous activities. For more advice and suggested pregame and workplace flexibility regimens, see **Chapter 16—Sports** and **Chapter 17—Work**. Many of these exercises may help ease the discomfort of minor stiffness or soreness in the various parts of your body. For more information and a list of suggested quick-relief stretches for each body part, see the appropriate chapter in **Part I**.

Finally, these exercises may also serve as part of a rehabilitation program for a wide range of problems. They should only be used for this purpose, however, under the supervision of a physical therapist.

Although each exercise should be repeated several times to be effective, there is no blanket rule for the number of repetitions appropriate for any particular individual in any particular case. If you are using these exercises as part of a regular maintenance regimen, pregame stretching routine, or quick-relief program, 3 to 5 repetitions for 10 seconds each is a good target number. You should stretch until you feel a gentle pull on the muscle(s) you are targeting, and then hold that position without forcing it.

If you are using these exercises as part of a rehabilitation program, the number of repetitions and their duration should be determined in consultation with your physical therapist.

Cautions

If you have pain (other than simple stiffness or soreness) in any part of your body, a history of health trouble, or an existing medical condition (including pregnancy), it is essential to check with your physical therapist before attempting any of these exercises. And if you experience pain, instability, tingling, or numbness in any part of your body—or if you feel dizzy—during any exercise, you should stop doing it at once to avoid the possibility of injury.

ANKLE/FOOT

BACK

DIAPHRAGMATIC BREATHING
Targets the muscles in the diaphragm and lower rib cage.

Note: *This exercise should be done facing a mirror.*

1. Sit all the way back on a sturdy, armless chair, feet up on a small footstool, with your shoulders down and relaxed (the back of the chair should be straight and positioned near a wall, if possible). Keep your stomach in, chin tucked, gaze forward, and head upright. Rest your hands on your abdomen.

2. Gently exhale through pursed lips, then begin a slow, deep inspiration through the nose. As you inhale, your lower rib cage will expand, and your hands will rise with the outward movement of your abdomen. Hold the deep breath for the count of 5. Gently exhale through pursed lips, applying light pressure over the abdomen. Exhale for a count of 10.

3. Repeat no more than 3 or 4 times per minute.

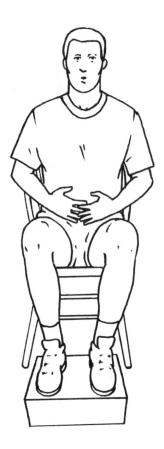

BACK • NECK

BASIC LOW BACK STRETCH
Targets the muscles in the low back.

1. Lie on your back with your knees bent and your feet flat on the floor. Keep your stomach tight, your neck straight, and the small of your back pressed toward the floor to maintain proper alignment. Keep your hands on your lower abdomen and your shoulders down and relaxed. Inhale.

2. Slowly tighten your stomach and pinch your buttocks gently together while flattening your back against the floor. Exhale as you stretch. Hold the stretch for 5 to 30 seconds, breathing evenly as you hold.

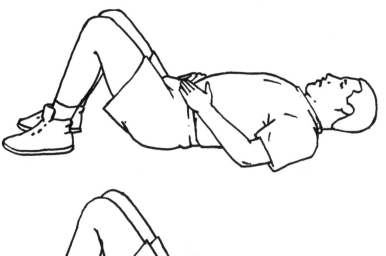

BACK

LOW BACK STRETCH
Targets the muscles in the low back
and buttocks.

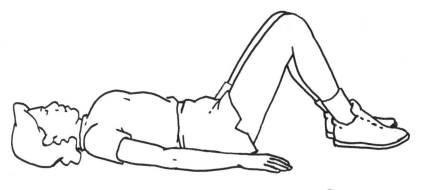

1. Lie on your back with your knees bent and your
feet flat on the floor. Keep your stomach tight, your
neck straight, and the small of your back pressed
toward the floor to maintain proper alignment. Inhale.

2. Slowly bring both knees to your chest, clasping
your hands under your thighs. Exhale as you stretch.
Hold the stretch for 5 to 30 seconds, breathing evenly
as you hold. Release one knee at a time back to the
starting position.

You may also bring in and release knees one at a time.

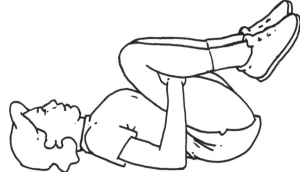

BACK

ADVANCED BACK STRETCH
Targets the muscles in the upper and low back
and buttocks.

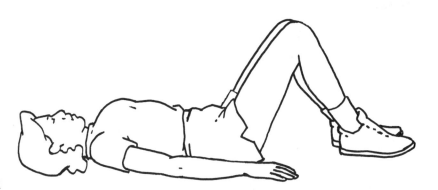

1. Lie on your back with your knees bent and your
feet flat on the floor. Keep your stomach tight,
your neck straight, and the small of your back pressed
toward the floor to maintain proper alignment. Inhale.

2. Slowly bring both knees to your chest, clasping your
hands under your thighs. Gently pull your thighs
toward your chest and lift your head and shoulders up
until your shoulder blades lift off the floor. Exhale as
you lift. Hold the stretch for 5 to 30 seconds, breathing
evenly as you hold. Release your shoulders and then
one knee at a time back to the starting position.

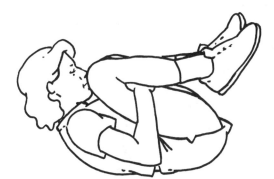

BACK

CAT STRETCH
Targets the muscles in the back.

1. Kneel down on your hands and knees. Keep your chin tucked and head and neck aligned and straight. Inhale.

2. Pull your stomach and chin in as you slowly round your back up. Inhale as you round up and don't let your back sag. Hold for 5 to 30 seconds, breathing evenly as you hold. Return slowly to the starting position.

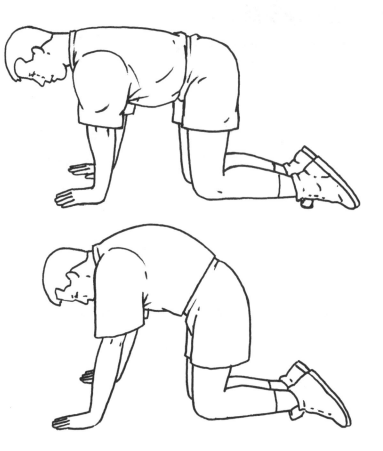

BACK

SEATED LOW BACK STRETCH
Targets the muscles in the low back, buttocks, and shoulders.

1. Sit all the way back on a sturdy, armless chair, with your arms at your sides and your shoulders down and relaxed (the back of the chair should be straight and positioned near a wall, if possible). Keep your stomach in, small of back pressed toward the back of the chair, chin tucked, gaze forward, and head upright. Inhale.

2. Bend your trunk down, allowing your hands to reach toward the floor and your head to rest on your knees. Exhale as you stretch down. Hold the stretch for 5 to 30 seconds, breathing evenly as you hold. Return to the starting position, uncurling slowly, one vertebra at a time, inhaling slowly as you sit up.

BACK

THE PRAYER

Targets the muscles in the upper and low back, front of the ankles, and lower legs.

1. Kneel down on your hands and knees. Keep your stomach in, chin tucked, and head and neck aligned and straight. Inhale.

2. Drop your buttocks back onto your heels while gently leaning your body backward and keeping your hands on the floor outstretched in front of you. Exhale as you stretch. Hold the stretch for 5 to 30 seconds, breathing evenly as you hold. Return slowly to the starting position.

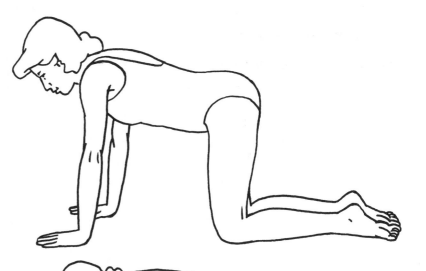

BACK • HIP • KNEE

CROSS-LEGGED SPINE STRETCH

Targets the muscles in the hips and back.

1. Sit cross-legged on the floor with your knees bent and your palms down at your sides. Keep your stomach in, chin tucked, gaze forward, and head upright. Inhale.

2. Curl your entire spine slowly, one vertebra at a time, sliding your hands forward along the floor. Exhale as you stretch forward, trying to touch the top of your head to the floor. Hold the stretch for 5 to 30 seconds, breathing evenly as you hold. Return to the starting position, slowly uncurling one vertebra at a time, inhaling as you sit up.

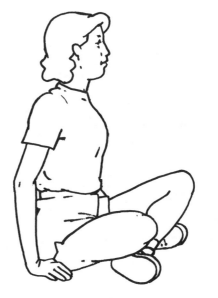

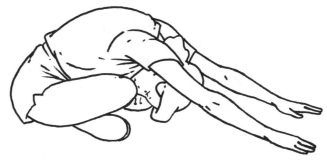

BACK • HIP • KNEE

LOW BACK HAMSTRING STRETCH
Targets the muscles in the low back, buttocks, and back of the thighs.

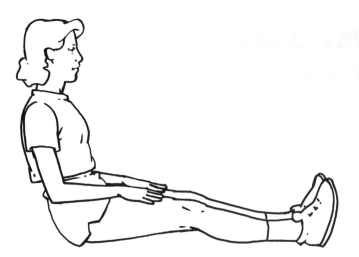

1. Sit with your legs out straight and your palms on your thighs. (If this does not feel comfortable at first, you may start by sitting with your legs straight out and your arms at your sides, with your hands on the floor behind your buttocks.) Keep your stomach in, chin tucked, gaze forward, head upright, and knees slightly bent. Inhale.

2. Curl your entire spine slowly, one vertebra at a time, sliding your hands forward along your legs. Exhale as you stretch forward, trying to touch the top of your head to your knees. Hold the stretch for 5 to 30 seconds, breathing evenly as you hold. Return to the starting position, uncurling slowly, one vertebra at a time, inhaling as you sit up.

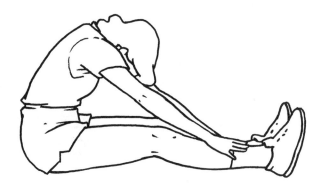

You may also stretch forward along one leg at a time, keeping the other leg out to the side and bent, or stretch forward while keeping the back straight.

BACK

STANDING LOW BACK STRETCH
Targets the muscles in the low back, buttocks, and back of the thighs.

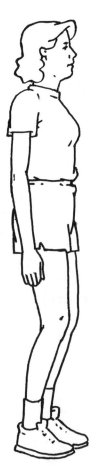

1. Stand with your knees straight or, if that's not comfortable, with your knees slightly bent. Keep your arms at your sides, your stomach in, chin tucked, gaze forward, and head upright. Inhale.

2. Slowly bend forward by rounding your neck, mid-back, and low back fully down into a relaxed position. Your arms should hang down loosely. Exhale as you stretch. Hold the stretch for 5 to 30 seconds, breathing evenly as you hold. Return to an upright position by uncurling your spine one vertebra at a time, keeping your chin and stomach in, inhaling as you stand up.

BACK

SEATED SPINAL TWIST
Targets the muscles in the sides of the torso.

1. Sit all the way back on a sturdy, armless chair, feet up on a small footstool, with your shoulders down and relaxed (the back of the chair should be straight and positioned near a wall, if possible). Keep your stomach in, small of back pressed toward the back of the chair, chin tucked, gaze forward, and head upright. Cross your arms over your chest. Inhale.

2. Gently twist your trunk to one side as far as you can comfortably go. Exhale as you twist. Hold the stretch for 5 to 30 seconds, breathing evenly as you hold. Return slowly to the starting position. Inhale as you return to the starting position.

3. Repeat on the opposite side.

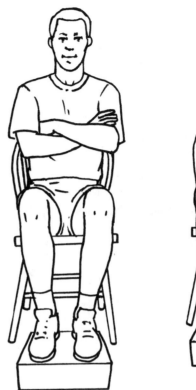
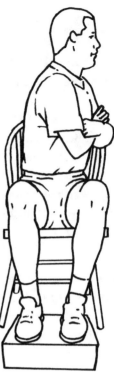

BACK

GENTLE SPINAL TWIST
Targets the muscles in the low back and buttocks.

1. Lie on the floor with your knees bent and your arms on the floor straight out to the sides at shoulder height. Press the small of your back toward the floor and keep your stomach tight and your neck straight to maintain proper alignment. Cross your right leg over your left leg and drop both legs to the left. Inhale.

2. Slowly rotate your head to the right. Keep both arms flat on the floor. Exhale as you stretch. Hold the stretch for 5 to 30 seconds, breathing evenly as you hold. Return slowly to the starting position.

3. Repeat on the opposite side.

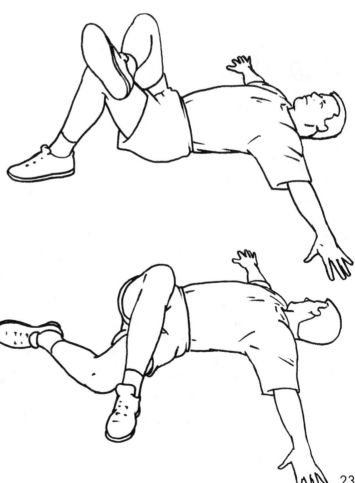

BACK

ADVANCED SPINAL TWIST
Targets the muscles in the buttocks and back.

1. Sit on the floor. Extend your right leg out straight in front of you. Bend your left leg and place your left foot on the floor at the outside of your right knee. Wrap your upper right arm around your left lower leg, keeping your elbow below your knee and your left hand behind your left buttock. Keep your stomach in, chin tucked, gaze forward, and head upright. Inhale.

2. Turn your head and shoulders to the left as you push your left leg over to the right. Exhale as you turn. Hold the stretch for 5 to 30 seconds, breathing evenly as you hold.

3. Repeat on the opposite side.

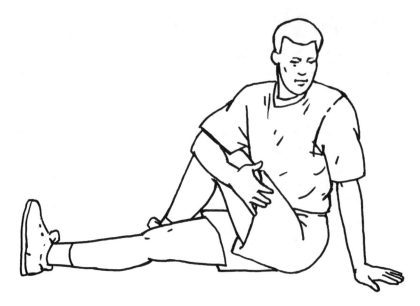

BACK • SHOULDER

SIDE STRETCH
Targets the muscles on the sides of the torso and shoulders.

1. Stand up straight or sit all the way back on a sturdy, armless chair, feet up on a small footstool, with your shoulders down and relaxed (the back of the chair should be straight and positioned near a wall, if possible). Keep your stomach in, chin tucked, gaze forward, and head upright. Inhale.

2. Gently lean your trunk over to one side as the opposite arm (kept straight, palm down) comes up overhead and reaches toward a point where the wall would meet the ceiling. Exhale as you stretch. Hold the stretch for 5 to 30 seconds, breathing evenly as you hold. Return slowly to the starting position.

3. Repeat on the opposite side.

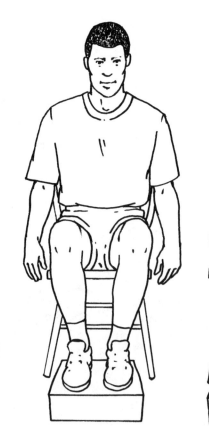
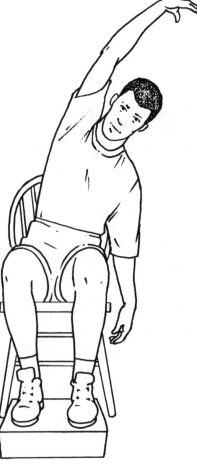

BACK

EXTENDED-ARM SIDE STRETCH

Targets the muscles in the outer thighs, hips, sides of the torso, back of the shoulders, and arms.

1. Stand with your legs spread a bit more than shoulder width apart, your feet facing forward and your knees straight, or if that's not comfortable, slightly bent. Keep your arms at your sides and your palms facing in. Inhale.

2. Raise your right arm up overhead with your palm facing the floor and slide your left hand down your leg to your ankle. Your head should stay aligned with your spine; do not bend forward at the hip. Exhale as you stretch down. Hold the stretch for 5 to 30 seconds, breathing evenly as you hold. Return slowly to the starting position.

3. Repeat on the opposite side.

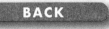

BACK

THE STRETCHER

Targets the muscles in the abdomen, chest, and arms.

1. Lie on your back with your legs out straight and your arms extended overhead. Keep your neck straight to maintain proper alignment. Point your toes straight ahead. Inhale.

2. Pull your arms and legs in opposite directions as much as possible. Exhale as you stretch. Hold the stretch for 5 to 30 seconds, breathing evenly as you hold.

BACK • SHOULDER

STRETCH AND REACH
Targets the muscles in the abdomen, upper chest, shoulders, and arms.

1. Stand in the yoga sun pose with your arms at your sides and your feet parallel. Keep your stomach in, chin tucked, gaze forward, head upright, and knees slightly bent. Inhale.

2. Raise your arms out to the sides and overhead, bringing your arms together so that your palms come together as you look up at your hands. Hold the stretch for 5 to 30 seconds, breathing evenly as you hold. Exhale as you return slowly to the starting position.

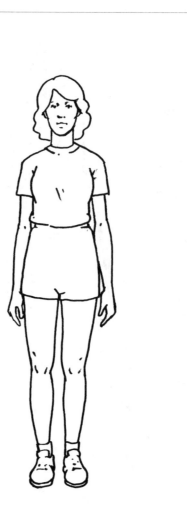
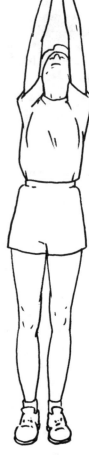

BACK

REVERSE CAT STRETCH
Targets the muscles in the upper and low back and abdomen.

1. Kneel down on your hands and knees. Keep your stomach in, chin tucked, and head and neck aligned and straight. Inhale.

2. In the on-knees position, drop your stomach and arch your back in a reverse cat stretch position. Exhale as you stretch. Hold the stretch for 5 to 30 seconds, breathing evenly as you hold. Return slowly to the starting position.

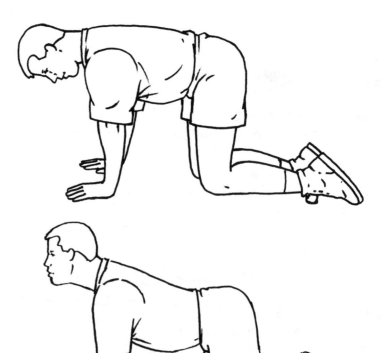

BACK

ABDOMINAL STRETCH
Targets the muscles in the abdomen.

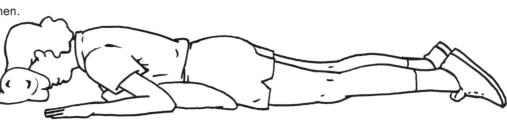

1. Lie on your stomach with your forehead resting on the floor. (You may use a towel roll under your forehead.) Place a large pillow under your stomach. Keep your hands flat on the floor at shoulder level. Inhale.

2. Keep your chin in and head, neck, and back aligned. Push up onto your elbows, arching your spine backward and exhaling as you push up. Keep your head, back, and neck aligned with each other and your hips in contact with the floor. Hold the stretch for 5 to 30 seconds, breathing evenly as you hold. Return slowly to the starting position.

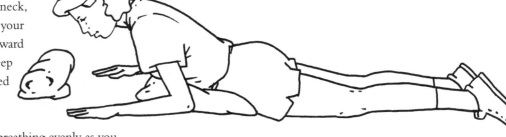

BACK • HIP

COBRA STRETCH
Targets the muscles in the abdomen and hips.

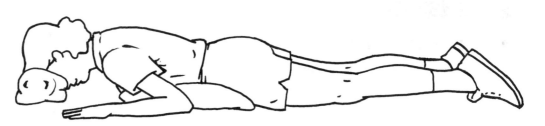

1. Lie on your stomach with your forehead resting on the floor. (You may use a towel roll under your forehead.) Place a large pillow under your stomach. Keep your hands flat on the floor at shoulder level. Inhale.

2. Keep your chin in and head, neck, and back aligned. Push up with extended arms until your chest is off the floor (your hips should remain in contact with the floor), exhaling as you push up. Hold the stretch for 5 to 30 seconds, breathing evenly as you hold. Return slowly to the starting position.

BACK • SHOULDER

CORNER STRETCH

Targets the muscles in the upper chest.

1. Stand up straight. With your feet parallel, face the corner of the wall. Keep your stomach in, chin tucked, gaze forward, head upright, and knees slightly bent. Bend your arms and raise them as close to shoulder height as you comfortably can. Place your arms on the wall (as if you're about to do a push-up) and point your fingers toward the ceiling. Inhale.

2. Slowly lean your body toward the corner. Be careful not to flex at your hips; you should press your hips slightly forward. Exhale as you lean into the wall. Hold the stretch for 5 to 30 seconds, breathing evenly as you hold. Inhale as you straighten up.

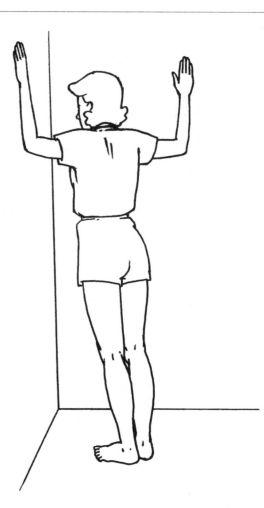

NECK

NECK LENGTHENER

Targets the muscles in the back of the neck.

1. Lie on your back with your knees bent and your feet flat on the floor. Keep your stomach tight, your neck straight, and the small of your back pressed toward the floor to maintain proper alignment. Keep your hands on your lower abdomen and your shoulders down and relaxed. Inhale.

2. Pull your chin in so the back of your neck flattens to the floor. Exhale as you pull your chin in. Hold the stretch for 5 to 30 seconds, breathing evenly as you hold, then gently release the pressure.

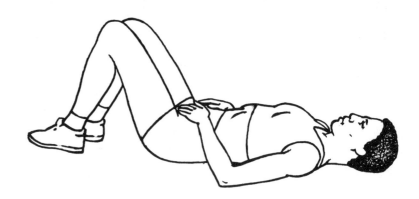

BACK • NECK

SPINE LENGTHENER
Targets the muscles in the back and neck.

1. Stand up straight. Keep your stomach in, chin tucked, gaze forward, head upright, and knees slightly bent. Inhale.

2. Pulling your chin back and in, pretend that a string is pulling you straight up from the top of your head, further tighten your stomach muscles, and pull your lower shoulder blades gently together. Feel the stretch in your back and neck. Exhale as you stretch. Hold the stretch for 5 to 30 seconds, breathing evenly as you hold.

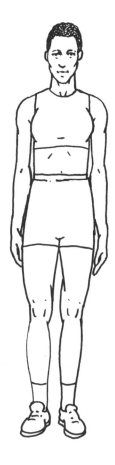

NECK

SEATED NECK NOD
Targets the muscles in the back and front of the neck.

1. Sit all the way back on a sturdy chair, feet up on a small footstool, with your arms supported on armrests and your shoulders down and relaxed (the back of the chair should be straight and positioned near a wall, if possible). Keep your stomach in, small of back pressed toward the back of the chair, chin tucked, gaze forward, and head upright. Inhale.

2. Flex (nod) your head forward, slowly bringing your chin down toward your chest and exhaling as you flex. Slowly stretch and hold for 5 to 30 seconds, breathing evenly as you hold. Inhale and raise your head back up, one vertebra at a time. Then extend your neck by moving your head backward to look at the ceiling, exhaling as you stretch. Return slowly to the starting position.

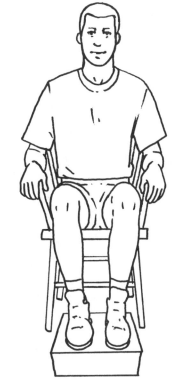

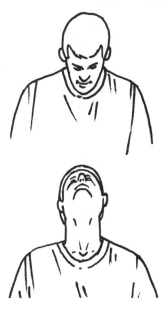

NECK

RAISED-ARM NECK FLEX
Targets the muscles in the back of the neck, upper back, and shoulders.

1. Sit all the way back on a sturdy chair, feet up on a small footstool, with your shoulders down and relaxed and your fingertips at the back of your head (the back of the chair should be straight and positioned near a wall, if possible). Keep your stomach in, small of back pressed toward the back of the chair, chin tucked, gaze forward, and head upright. Inhale.

2. Keeping your shoulders level, gently bring your chin to your chest, allowing the weight of your hands to increase the stretch. Do not let your upper back or spine lean forward; the movement takes place only in your neck, and you may feel a pull between your shoulder blades. Exhale as you stretch. Hold the stretch for 5 to 30 seconds, breathing evenly as you hold.

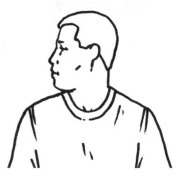

NECK

SEATED NECK TWIST
Targets the muscles in the sides and back of the neck.

1. Sit all the way back on a sturdy chair, feet up on a small footstool, with your arms supported on armrests and your shoulders down and relaxed (the back of the chair should be straight and positioned near a wall, if possible). Keep your stomach in, small of back pressed toward the back of the chair, chin tucked, gaze forward, and head upright. Inhale.

2. Slowly rotate your head through its maximum range of motion to the right, then to its maximum range of motion to the left (as if shaking your head "no"). Exhale as you turn. Hold the stretch for 5 to 10 seconds in each position. Inhale as you turn your head back to face forward.

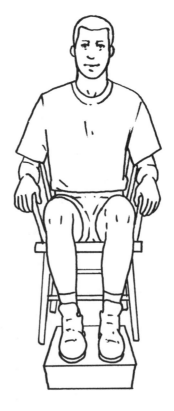

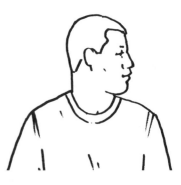

NECK

NECK ROTATION

Targets the muscles in the back and the sides of the neck.

1. Sit all the way back on a sturdy chair, feet up on a small footstool, with your arms supported on armrests, your shoulders down and relaxed (the back of the chair should be straight and positioned near a wall, if possible). Keep your stomach in, small of back pressed toward the back of the chair, and chin tucked. Inhale.

2. Keeping your shoulders level, gently turn your chin up to your right shoulder, then back across your chest to your left shoulder. (Be sure to keep your chin on your chest throughout the exercise.) Exhale as you rotate.

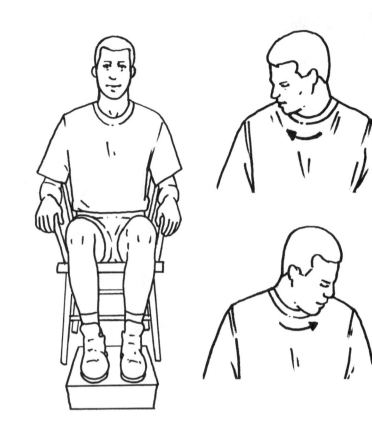

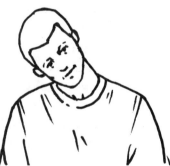

NECK

SEATED NECK SIDE BEND

Targets the muscles on the sides of the neck.

1. Sit all the way back on a sturdy chair, feet up on a small footstool, with your arms supported on armrests and your shoulders down and relaxed (the back of the chair should be straight and positioned near a wall, if possible). Keep your stomach in, small of back pressed toward the back of the chair, chin tucked, gaze forward, and head upright. Inhale.

2. Keeping your shoulders level, pull your chin back and in and keep the top of your head toward the ceiling. Slowly bend your head to the side (right ear lobe goes toward your right shoulder; be sure not to rotate neck) and gently pull your opposite shoulder down. Exhale while you stretch. Hold the stretch for 5 to 10 seconds, breathing evenly as you hold. Then inhale as you move your head back up and then bend to the left as far as you can comfortably go. Exhale as you stretch. Hold the stretch for 5 to 10 seconds, breathing evenly as you hold.

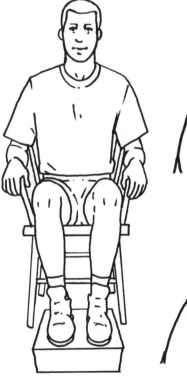

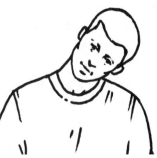

NECK

LATERAL NECK SIDE BEND
Targets the muscles in the sides of the neck.

1. Sit all the way back on a sturdy chair, feet up on a small footstool, with your arms supported on armrests and your shoulders down and relaxed (the back of the chair should be straight and positioned near a wall, if possible). Keep your stomach in, small of back pressed toward the back of the chair, chin tucked, gaze forward, and head upright. Inhale.

2. Keeping your shoulders level, pull your chin back and in and keep the top of your head toward the ceiling. Slowly bend your head to the side (right ear lobe goes toward your right shoulder; be sure not to rotate neck) as far as you can comfortably go and, at the same time, reach your left hand down toward the floor. Hold for 5 to 10 seconds and exhale during the stretch. Then inhale as you move your head back up.

3. Repeat on the opposite side.

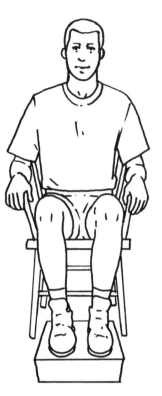
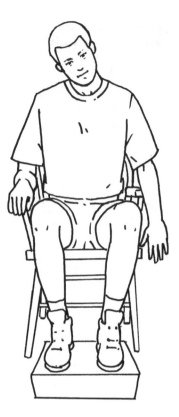

NECK

ASSISTED LATERAL NECK STRETCH
Targets the muscles in the sides of the neck.

1. Sit all the way back on a sturdy chair, feet up on a small footstool, with your arms supported on armrests and your shoulders down and relaxed (the back of the chair should be straight and positioned near a wall, if possible). Keep your stomach in, small of back pressed toward the back of the chair, chin tucked, gaze forward, and head upright. Inhale.

2. Keeping your shoulders level, pull your chin back and in and keep the top of your head toward the ceiling. Slowly bend your head to the side (right ear lobe goes toward your right shoulder; be sure not to rotate neck) as far as you can comfortably go and, at the same time, reach your left hand down toward the floor. Reach your right hand up and over your head, placing it gently on the left side of your head as you allow the weight of your hand to increase the stretch over to your right side. Hold for 5 to 10 seconds and exhale during the stretch. Then inhale as you move your head back up.

3. Repeat on the opposite side.

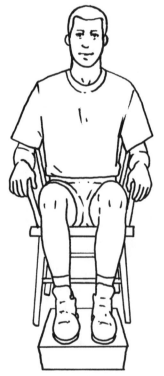
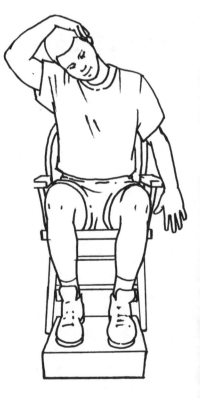

NECK

NECK CIRCLES
Targets the muscles in the neck.

1. Sit all the way back on a sturdy chair, feet up on a small footstool, with your arms supported on armrests, your shoulders down and relaxed, and your chin resting on your chest (the back of the chair should be straight and positioned near a wall, if possible). Keep your stomach in, small of back pressed toward the back of the chair, and chin tucked. Inhale.

2. Rotate your head slowly by "drawing" a large circle in front of you with your chin. Begin the circle by sliding your chin up and over your right shoulder, exhaling as you go. As you reach the top of your shoulder, let your head gently drop back and your chin point to the ceiling. Inhale and then continue the circle down and over the left shoulder, returning your chin to the chest position.

3. Gently rotate your head in a clockwise direction and then in a counterclockwise direction.

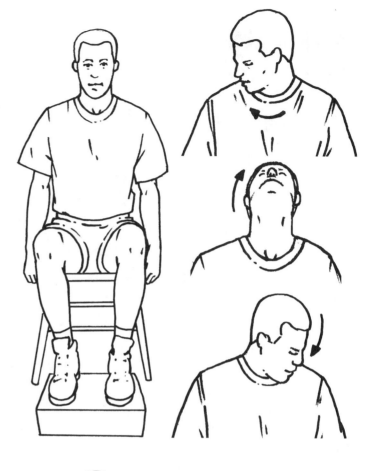

JAW

JAW RELAXER
Targets the muscles in the jaw.

Note: *This exercise should be done facing a mirror.*

1. Sit all the way back on a sturdy, armless chair, feet up on a small footstool, with your shoulders down and relaxed (the back of the chair should be straight and positioned near a wall, if possible). Keep your stomach in, small of back pressed toward the back of the chair, chin tucked, gaze forward, and head upright.

2. Keep the tip of your tongue on the roof of your mouth and your jaw relaxed (not clenched). Open and close your mouth several times, being sure that your chin is moving perfectly straight up and down. Breathe in and out through your nose during the entire stretch.

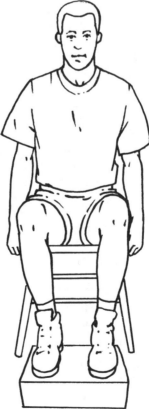
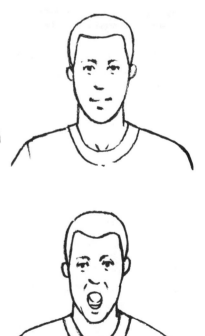

JAW

LATERAL JAW RELAXER
Targets the muscles in the jaw.

Note: *This exercise should be done facing a mirror.*

1. Sit all the way back on a sturdy, armless chair, feet up on a small footstool, with your shoulders down and relaxed (the back of the chair should be straight and positioned near a wall, if possible). Keep your stomach in, small of back pressed toward the back of the chair, chin tucked, gaze forward, and head upright.

2. Keep your jaw relaxed (not clenched). Slowly move your jaw from side to side. Breathe in and out through your nose during the entire stretch.

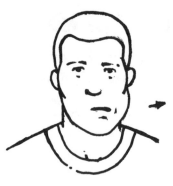

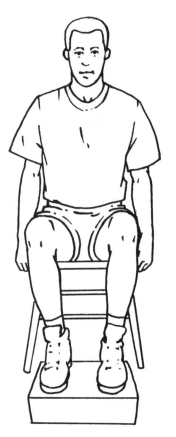

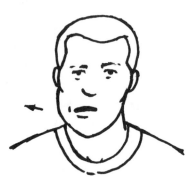

SHOULDER • BACK

UPPER BACK STRETCH
Targets the upper back and shoulders.

1. Sit all the way back on a sturdy, armless chair, feet up on a small footstool, with your shoulders down and relaxed (the back of the chair should be straight and positioned near a wall, if possible). Keep your stomach in, small of back pressed toward the back of the chair, chin tucked, gaze forward, and head upright. Raise your arms straight out in front of you at shoulder height. Clasp your hands together with your palms facing toward you. Inhale.

2. Keeping your fingers clasped, turn your palms away from you and bring your chin to chest as you push your hands away from you. Exhale as you stretch. Hold the stretch for 5 to 30 seconds, breathing evenly as you hold. Inhale as you return your head and hands back to the starting position.

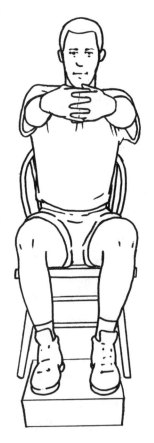

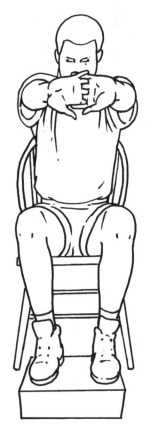

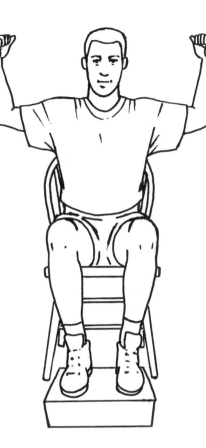
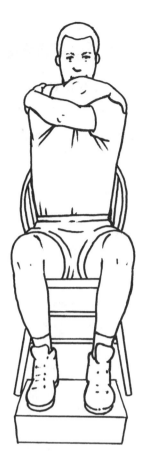

SHOULDER · BACK

UPPER BACK/SHOULDER STRETCH

Targets the muscles in the upper back and shoulders.

1. Sit all the way back on a sturdy, armless chair, feet up on a small footstool, with your shoulders down and relaxed (the back of the chair should be straight and positioned near a wall, if possible). Keep your stomach in, small of back pressed toward the back of the chair, chin tucked, gaze forward, and head upright. Raise your arms to your sides (parallel to the floor) with your forearms bent so your fists point upward. Inhale.

2. Keeping your elbows at shoulder height, draw your arms across your body and reach around your back with each opposing hand as far as possible, giving yourself a bear hug. Exhale as you reach and stretch. Hold the stretch for 5 to 30 seconds, breathing evenly as you hold.

SHOULDER

SHOULDER ROLL

Targets the muscles in the shoulders, upper back, and chest.

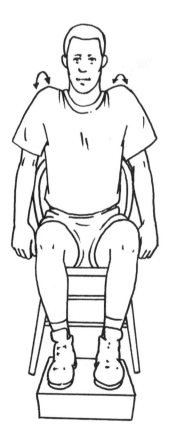

1. Sit all the way back on a sturdy, armless chair, feet up on a small footstool, with your shoulders down and relaxed (the back of the chair should be straight and positioned near a wall, if possible). Keep your stomach in, small of back pressed toward the back of the chair, chin tucked, gaze forward, and head upright. Inhale.

2. Roll your shoulders backward by lifting your shoulders up toward your ears and then rolling them back down as you pinch your shoulder blades together. Pause and then reverse the direction. Exhale as you roll your shoulders backward, inhale as you roll your shoulders forward.

SHOULDER

ARM SWING

Targets the muscles in the shoulders.

Note: *This exercise may also be done with a light hand weight.*

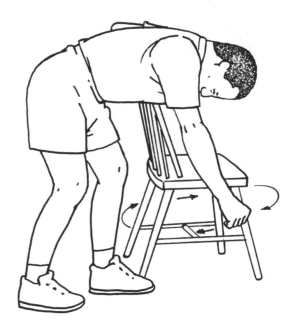

1. Stand with your left hand on the top of the back rest of a chair (which should be placed to your left side), your stomach in, chin tucked, gaze forward, and head upright. Stand with your feet shoulder-width apart, with one foot forward and your knees slightly bent. With your stomach tight and your neck straight to maintain proper alignment, lean your trunk forward and let your free arm hang down. Inhale.

2. Gently swing your arm very loosely like a pendulum: (a) back and forth in front of your body; (b) back and forth along the side of your body; (c) in as big a circle clockwise as possible; and (d) in as big a circle counter-clockwise as possible. Breathe evenly throughout. *If you use a weight, inhale before and exhale as you complete each movement.*

3. Repeat on the opposite side.

SHOULDER

OVERHEAD SHOULDER STRETCH

Targets the muscles in the chest and shoulders.

1. Lie on your back with your knees bent and your feet flat on the floor. Keep your hands on your lower abdomen, shoulders down and relaxed, chin tucked, stomach muscles tightened, and back flat against the floor. Inhale.

2. Straighten your arms and then raise them up overhead, attempting to touch the back of your upper arms to the floor. Exhale as you stretch. Hold the stretch for 5 to 30 seconds, breathing evenly as you hold. Return slowly to the starting position.

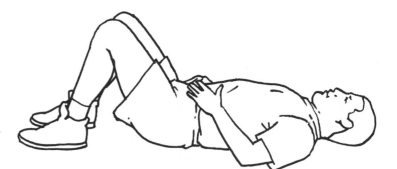

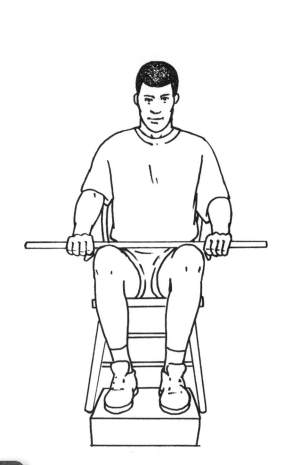
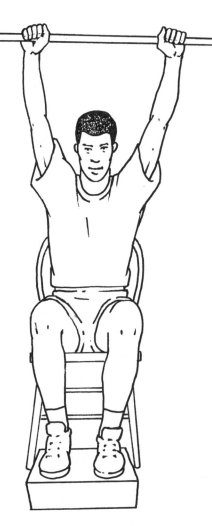

SHOULDER

OVERHEAD LIFT

Targets the muscles in the chest, shoulders, and sides of the torso.

Note: *This exercise uses a stick.*

1. Sit all the way back on a sturdy, armless chair, feet up on a small footstool, with your shoulders down and relaxed (the back of the chair should be straight and positioned near a wall, if possible). Keep your stomach in, small of back pressed toward the back of the chair, chin tucked, gaze forward, and head upright. Hold a stick in both hands and rest it across your knees. Inhale.

2. Raise both your arms up overhead as far as you can comfortably go. Exhale as you lift. Hold the stretch for 5 to 30 seconds, breathing evenly as you hold. Return slowly to the starting position.

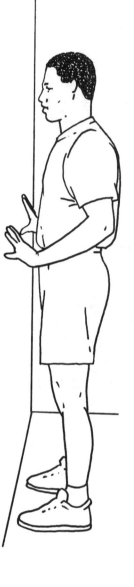
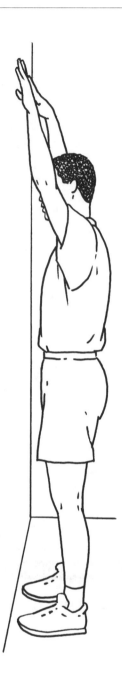

SHOULDER

FRONT FINGER WALK
Targets the muscles in the chest and shoulders.

1. Stand up straight and have your toes almost touching a wall. Keep your stomach in, chin tucked, gaze forward, head upright, and knees slightly bent. Place your hands at waist level with your palms facing the wall and your fingertips touching the wall. Inhale.

2. Use your fingers to walk both arms up overhead as far as you can comfortably go. Exhale as you stretch. Hold the stretch for 5 to 30 seconds, breathing evenly as you hold. Walk your arms slowly back down to the starting position.

SHOULDER

REVERSE BUTTERFLY STRETCH

Targets the muscles in the front and back of the shoulders, under the shoulder blades, and chest.

1. Lie on your back with your knees bent and your feet flat on the floor. Keep your shoulders down and relaxed, chin tucked, stomach muscles tightened, and back flat against the floor. Place your hands over your ears and point your elbows toward the ceiling. Inhale.

2. Push your elbows back toward the floor. Exhale as you stretch. Hold the stretch for 5 to 30 seconds, breathing evenly as you hold.

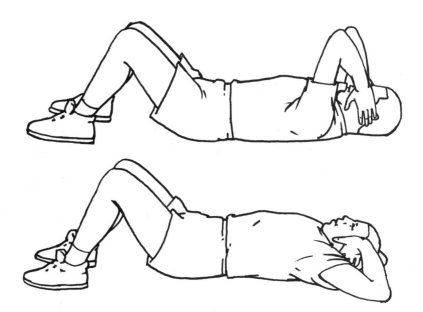

SHOULDER

FAN STRETCH

Targets the muscles in the chest, shoulders, and sides of the torso.

1. Lie on your back with your knees bent and your feet flat on the floor. Keep your hands on your lower abdomen, shoulders down and relaxed, chin tucked, stomach muscles tightened, and back flat against the floor. Inhale.

2. Place both your arms out to your sides at shoulder height. Turn your palms up so that they are facing the ceiling and move your arms up toward your ears, being sure to keep them on the floor. Exhale as you stretch. Hold the stretch for 5 to 30 seconds, breathing evenly as you hold. Return slowly to the starting position.

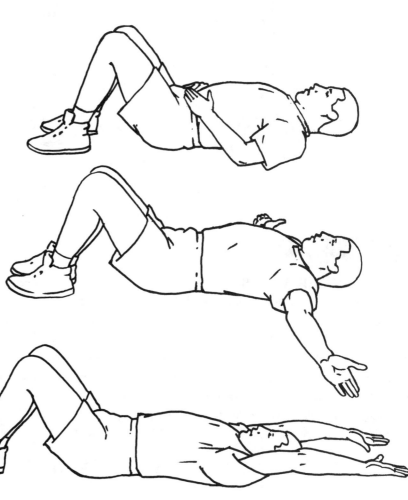

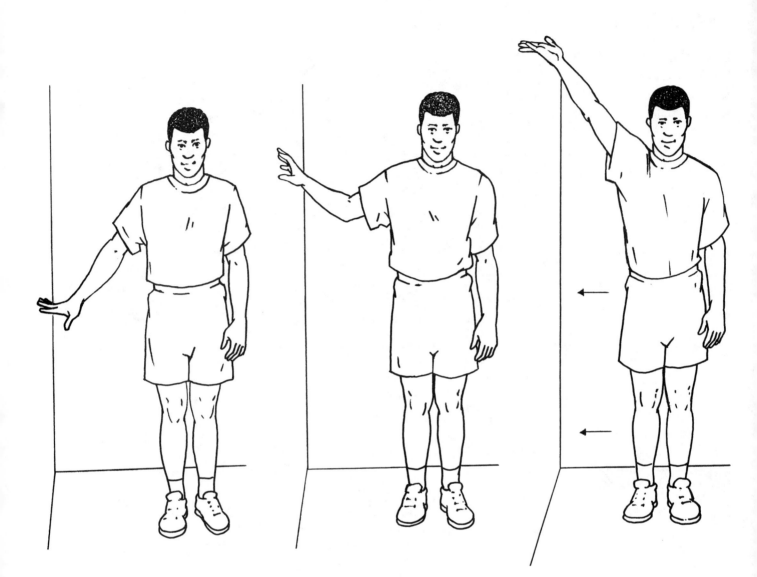

SIDE FINGER WALK
Targets the muscles in the shoulders and sides of the torso.

1. Stand up straight with one side pointed toward the wall and your feet about 2 feet from the wall. Keep your stomach in, chin tucked, gaze forward, head upright, and knees slightly bent. With your palms facing down, place your fingertips on the wall. Inhale.

2. Walk your hand up the wall to shoulder height, then turn your palm up and continue sliding it up the wall as far as you can comfortably go, moving your body closer to the wall as you go up. Exhale as you stretch. Hold the stretch for 5 to 30 seconds, breathing evenly as you hold. Walk your arm slowly back down to the starting position. (You may lift the opposite arm simultaneously to keep the body in correct upright alignment so you don't lean away from the wall.)

3. Repeat on the opposite side.

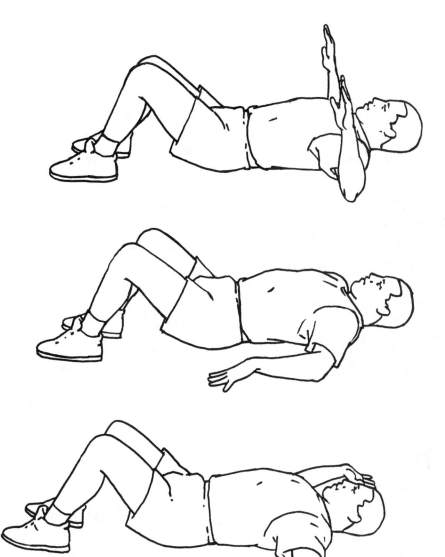

SHOULDER

FOREARM ROLL

Targets the muscles in the shoulders.

1. Lie on your back with your knees bent and your feet flat on the floor. With your shoulders down and relaxed, chin tucked, stomach muscles tightened, and back flat against the floor, place both your arms out to your sides at shoulder height and bend your elbows so your fingers point toward the ceiling. Inhale.

2. Roll your forearms forward and back, attempting to touch your forearms to the floor. Exhale as you stretch. Hold the stretch for 5 to 30 seconds in each direction, breathing evenly as you hold.

You may also roll the forearms one at a time.

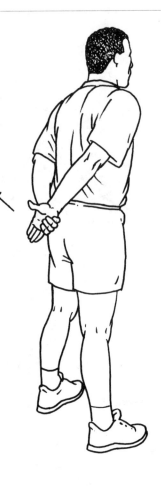

SHOULDER

CLASPED-HANDS STRETCH
Targets the muscles in the front of the shoulders and the upper chest.

1. Stand up straight or sit on a sturdy, armless chair, feet up on a small footstool, with your shoulders down and relaxed (the back of the chair should be straight and positioned near a wall, if possible). Keep your stomach in, chin tucked, gaze forward, and head upright. Be sure not to arch your back. Inhale.

2. Clasp your hands together behind your back. Keeping your stomach tight and your neck straight to maintain good alignment, raise your arms as high up in back as you can comfortably go. Exhale as you stretch. Hold the stretch for 5 to 30 seconds, breathing evenly as you hold.

SHOULDER

OUTER SHOULDER STRETCH
Targets the muscles in the shoulders.

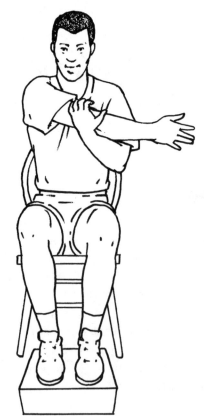

1. Stand up straight or sit all the way back on a sturdy, arm-less chair, feet up on a small footstool, with your shoulders down and relaxed (the back of the chair should be straight and positioned near a wall, if possible). Keep your stomach in, small of back pressed toward the back of the chair, chin tucked, gaze forward, and head upright. Inhale.

2. Reach your right arm across the front of your body as close to shoulder height as comfortably possible, making sure you keep your shoulders down. Reach your left hand under your right arm, grasp it above your elbow, and gently stretch your right arm farther across the front of your body. Be sure to keep your shoulders down, your stomach tight, and your neck straight to maintain good alignment during the stretch. Exhale as you stretch. Hold the stretch for 5 to 30 seconds, breathing evenly as you hold.

3. Repeat on the opposite side.

SHOULDER

ARM CIRCLES
Targets the muscles in the upper back and chest.

1. Sit all the way back on a sturdy, armless chair, feet up on a small footstool, with your shoulders down and relaxed (the back of the chair should be straight and positioned near a wall, if possible). Keep your stomach in, small of back pressed toward the back of the chair, chin tucked, gaze forward, and head upright. Raise both arms out to the sides to shoulder height. Inhale.

2. Slowly and smoothly circle both arms in as big an arc as you can comfortably do and then reverse the direction. Inhale as you circle your arms up, exhale slowly through two circles, and repeat the breathing sequence.

You may also circle one arm at a time.

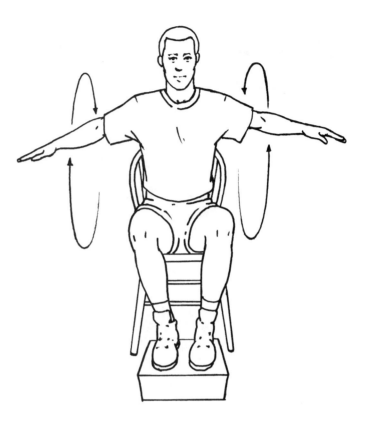

SHOULDER

SHOULDER ROTATOR
Targets the muscles in the shoulders and chest.

Note: *This exercise uses a towel.*

1. Stand up straight or sit all the way back on a sturdy, armless chair, feet up on a small footstool, with your shoulders down and relaxed (the back of the chair should be straight and positioned near a wall, if possible). Keep your stomach in, chin tucked, gaze forward, and head upright. Hold a towel in one hand and drop it over your shoulder. Place the back of the other hand against your lower back and grasp the lower end of the towel with it. Be sure not to arch your back. Inhale.

2. Keeping your stomach tight and your neck straight to maintain proper alignment, gently pull the towel with your uppermost arm, raising the lowermost arm as high as you comfortably can. Exhale as you stretch. Hold the stretch for 5 to 30 seconds, breathing evenly as you hold. Then pull the towel with your lowermost arm, pulling the uppermost arm as low as you comfortably can. Exhale as you stretch. Hold the stretch for 5 to 30 seconds, breathing evenly as you hold.

3. Repeat on the opposite side.

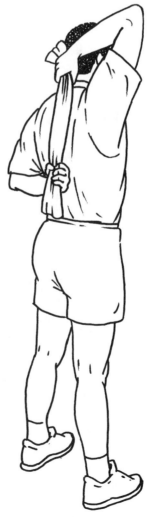

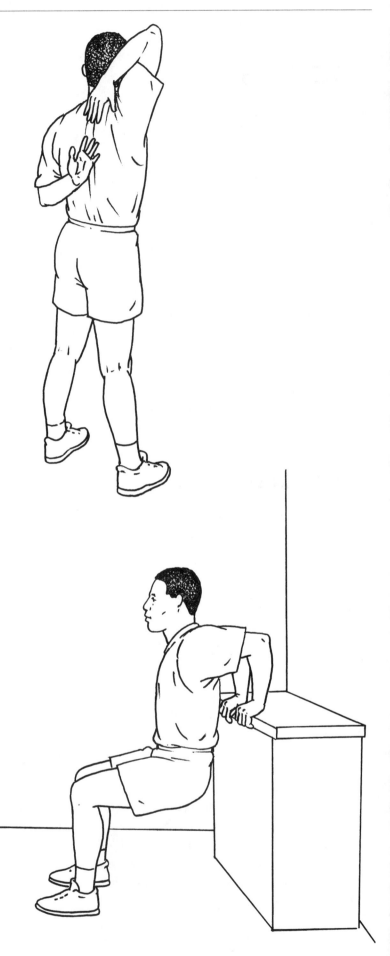

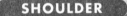

SHOULDER

SHOULDER RELEASE

Targets the muscles in the shoulders.

1. Stand up straight or sit forward on a sturdy, armless chair, feet up on a small footstool, with your shoulders down and relaxed (the back of the chair should be straight and positioned near a wall, if possible). Keep your stomach in, chin tucked, gaze forward, and head upright. Be sure not to arch your back.

2. Bring one arm behind your low back and the opposite arm up over your shoulder as you try to make your fingers meet. Inhale. Do not let your upper back or spine lean forward. Exhale as you stretch. Hold the stretch for 5 to 30 seconds, breathing evenly as you hold.

3. Repeat, switching arms in the upper and lower positions

SHOULDER

SHOULDER DIP

Targets the muscles in the shoulders, front of the upper arms, and chest.

1. Stand with your back toward a desk or table that is pushed against a wall, with your feet about 3 feet away from the desk and your hands clasped on the edge of it. Keep your stomach in, chin tucked, gaze forward, head upright, and knees slightly bent. Inhale.

2. Bend your knees as far as you comfortably can, bending your elbows, and lower your body with the weight on your arms. (Be sure your knees stay behind or just over your ankles. If you do not feel a shoulder stretch, move your feet farther away from the desk.) Exhale as you stretch. Hold the stretch for 5 to 30 seconds, breathing evenly as you hold.

ELBOW

ELBOW STRETCH

Targets the muscles in the front of the upper arms.

1. Sit all the way back on a sturdy, armless chair, feet up on a small footstool, with your shoulders down and relaxed (the back of the chair should be straight and positioned near a wall, if possible). Keep your stomach in, small of back pressed toward the back of the chair, chin tucked, gaze forward, and head upright. Bend your elbows all the way up, bringing your hands toward your chin. Inhale.

2. Lower your forearms, straightening your elbows completely. Extend your arms behind your body and rotate your forearms in so that your palms are facing away from your body. Exhale as you stretch. Hold the stretch for 5 to 30 seconds, breathing evenly as you hold. Inhale as you return slowly to starting position.

You may also do the exercise one elbow at a time.

ELBOW · SHOULDER

TRICEPS STRETCH

Targets the muscles in the back of the upper arms, shoulders, and chest.

1. Stand up straight or sit all the way back on a sturdy, armless chair, feet up on a small footstool, with your shoulders down and relaxed (the back of the chair should be straight and positioned near a wall, if possible). Keep your stomach in, chin tucked, gaze forward, and head upright. Inhale.

2. Place one hand behind your head (upper arm close to your ear), reaching your fingers down toward the middle of your upper back (your elbow points to the ceiling). Keeping your stomach tight and your neck straight to maintain proper alignment, place your opposite hand on the top of your elbow and gently push your upper arm back and down. Be sure not to arch your back. Exhale as you stretch. Hold the stretch for 5 to 30 seconds, breathing evenly as you hold.

3. Repeat on the opposite side.

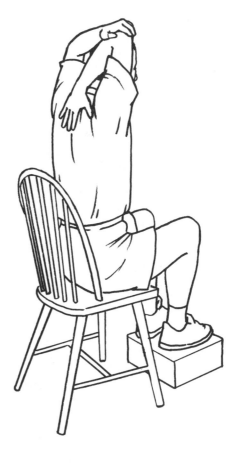

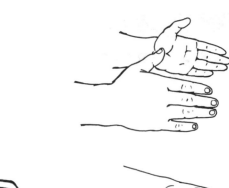

WRIST/HAND

FOREARM PRONATION-SUPINATION
Targets the muscles in the forearms.

1. Sit all the way back on a sturdy, armless chair, feet up on a small footstool, with your shoulders down and relaxed (the back of the chair should be straight and positioned near a wall, if possible). Keep your stomach in, small of back pressed toward the back of the chair, chin tucked, gaze forward, and head upright. Keep your elbows at the sides of your body and bend them at a right angle. Keep your forearms in a neutral position with your thumbs pointing up. Inhale.

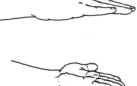

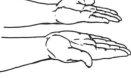

2. Gently turn your palms down as far as you can comfortably go, then turn your palms all the way up as far as you can comfortably go. Exhale as you turn your palms. Hold the stretch for 5 to 30 seconds in each position, breathing evenly as you hold.

You may also turn the palms up and down one at a time.

WRIST/HAND

WRIST FLEXION-EXTENSION
Targets the muscles in the wrists.

1. Sit all the way back on a sturdy, armless chair, feet up on a small footstool, with your shoulders down and relaxed (the back of the chair should be straight and positioned near a wall, if possible). Keep your stomach in, small of back pressed toward the back of the chair, chin tucked, gaze forward, and head upright. Keep your elbows at the sides of your body and bend them at a right angle with your wrists straight, palms facing down, and fingers relaxed. Inhale.

2. With your fingers relaxed, bend your wrists all the way down, then bring them all the way up. Exhale as you stretch. Hold the stretch 5 to 30 seconds in each position, breathing evenly as you hold.

You may also bend the wrists up and down one at a time.

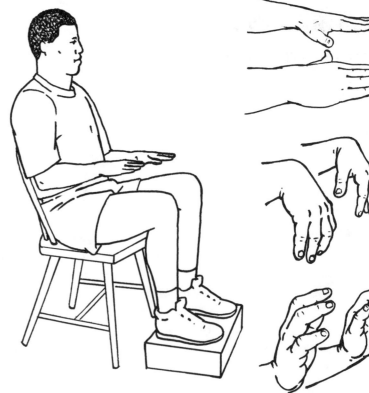

WRIST/HAND

PALM-UP WRIST/FINGER EXTENSION

Targets the muscles in the wrists, hands, and forearms.

1. Sit all the way back on a sturdy, armless chair, feet up on a small footstool, with your shoulders down and relaxed (the back of the chair should be straight and positioned near a wall, if possible). Keep your stomach in, small of back pressed toward the back of the chair, chin tucked, gaze forward, and head upright. Place one arm out straight in front of you at shoulder level with your palm up and your fingertips pointing toward the floor. Inhale.

2. With your other hand, gently press your fingertips toward you. Exhale as you stretch. Hold the stretch for 5 to 30 seconds, breathing evenly as you hold.

3. Repeat on the opposite side.

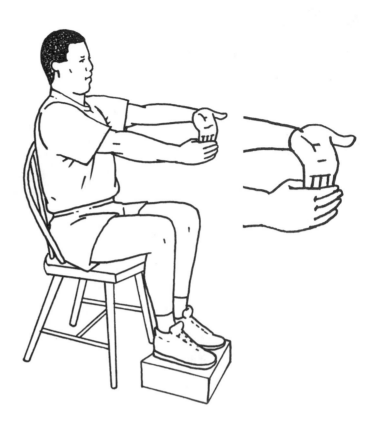

WRIST/HAND

PALM-DOWN WRIST/FINGER FLEXION

Targets the muscles in the wrists, hands, and forearms.

1. Sit all the way back on a sturdy, armless chair, feet up on a small footstool, with your shoulders down and relaxed (the back of the chair should be straight and positioned near a wall, if possible). Keep your stomach in, small of back pressed toward the back of the chair, chin tucked, gaze forward, and head upright. Place one arm out straight in front of you at shoulder level with your palm down and your fingertips pointing toward the floor. Inhale.

2. With your other hand, gently press the back of your hand toward you. Exhale as you stretch. Hold the stretch for 5 to 30 seconds, breathing evenly as you hold.

3. Repeat on the opposite side.

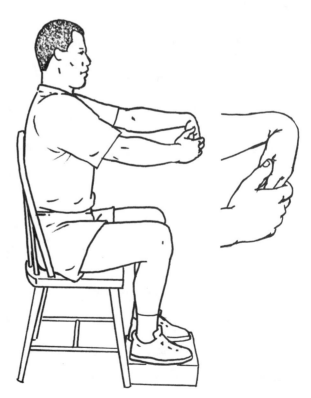

WRIST/HAND

FLAT HAND STRETCH
Targets the muscles in the wrists and fingers.

1. Stand up straight and place your hands flat on a desk or table. Keep your stomach in, head upright, chin tucked, gaze forward, and knees slightly bent. Spread your hands as far apart as possible and keep your elbows straight but soft. Inhale.

2. Gently lean your body forward over your elbow and wrist joints. Exhale as you stretch forward. Hold the stretch for 5 to 30 seconds, breathing evenly as you hold.

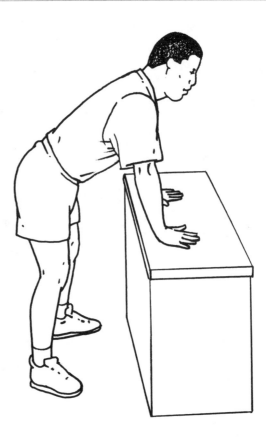

WRIST/HAND

WRIST ABDUCTION-ADDUCTION
Targets the muscles in the forearms and wrists.

1. Sit all the way back on a sturdy, armless chair, feet up on a small footstool, with your shoulders down and relaxed (the back of the chair should be straight and positioned near a wall, if possible). Keep your stomach in, small of back pressed toward the back of the chair, chin tucked, gaze forward, and head upright. Keep your elbows at the sides of your body and bend them at a right angle with your forearms in a neutral position, thumbs pointing up, and palms facing in. Inhale.

2. With your fingers relaxed, bend your wrists all the way down, then bring them all the way up. Exhale as you stretch. Hold the stretch 5 to 30 seconds in each position, breathing evenly as you hold.

You may also move the wrists up and down one at a time.

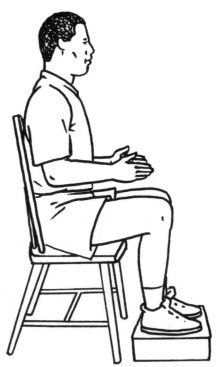
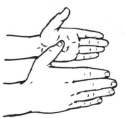
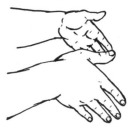
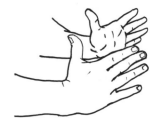

WRIST/HAND

FIST FLEX
Targets the muscles in the fingers and thumb.

1. Sit all the way back on a sturdy, armless chair, feet up on a small footstool, with your shoulders down and relaxed (the back of the chair should be straight and positioned near a wall, if possible). Keep your stomach in, small of back pressed toward the back of the chair, chin tucked, gaze forward, and head upright. Keep your elbows at the sides of your body and bend them at a right angle with your fingers out straight and palms facing each other. Inhale.

2. Make full fists, clenching your fingers and exhaling as you stretch. Hold the stretch for 5 to 30 seconds, breathing evenly as you hold.

You may also clench the fingers of one hand at a time.

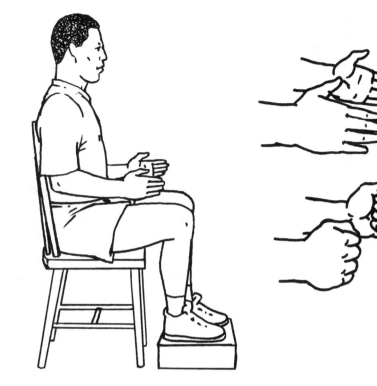

WRIST/HAND

WRIST/FINGER FLEXION
Targets the muscles in the wrists and hands.

1. Sit all the way back on a sturdy, armless chair, feet up on a small footstool, with your shoulders down and relaxed (the back of the chair should be straight and positioned near a wall, if possible). Keep your stomach in, small of back pressed toward the back of the chair, chin tucked, gaze forward, and head upright. Keep your elbows at the sides of your body and bend them at a right angle with your hands out, palms facing each other. Inhale.

2. Make full fists with your fingers clenched, bending your wrists inward at the same time. Exhale as you stretch. Hold the stretch for 5 to 30 seconds, breathing evenly as you hold.

You may also clench the fingers of one hand at a time.

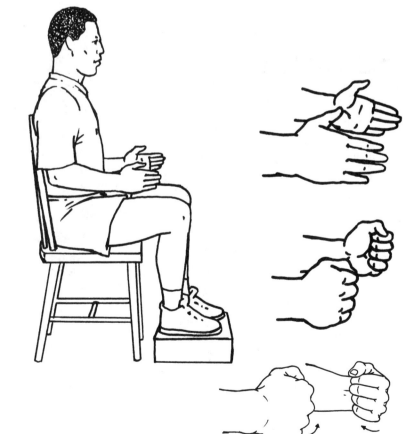

WRIST/HAND

FINGER PRESS
Targets the muscles in the fingers.

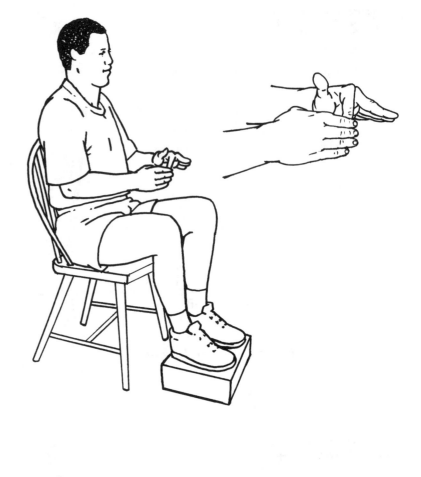

1. Sit all the way back on a sturdy, armless chair, feet up on a small footstool, with your shoulders down and relaxed (the back of the chair should be straight and positioned near a wall, if possible). Keep your stomach in, small of back pressed toward the back of the chair, chin tucked, gaze forward, and head upright. Keep your elbows at the sides of your body and bend them at a right angle with your hands out, palms down. Your wrists should be straight and the bottom knuckles bent, with the rest of each finger straight (like a table top). Inhale.

2. Using one hand, gently press down one finger (just below the knuckle) at a time on your other hand. Exhale as you stretch each finger. Hold the stretch for 5 to 30 seconds for each finger, breathing evenly as you hold.

3. Repeat on the opposite side.

WRIST/HAND

FINGER EXTENSION
Targets the muscles in the fingers.

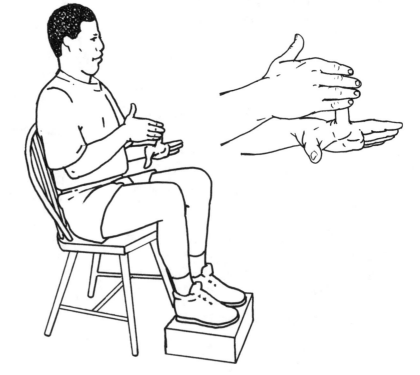

1. Sit all the way back on a sturdy, armless chair, feet up on a small footstool, with your shoulders down and relaxed (the back of the chair should be straight and positioned near a wall, if possible). Keep your stomach in, small of back pressed toward the back of the chair, chin tucked, gaze forward, and head upright. Keep your elbows at the sides of your body and bend them at a right angle with your hands out, palms down, and fingers as wide apart as possible. Inhale.

2. Using one hand, gently pull back one finger on your other hand at a time. Exhale as you stretch each finger. Hold the stretch for 5 to 30 seconds for each finger, breathing evenly as you hold.

3. Repeat on the opposite side.

WRIST/HAND

FINGER TOUCH
Targets the muscles in the fingers.

1. Sit all the way back on a sturdy, armless chair, feet up on a small footstool, with your shoulders down and relaxed (the back of the chair should be straight and positioned near a wall, if possible). Keep your stomach in, small of back pressed toward the back of the chair, chin tucked, gaze forward, and head upright. Keep your elbows at the sides of your body and bend them at a right angle with your hands out, palms down. Inhale.

2. Bring the tips of your fingers in and let them touch the edge of your palms (working up to bringing the tips of the fingers to just touch the heel of your palm). Exhale as you stretch your fingers. Hold the stretch for 5 to 30 seconds, breathing evenly as you hold.

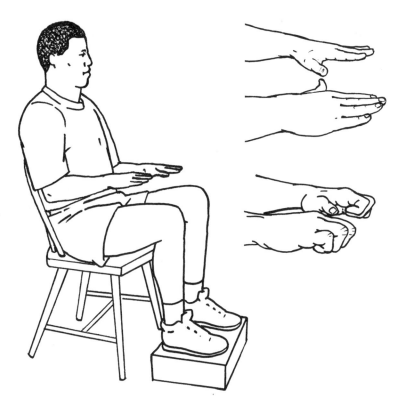

WRIST/HAND

THUMB FLEXION
Targets the muscles in the thumbs.

1. Sit all the way back on a sturdy, armless chair, feet up on a small footstool, with your shoulders down and relaxed (the back of the chair should be straight and positioned near a wall, if possible). Keep your stomach in, small of back pressed toward the back of the chair, chin tucked, gaze forward, and head upright. Keep your elbows at the sides of your body and bend them at a right angle with your hands out, palms down. Inhale.

2. Slowly and gently reach your thumbs toward the palms of your hands. Exhale as you stretch. Hold the stretch for 5 to 30 seconds, breathing evenly as you hold.

You may also stretch the thumbs one at a time.

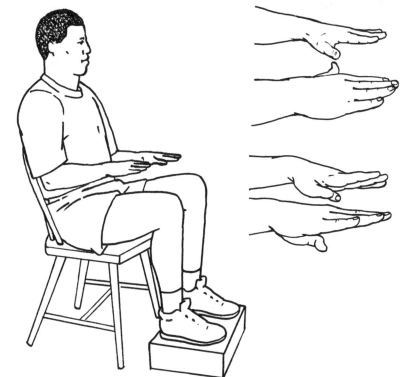

WRIST/HAND

THUMB EXTENSION
Targets the muscles in the thumbs.

1. Sit all the way back on a sturdy, armless chair, feet up on a small footstool, with your shoulders down and relaxed (the back of the chair should be straight and positioned near a wall, if possible). Keep your stomach in, small of back pressed toward the back of the chair, chin tucked, gaze forward, and head upright. Keep your elbows at the sides of your body and bend them at a right angle with your hands out, palms down. Inhale.

2. With one hand, gently press the thumb of your other hand upward toward your wrist and the back of your hand. Exhale as you stretch. Hold the stretch for 5 to 30 seconds, breathing evenly as you hold.

3. Repeat on the opposite side.

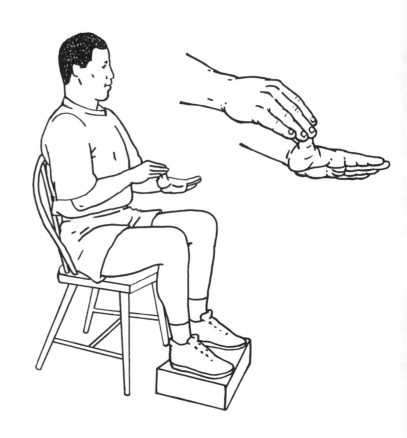

WRIST/HAND

THUMB CIRCLES
Targets the muscles in the thumbs.

1. Sit all the way back on a sturdy, armless chair, feet up on a small footstool, with your shoulders down and relaxed (the back of the chair should be straight and positioned near a wall, if possible). Keep your stomach in, small of back pressed toward the back of the chair, chin tucked, gaze forward, and head upright. Keep your elbows at the sides of your body and bend them at a right angle with your hands out, palms down. Inhale.

2. Slowly circle your thumbs as widely as possible clockwise and counterclockwise. Exhale as you circle your thumbs.

You may also circle the thumbs one at a time.

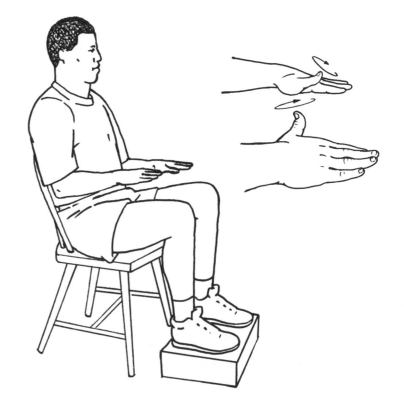

HIP

HIP CIRCLES
Targets the muscles in the hip.

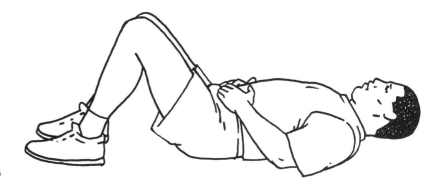

1. Lie on your back with your knees bent and your feet flat on the floor. Keep your stomach tight, your neck straight, and the small of your back pressed toward the floor to maintain proper alignment. Keep your hands on your lower abdomen and your shoulders down and relaxed. Inhale.

2. Pull one knee up toward your chest, keeping your knee bent. Place your hand on top of your knee and gently "draw" as big a circle as possible with your knee, clockwise and counterclockwise. Exhale as you stretch.

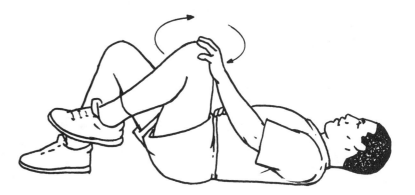

3. Repeat on the opposite side.

HIP

LYING HIP FLEXOR STRETCH
Targets the muscles in the hips.

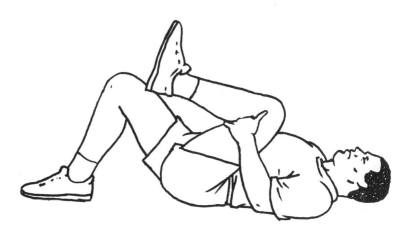

1. Lie on your back with your knees bent and your feet flat on the floor. Keep your stomach tight, your neck straight, and the small of your back pressed toward the floor to maintain proper alignment. Bring one knee up to your chest and wrap your hands under your thigh. Inhale.

2. Slowly slide your opposite leg down along the floor (do not arch your back). Exhale as you stretch. Hold the stretch for 5 to 30 seconds, breathing evenly as you hold. Return your legs slowly to the starting position.

3. Repeat on the opposite side.

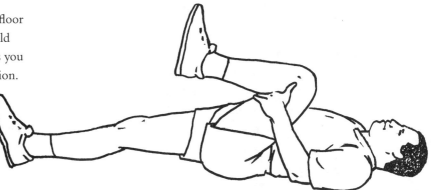

HIP

LUNGE STRETCH

Targets the muscles in the front of the upper thighs.

1. Stand with your feet a few inches apart. Keep your stomach in, chin tucked, gaze forward, and head upright. Inhale.

2. Step forward ("lunge") with one foot, being sure that your forward knee is directly over your ankle joint. Step as far forward as you can safely and comfortably go. Lower the knee of your back leg slowly toward the floor. Straighten your back leg out behind you and gently lean forward, keeping your body straight. Do not arch your back. Exhale as you stretch.

3. Repeat on the opposite side.

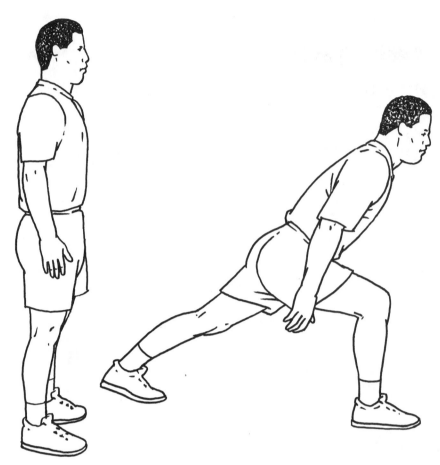

HIP

HIP OPENER

Targets the muscles in the inner thigh.

1. Lie on your back with your knees bent and your feet flat on the floor. Keep your stomach tight, your neck straight, and the small of your back pressed toward the floor to maintain proper alignment. Keep your hands on your lower abdomen and your shoulders down and relaxed. Straighten one leg out on the floor. Inhale.

2. Making sure that your leg does not roll in or out, slide your heel across the floor, moving your leg out to the side as far as comfortably possible (be sure that your leg stays on the supporting surface and your knee is straight). Exhale as you stretch. Hold the stretch for 5 to 30 seconds, breathing evenly as you hold. Return slowly to the starting position.

3. Repeat on the opposite side.

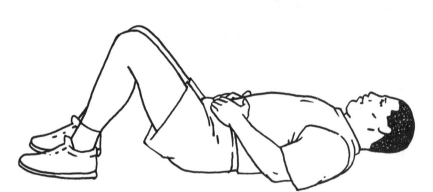

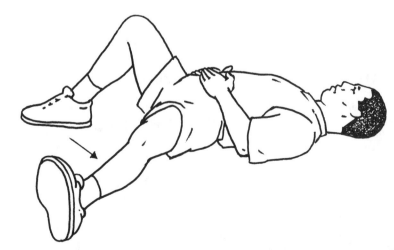

HIP

BUTTERFLY STRETCH
Targets the muscles in the groin, inner thigh, and hip.

1. Sit on the floor with the bottoms of your feet together and your hands on the inner sides of your thighs. Keep your stomach in, chin tucked, gaze forward, and head upright. Inhale.

2. Slowly and gently move your feet toward your buttocks. With your stomach tucked in and your head and neck straight, simultaneously lean forward. (For increased stretch, gently push your thighs to the floor.) Exhale as you stretch forward. Hold the stretch for 5 to 30 seconds, breathing evenly as you hold. Inhale as you straighten up.

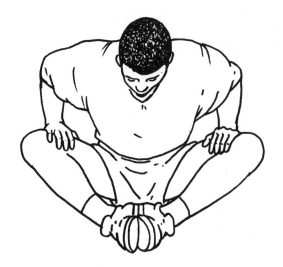

HIP • BACK

V-SIT STRETCH
Targets the muscles in the inner thighs and low back.

1. Sit with your legs out straight and placed as far apart as possible. Keep your knees slightly bent, your stomach tight, and your neck straight to maintain good alignment. Inhale.

2. Gently lean your trunk forward between your legs. Reach forward, sliding your hands across the floor, as you attempt to touch your head to the floor. Exhale as you stretch forward. Hold the stretch for 5 to 30 seconds, breathing evenly as you hold. Return slowly to the starting position, inhaling as you sit up.

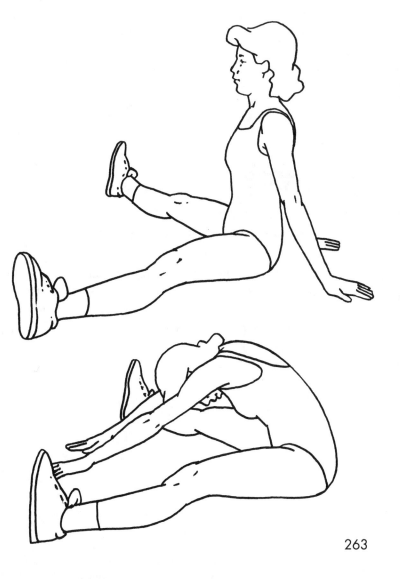

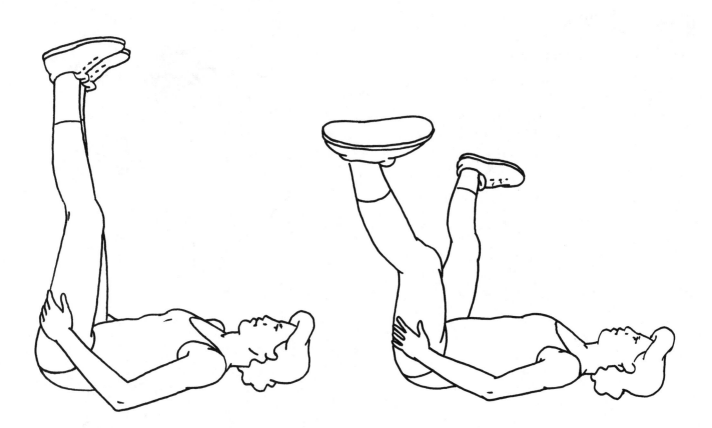

HIP

LYING V-STRETCH
Targets the muscles in the inner thighs and hips.

1. Lie on your back with your legs straight up in the air. Keep your stomach tight, your neck straight, and the small of your back pressed toward the floor to maintain proper alignment. Place your hands on the outsides of your thighs, keeping your shoulders down and relaxed. Inhale.

2. Gently lower your legs as far out to the sides as is comfortably possible. Exhale as you stretch. Hold the stretch for 5 to 30 seconds, breathing evenly as you hold. Slowly bring your legs back to center.

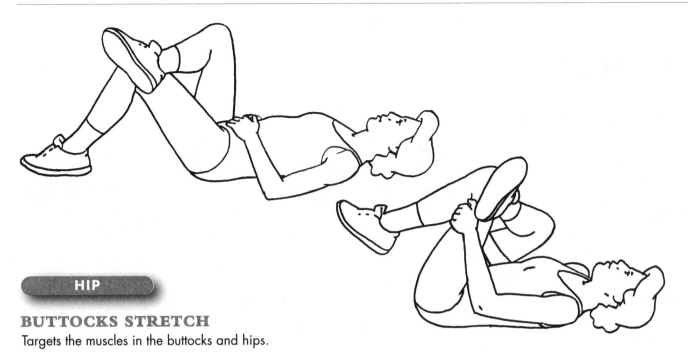

HIP

BUTTOCKS STRETCH
Targets the muscles in the buttocks and hips.

1. Lie on your back with your knees bent and your feet flat on the floor. Keep your stomach tight, your neck straight, and the small of your back pressed toward the floor to maintain proper alignment. Place the ankle of one leg on top of the opposite thigh (just above your knee). Inhale.

2. Bring your legs toward your chest as you clasp your hands under the thigh of the leg that was resting on the floor. Exhale as you stretch. Hold the stretch for 5 to 30 seconds, breathing evenly as you hold.

3. Repeat on the opposite side.

HIP • KNEE

HIP ABDUCTOR STRETCH
Targets the muscles in the outer hips, thighs, sides of the torso, and upper arms.

1. Stand up straight and face sideways toward a wall. Keep your stomach in, chin tucked, gaze forward, head upright, and knees slightly bent. Keeping your arms straight, raise your right arm overhead and place on the wall. Inhale.

2. Cross your right foot behind your left ankle. Keeping your knee straight, slowly lean into the wall. Feel the stretch on the outside of your right thigh. Exhale as you stretch. Hold the stretch for 5 to 30 seconds, breathing evenly as you hold.

3. Reverse sides and repeat.

HIP

LEG ROLL
Targets the muscles in the hip.

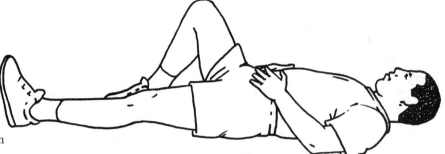

1. Lie on your back with your knees bent and your feet flat on the floor. Keep your stomach tight, your neck straight, and the small of your back pressed toward the floor to maintain proper alignment. Keep your hands on your lower abdomen and your shoulders down and relaxed. Straighten one leg out on the floor. Inhale.

2. Roll your straight leg inward as far as comfortably possible, then roll it outward as far as comfortably possible. Exhale as you stretch. Hold the stretch for 5 to 30 seconds in each position, breathing evenly as you hold.

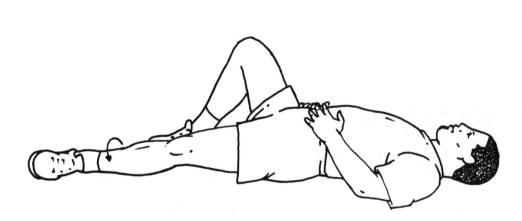

3. Repeat on the opposite side.

HIP • BACK • KNEE

HAMSTRING STRETCH WITH STRAIGHT LEG

Targets the muscles in the buttocks, back of the upper thighs, and calves.

Note: *This exercise may be done using a towel.*

1. Lie on your back with your knees bent and your feet flat on the floor. Keep your stomach tight, your neck straight, and the small of your back pressed toward the floor to maintain proper alignment. Keep your hands on your lower abdomen and your shoulders down and relaxed. Inhale.

2. Straighten one leg out in the air at the same level as your opposite knee (at a 45-degree angle). Hold your knee straight and flex your foot down toward you (pointing your toes toward the ceiling). Slowly raise your leg as high as comfortably possible, exhaling as you stretch. (You may hold a towel in your hands and wrap it around your foot to gently increase the stretch.) Hold the stretch for 5 to 30 seconds, breathing evenly as you hold. Bend your knee and return slowly to the starting position.

3. Repeat on the opposite side.

HIP • BACK • KNEE

BENT-KNEE HAMSTRING STRETCH

Targets the muscles in the buttocks, the back of the upper thighs, and calves.

Note: *This exercise may be done using a towel.*

1. Lie on your back with your knees bent and your feet flat on the floor. Keep your stomach tight, your neck straight, and the small of your back pressed toward the floor to maintain proper alignment. Keep your hands on your lower abdomen and your shoulders down and relaxed. Inhale.

2. Bend one knee toward your chest. Grasp the back of your thigh with your hands and gently raise your leg up, knee bent slightly, as high as comfortably possible. Hold the stretch for 5 to 30 seconds, breathing evenly as you hold. Return slowly to the starting position.

3. Repeat on the opposite side.

267

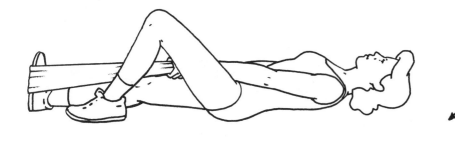

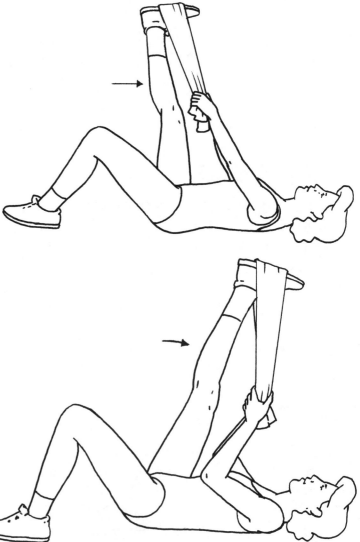

HIP • KNEE

HAMSTRING/HIP STRETCH

Targets the muscles in the buttocks, back of the thighs, calves, and inner thighs.

Note: *This exercise uses a towel.*

1. Lie on your back with one knee bent and the other leg flat on the floor. Keep your stomach tight, your neck straight, and the small of your back pressed toward the floor to maintain proper alignment. Keep your shoulders down and relaxed. Loop a towel under the foot of the extended leg. Inhale.

2. Use the towel to slowly raise your straight leg as high as comfortably possible, exhaling as you stretch. Flex your foot down toward you. Inhale.

3. Stretch your straight leg toward your other leg, crossing over the midline of your body and exhaling as you stretch. Use the towel to guide the stretch. Be sure your buttocks stay on the floor.

4. Slowly bring your leg back up and gently try to move it up higher, exhaling as you stretch. Hold the stretch for 5 to 30 seconds, breathing evenly as you hold.

5. Stretch your straight leg away from your body, exhaling as you stretch; buttocks stay on the floor.

6. Slowly bring your leg back up and gently try to move it up higher, exhaling as you stretch. Hold the stretch for 5 to 30 seconds, breathing evenly as you hold.

7. Bend your knee slowly and return to the starting position.

8. Repeat on the opposite side.

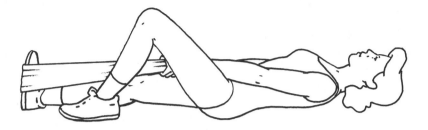

HIP • KNEE

HAMSTRING/HIP CIRCLES

Targets the muscles in the buttocks, back of the thighs, calves, and outer thighs.

Note: *This exercise uses a towel.*

1. Lie on your back with one knee bent and the other leg flat on the floor. Keep your stomach tight, your neck straight, and the small of your back pressed toward the floor to maintain proper alignment. Keep your shoulders down and relaxed. Loop a towel under the foot of the extended leg. Inhale.

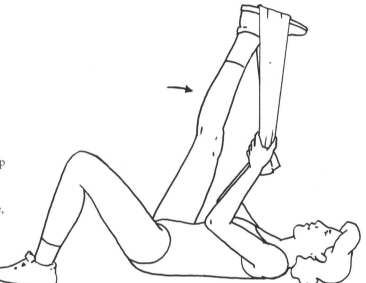

2. Slowly raise your straight leg as high as comfortably possible, exhaling as you stretch. Flex your foot down toward you. Inhale.

3. Make small circles with your leg as you bring it down to the floor, using the towel to guide the stretch. Be sure your buttocks stay on the floor. Inhale.

4. Slowly bring your leg back up and gently try to move it up higher, exhaling as you stretch. Hold the stretch for 5 to 30 seconds, breathing evenly as you hold.

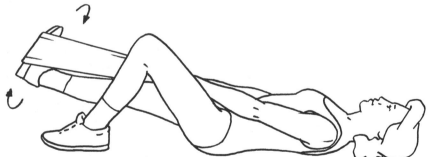

5. Bend your knee slowly and return to the starting position.

6. Repeat on the opposite side.

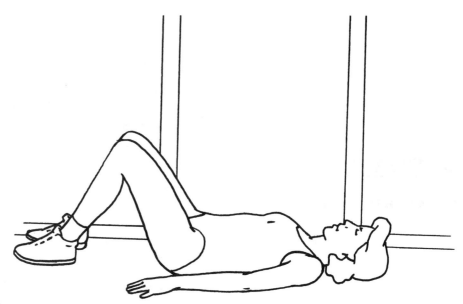

HIP • KNEE

ASSISTED HAMSTRING STRETCH

Targets the muscles in the back of the upper thighs.

1. Lie on your back with your knees bent and your feet flat on the floor. Keep your stomach tight, your neck straight, and the small of your back pressed toward the floor to maintain proper alignment. Place one hip up against the inside of a doorway frame. Inhale.

2. Raise the leg closest to the doorway into the air and hook it against the outside of the doorway frame. Exhale as you stretch. Hold the stretch for 5 to 30 seconds, breathing evenly as you hold.

3. Repeat on the opposite side.

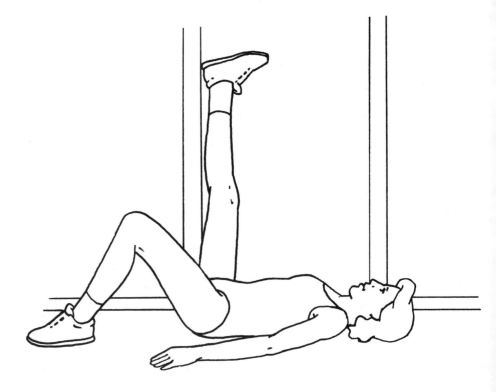

HIP • KNEE • BACK

STANDING HAMSTRING STRETCH

Targets the muscles in the back of the upper thighs, hips, and back.

1. Stand up straight, lift one leg, and place the heel of that leg on the edge of a table (or a lower surface, such as a stepstool or coffee table). Bend your other knee slightly and turn your standing foot so that it's slightly pointing out (use a nearby wall or chair for support if necessary). Inhale.

2. Tighten your stomach and keep your neck straight to maintain proper alignment, then put your right hand on your right thigh and slowly lean your body forward. Exhale as you stretch. Hold the stretch for 5 to 30 seconds, breathing evenly as you hold. Return slowly to the starting position.

3. Repeat on the opposite side.

You may also do this stretch by simply putting one leg out in front, heel on the floor, and gently leaning as far forward as you can, with your back knee bent and your hands on your thighs.

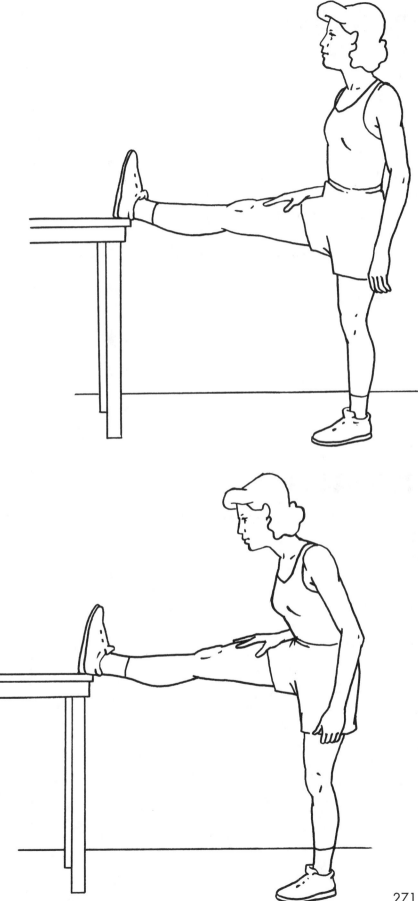

HIP • KNEE

BENT-KNEE QUAD STRETCH
Targets the muscles in the front of the thighs and hips.

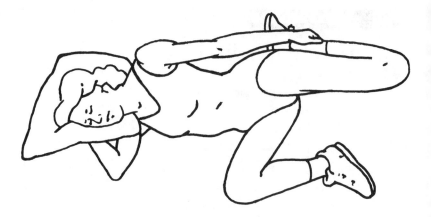

1. Lie on your right side with a pillow under your head. Inhale.

2. Bend your right knee toward your chest and place it on the floor. Straighten your left leg out, then bend that knee, grasping your left ankle with your hand and gently pulling your knee and hip backward. Exhale as you stretch. Hold the stretch for 5 to 30 seconds, breathing evenly as you hold.

3. Repeat on the opposite side.

HIP • KNEE

STANDING QUAD STRETCH
Targets the muscles in the front of the thighs and hips.

1. Stand up straight and face a wall about arm's distance away. Keep your stomach in, chin tucked, gaze forward, head upright, and knees slightly bent. Place your right palm against the wall for balance. Inhale.

2. Grasp your left ankle with your left hand and gently pull your knee backward, keeping your thighs even. (To increase the stretch, press your knee toward the floor at the same time as you press your hip slightly forward, but do not arch your back.) Exhale as you stretch. Hold the stretch for 5 to 30 seconds, breathing evenly as you hold.

3. Repeat on the opposite side.

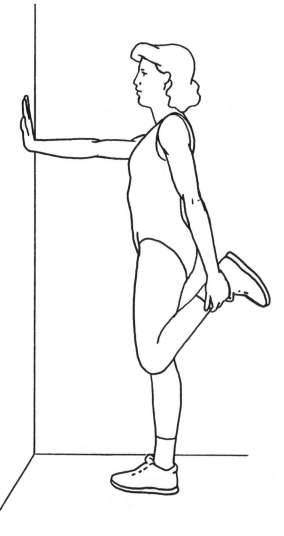

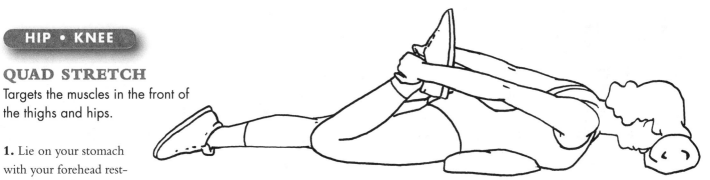

HIP • KNEE

QUAD STRETCH
Targets the muscles in the front of the thighs and hips.

1. Lie on your stomach with your forehead resting on the floor. (You may use a towel roll under your forehead.) Place a large pillow under your stomach. Keep your stomach tight and your neck straight to maintain proper alignment. Bring one of your heels toward your buttocks, grasping your ankle with your hands. Inhale.

2. Keeping your thighs together and your body straight, gently pull your ankle toward your buttock as you press your hip to the floor. Exhale as you stretch. Hold the stretch for 5 to 30 seconds, breathing evenly as you hold.

3. Repeat on the opposite side.

HIP • KNEE

CROSS THIGH STRETCH
Targets the muscles in the front of the thighs.

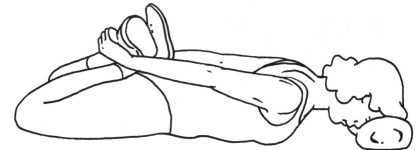

1. Lie on your stomach with your forehead resting on the floor. (You may use a towel roll under your forehead.) Place a large pillow under your stomach. Keep your stomach tight and your neck straight to maintain proper alignment and bend both knees. Inhale.

2. Cross one ankle over the other and bring your heels as close to your buttocks as possible. Exhale as you stretch. Hold the stretch for 5 to 30 seconds, breathing evenly as you hold.

3. Reverse your ankle position and repeat.

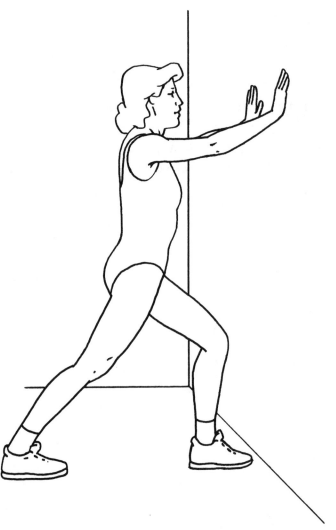

ANKLE/FOOT

FLEXED-FOOT STRETCH
Targets the muscles in the calves, arches of the feet, and back of the upper thighs.

Note: *This exercise may be done using a towel.*

1. Sit on the floor with your legs outstretched and your hands on the floor behind your buttocks. Keep your stomach in, chin tucked, gaze forward, head upright, and knees slightly bent. Inhale.

2. Flex your feet toward you. (To gently increase the stretch, you may hold a towel in your hands, loop it around your foot, and pull forward gently.) Exhale as you stretch. Hold the stretch for 5 to 30 seconds, breathing evenly as you hold.

ANKLE/FOOT • KNEE

RUNNER'S STRETCH
Targets the muscles in the calves.

1. Stand about arm's length away from a wall. Keep your stomach in, chin tucked, gaze forward, head upright, and knees slightly bent. Place your hands on the wall with your palms at shoulder level. Place one foot forward with the knee bent (be sure the knee of the forward leg is just above or behind the ankle) and your other leg straight back as far as possible with your heel on the floor. Inhale.

2. With your stomach tight and your neck straight, gently lean into the wall, increasing the bend of your forward leg and keeping heel of your other leg on the floor. Exhale as you stretch. Hold the stretch for 5 to 30 seconds, breathing evenly as you hold.

3. Repeat with reverse leg positions.

ANKLE/FOOT

CALF STRETCH WITH FLEXED KNEE
Targets the muscles in the calves.

1. Stand about arm's length away from a wall. Keep your stomach in, chin tucked, gaze forward, head upright, and knees slightly bent. Place your hands on the wall with your palms at shoulder level. Place one leg forward with the knee bent (be sure the knee of the forward leg is directly over the ankle joint) and the other leg behind with the knee bent. Keep both feet flat on the floor. Inhale.

2. Bend the front leg, keeping the back foot on the floor with knee bent, until you feel a stretch in the lower calf area of the front leg. Exhale as you stretch. Hold the stretch for 5 to 30 seconds, breathing evenly as you hold.

3. Repeat with reverse leg positions.

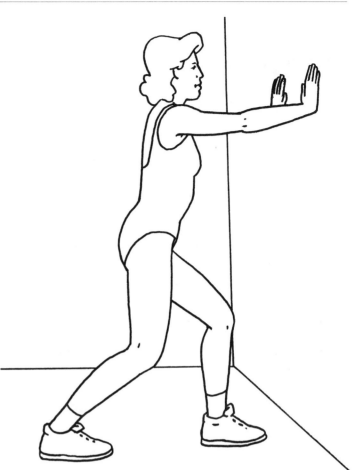

ANKLE/FOOT

HEEL STRETCH
Targets the muscles in the calves.

1. Stand on a step and hold onto the handrail. Keep your stomach in, chin tucked, gaze forward, head upright, and knees straight but not rigid. Let both heels hang down over the edge of the step. Inhale.

2. Keeping your legs straight, lower your heels down as far as possible until you feel a stretch in the back of your calves. Exhale as you stretch. Hold the stretch for 5 to 30 seconds, breathing evenly as you hold.

You may also lower one heel at a time, keeping the other foot planted on the step.

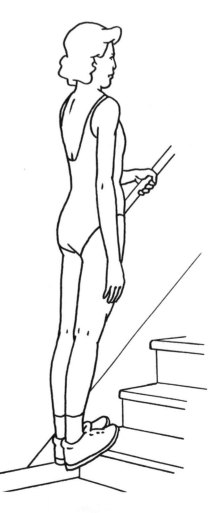

ANKLE/FOOT

BENT-KNEE HEEL STRETCH
Targets the muscles in the calves.

1. Stand on a step and hold onto the handrail. Keep your stomach in, chin tucked, gaze forward, head upright, and knees slightly bent. Bend your knees and let both heels hang down over the edge of the step. Inhale.

2. Keeping your knees bent, lower your heels down as far as possible until you feel a stretch in your lower calves. Exhale as you stretch. Hold the stretch for 5 to 30 seconds, breathing evenly as you hold.

You may also lower one heel at a time, keeping the other foot planted on the step.

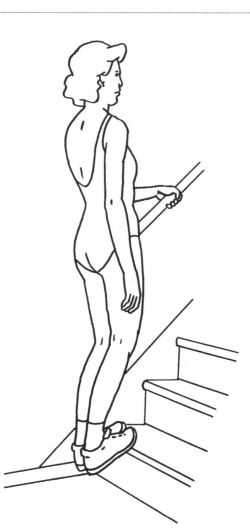

ANKLE/FOOT

POINTED-TOE STRETCH
Targets the muscles in the front of the shins, ankles, and toes.

1. Sit on the floor with your legs outstretched and your hands on the floor behind your buttocks. Keep your stomach in, chin tucked, gaze forward, head upright, and knees slightly bent. Inhale.

2. Point your toes away from you. Exhale as you stretch. Hold the stretch for 5 to 30 seconds, breathing evenly as you hold.

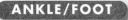

ANKLE/FOOT

LOWER LEG LENGTHENER

Targets the muscles in the front of the lower legs.

1. Stand about 2 feet away from a wall. Keep your stomach in, chin tucked, gaze forward, head upright, and knees slightly bent. Place your hands on the wall with your palms at shoulder level. With your back straight, place one leg forward with your foot flat on the floor, and place the other leg behind it with your toes pointing backward on the floor. Inhale.

2. Bend both knees until you feel, stretch in the front of your back lower leg (shin area). Exhale as you stretch. Hold the stretch for 5 to 30 seconds, breathing evenly as you hold.

3. Repeat with reverse leg positions.

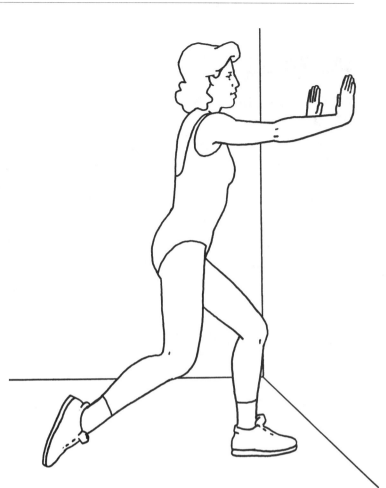

ANKLE/FOOT

FOOT SUPINATION AND INVERSION

Targets the muscles in the inside and outside of the lower legs and feet.

1. Sit on the floor with your legs out-stretched and your hands on the floor behind your buttocks. Keep your stomach in, chin tucked, gaze forward, head upright, and knees slightly bent. Inhale.

2. Turn your feet inward and toward you, pointing your toes to increase the stretch. Roll only your foot, not your whole leg. Exhale as you stretch. Hold the stretch for 5 to 30 seconds, breathing evenly as you hold.

ANKLE/FOOT

FOOT PRONATION AND EVERSION

Targets the muscles in the inside and outside of the lower legs and feet.

1. Sit on the floor with your legs outstretched and your hands on the floor behind your buttocks. Keep your stomach in, chin tucked, gaze forward, head upright, and knees slightly bent. Inhale.

2. Turn your feet downward and outward. Roll only your foot, not your whole leg. Exhale as you stretch. Hold the stretch for 5 to 30 seconds, breathing evenly as you hold.

ANKLE/FOOT

FOOT CIRCLES

Targets the muscles in the ankles and feet.

1. Sit on the floor with your legs outstretched and your hands on the floor behind your buttocks. Keep your stomach in, chin tucked, gaze forward, head upright, and knees slightly bent. Inhale.

2. With your toes in a neutral position, circle your feet clockwise and counterclockwise, making sure your whole leg does not move. Exhale as you stretch.

ANKLE/FOOT

TOE FLEXOR
Targets the muscles in the toes.

1. Sit on the floor barefoot with your legs outstretched and your hands on the floor behind your buttocks. Keep your stomach in, chin tucked, gaze forward, head upright, and knees slightly bent. Inhale.

2. Pull only your toes toward you and then curl them down. Exhale as you stretch. Hold the stretch for 5 to 30 seconds in each position, breathing evenly as you hold.

ANKLE/FOOT

TOE EXTENSION AND SPREAD
Targets the muscles in the toes.

1. Sit on the floor barefoot with your legs outstretched and your hands on the floor behind your buttocks. Keep your stomach in, chin tucked, gaze forward, head upright, and knees slightly bent. Inhale.

2. Pull your toes up and spread them as far apart as possible. Exhale as you stretch. Hold the stretch for 5 to 30 seconds, breathing evenly as you hold.

First Aid Basics

A traumatic injury to the body caused by a fall or an accident, or any injury resulting in intense pain, has the potential to be very serious and should be treated with extreme care. Even if an injury doesn't seem too severe, it's always best to err on the side of caution; without medical training, it's easy to misdiagnose a problem.

If such an injury strikes, it is important to know and apply basic first aid techniques. Below is a brief, useful survey of immobilization techniques as they might apply to the various body parts discussed in this book. The goal is to ensure safety and keep the injured part stable to prevent further injury.

Most of the advice in this section is meant to help you assist another person who has been injured, although in some instances you may be able to attend to an injury of your own—or at least give someone guidance in helping you.

Of course, a few short paragraphs cannot contain enough advice to cover every emergency situation that may arise. So while the information below is a good place to start, it is highly recommended for your own and others' sake that you receive a more thorough education in first aid, including cardiopulmonary resuscitation (CPR), through organizations such as the American Red Cross.

Back

Because of the risk of life-threatening damage to the spinal cord, any traumatic injury to the back should be considered a major medical emergency. Never attempt to move a person who has suffered back trauma. Tell the injured person to lie still. Call for medical treatment immediately. It's also a good idea to cover the person with a blanket so that he or she stays warm.

Neck

As with the back, any traumatic injury to the neck may result in life-threatening damage to the spinal cord. For this reason, it's important not to move the injured person at any time; also, make sure the person lies as still as possible. Check right away to make sure that the injured person is breathing. If not, the individual will require immediate CPR; the airway must be maintained before any other first aid is performed. If you are unable to administer CPR, quickly find someone who can, if possible. And call at once for medical treatment. It's also a good idea to cover the person with a blanket so that he or she stays warm.

Jaw

Traumatic injuries to the jaw usually take the form of fracture or dislocation, often as the result of a blow to the face. The jaw may be hanging loosely and will need to be supported while you seek medical treatment. The jaw can be supported manually by placing the fingers of one or both hands in the mouth, "hooking" the fingers over the teeth of the lower jaw, and supporting the chin with the thumbs or the heel of the hand. Or secure the jaw as comfortably as possible and without increasing the pain by placing a cravat bandage made of cloth under the chin and tying it at the top of the head.

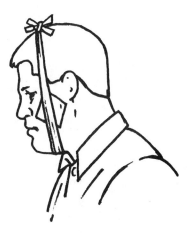

Cravat bandage for jaw

Shoulder

An injury to the shoulder will usually occur to the humerus—the upper arm bone—or collarbone. With any shoulder injury, it's essential to immobilize the shoulder with a sling and a swath. It's generally best to immobilize the shoulder in the position you found it. A sling can be fashioned out of a scarf or any triangular piece of fabric. Carefully loop the fabric under the injured arm and tie the fabric around the back of the neck. An additional swath (cloth or bandage) can be wrapped around the body to secure the arm to the body. If material for a sling cannot be found, the arm can also be immobilized by simply pinning the sleeve of the injured arm in place. Make sure that the bandages and tape aren't so tight that they cut off circulation. Check for a pulse at the wrist on the affected side. If there is no pulse or if the arm is cold, numb, or discolored, the situation calls for emergency medical care. In case of swelling, remove any watch or other jewelry. With any shoulder injury, it's important to seek treatment as soon as possible. If the injury seems major, it's also a good idea to cover the person with a blanket so that he or she stays warm.

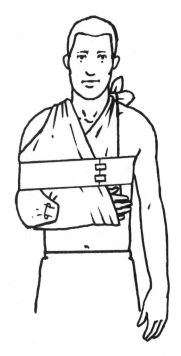

Sling and swath for shoulder

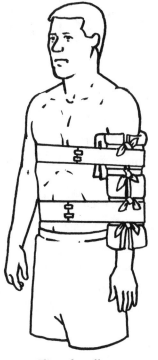

Sling for elbow

Elbow

An elbow injury can include a fractured and/or dislocated bone. As with a shoulder injury, the injured arm should be secured to the body in a sling or the sleeve pinned up against the body (see "Shoulder," above). It is usually best to immobilize the elbow in the position it was found. Secure the arm to the body with large bandages that encircle the entire midsection. Make sure that the bandages and tape aren't so tight that they cut off circulation. Check for a pulse at the wrist on the affected side. If there is no pulse or if the arm is cold, numb, or discolored, the situation calls for emergency medical care. In case of swelling, remove any watch or other jewelry. Follow the RICE recommendations (see the box, **"RICE,"** on page 284) and seek treatment.

Wrist

It's often impossible to determine whether a wrist injury is a sprain, a fracture, or something else entirely. When an injury occurs, immobilize the wrist with a splint. A splint can easily be fashioned by securing rolled up newspapers or towels to the injured wrist with bandages. Make sure that the bandages and tape aren't so tight that they cut off circulation. A sling should also be used to keep the wrist elevated and reduce the blood flow to the injured body part (see "Shoulder," above). Check for a pulse at the affected wrist. If there is no pulse or if the hand is cold, numb, or discolored, the situation calls for emergency medical care. In case of swelling, remove any watch or other jewelry. Follow the RICE recommendations (see the box, **"RICE,"** on page 284) and seek treatment.

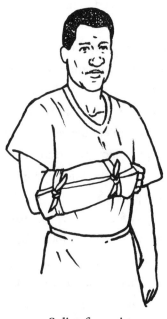

Splint for wrist

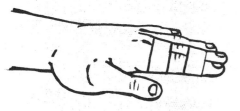

Buddy taping of injured finger

Hand

The delicate nature of the small bones in the hand and the frequency with which we need to use our hands makes any hand injury potentially serious. An injured finger may require a splint for immobilization or may simply be taped to the finger next to it for support ("buddy taping"). Make sure that the bandages and tape aren't so tight that they cut off circulation. Check whether the fingers are cold, numb, or discolored; if so, the situation calls for emergency medical care. With any finger injury, follow the RICE recommendations (see the box, **"RICE,"** on page 284) and seek treatment as soon as possible.

Hip

A traumatic injury to the hip should be considered a serious medical condition. The injured person should not be moved or allowed to move, because a hip fracture or dislocation has the potential to cause serious internal damage. Instruct the injured person to lie still. If the injury seems major, it's also a good idea to cover the person with a blanket so that he or she stays warm. Call for medical treatment immediately.

Knee

A traumatic injury to the knee resulting from an accident or fall requires immediate medical attention. The injured person should be instructed to lie still, and the injured knee should be secured. Secure a splint with bandages to the injured knee in the position you found it—do not make an attempt to straighten it if it's bent. To immobilize a bent knee, secure it to the uninjured leg (also bent), setting rolled newspapers or towels between the legs. Make sure that the bandages and tape aren't so tight that they cut off circulation. Check for a pulse at the ankle of the affected leg. If there is no pulse or if the lower leg is cold, numb, or discolored, the situation may be especially serious. If at all possible, follow the RICE recommendations (see the box, **"RICE,"** on page 284) while awaiting medical treatment. If the injury seems major, it's also a good idea to cover the person with a blanket so that he or she stays warm.

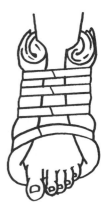

Ankle splinted with newspaper

Ankle

The ankle is susceptible to sprains, tears, and fractures, among other injuries. When an ankle injury occurs, carefully remove the injured person's shoe and sock and immobilize the injured ankle with a splint. A splint can be fashioned out of newspapers or towels rolled up so that they form a cylinder shape around the ankle. They should be secured with bandages on the bottom of the foot and both sides of the ankle for support. Make sure that the bandages and tape aren't so tight that they cut off circulation.

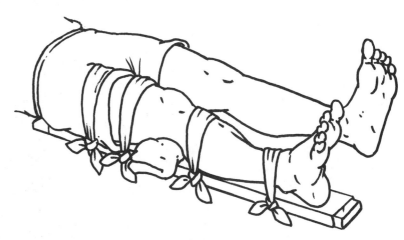

Straight knee splint

Check for a pulse at the affected ankle. If there is no pulse or if the foot is cold, numb, or discolored, the situation calls for emergency medical care. With any ankle injury, follow the RICE recommendations (see the box, "RICE," below) and seek treatment.

Foot

The small bones in the foot require immediate medical attention when an injury occurs. As with an ankle injury, carefully remove the injured person's shoe and sock and immobilize the entire foot and ankle area in a splint (see "Ankle," above). If an injury to a toe is suspected, the toe can be immobilized by simply taping it to the next toe for support ("buddy taping"). Make sure that the bandages and tape aren't so tight that they cut off circulation. If the toes are cold, numb, or discolored, the situation may be serious. Follow the RICE recommendations (see the box, "RICE," below) while awaiting medical treatment.

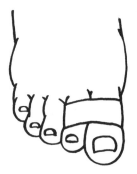

Buddy taping of injured toe

RICE

"RICE" is an acronym that stands for Rest, Ice, Compression, and Elevation. These four components make up one of the most fundamental first aid procedures in the case of many traumatic injuries. The RICE method is an integral part of the healing process because it may reduce or prevent swelling and pain and minimize the chance of further damage before medical professionals can attend to the injury. RICE is not, however, a substitute for proper treatment.

As soon as an injury occurs, the affected body part should be allowed to rest. Don't move or put pressure on the area. Apply ice to the affected area on a 20-minutes-on/20–40-minutes-off schedule continuously for a day or two. A convenient way to apply ice is to use crushed ice in a plastic bag covered with a moistened towel, or a bag of frozen vegetables, which easily conforms to the injured body part. Compress the injured body part by wrapping an elastic bandage around it. This bandage should be supportive but should not cut off circulation. (If the injured area feels numb, the bandage is too tight.) Unless it increases pain, elevate the injured body part by raising it up higher than heart level and placing it on piles of secured pillows or cushions, and keep the area stabilized.

Cardiovascular Conditioning

As valuable as a regimen of exercises designed to build and maintain strength, endurance, and flexibility may be, no fitness program can be considered complete if it does not include cardiovascular conditioning. Aerobic activities—like walking, running, water aerobics, and cycling—that get the heart pumping and the lungs working are absolutely essential to your overall health and well-being.

This point was reaffirmed in a recent U.S. Surgeon General report that concluded that Americans can substantially improve their health and quality of life by including moderate amounts of physical activity in their daily lives. The Surgeon General also noted that regular physical activity helps prevent cardiovascular disease.

It is highly recommended that you consult a professional to learn more about this subject and make cardiovascular conditioning part of your body maintenance regimen. Be sure to consult a physician before beginning any cardiovascular conditioning program.

The overall goal of cardiovascular conditioning is to receive the benefits of being physically active without tiring too quickly. Pacing yourself is especially important if you have been inactive. Monitoring your heart rate (beats per minute) during exercise using a watch with a second hand can help you measure your fitness level.

The American Heart Association (AHA) recommends using target heart rate zones to measure fitness level. This target rate is derived from your maximum heart rate—a figure that can be loosely calculated by starting with the number 220 and subtracting your age. The average maximum heart rate of a healthy 32-year-old, for example, is 188 beats per minute.

Your target zone falls between 50 and 75 percent of your maximum heart rate. So in the case of the healthy average 32-year-old, the target zone would be between 94 and 141 beats per minute.

For quick reference, you may use the Average Maximum Heart Rate Chart below, which is based on these formulas. Because these figures are averages, however, they should only be used as general guidelines.

The AHA recommends that during the first few weeks of an exercise program, you should aim for the low end of your target zone, then gradually build up to the high end.

Average Maximum Heart Rate Chart

AGE	MAXIMUM RATE (BEATS PER MINUTE)	TARGET RATE (BEATS PER MINUTE)
20	200	100 to 150
25	195	98 to 146
30	190	95 to 142
35	185	93 to 138
40	180	90 to 135
45	175	88 to 131
50	170	85 to 127
55	165	83 to 123
60	160	80 to 120
65	155	78 to 116
70	150	75 to 113

Index

Page numbers in **boldface** indicate illustrations.